Small Animal Dental, Oral & Maxillofacial Disease

A Color Handbook

Brook A. Niemiec

**Diplomate, American Veterinary Dental College,
Fellow, Academy of Veterinary Dentistry**

Southern California Veterinary Dental Specialties, San Diego, USA
vetdentalrad.com

T0383118

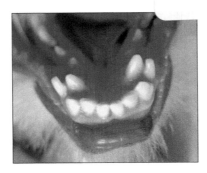

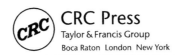

CRC Press
Taylor & Francis Group
Boca Raton London New York

CRC Press is an imprint of the
Taylor & Francis Group, an **informa** business

This book is dedicated to all who have helped me to become someone who could write/edit a book worth reading.

There are numerous veterinarians who have influenced my life and my career. From my first dental mentor, Dr. Michael Floyd, I learned not only dentistry, but also how to practice while still enjoying a balance of fun in life. Special thanks to my true mentor and founding member of the AVDC, Dr. Thomas Mulligan. Fortunately, you saw promise in me and worked diligently to bring it out, even if I was reluctant initially. Thank you for taking me under your wing and teaching me to be my best, through all those late nights at Main Street. However, veterinary medicine is more than dentistry. I would like to thank Dr. Barry Neichin, my first employer and the best general practitioner I know, for teaching me the basics of veterinary medicine. Drs. Michael Kelly and Robert Tugend continued that training and taught me that working in a team is rewarding. Finally, I would like to thank Dr. Robert Rooks, from whom I gained skills in marketing and client communications.

In addition to the veterinarians who have helped me along the way, I have benefited from working with a great group of technicians and assistants. First and foremost in this group is Dawn Sabatino, my right hand (and occasionally my left) for the last decade. So much of my practice would not be possible without you; thanks for all that you do. I owe many thanks to Robert Furman (soon to be a veterinarian) who was instrumental in starting my dental practice as well as making my life easier with his computer and electrical and handy man skills. A note of thanks is also due for my assistants who went above and beyond in years past: Teresa, Wendy, Tia, and Diane.

Outside of veterinary medicine, I would like to thank and recognize my original inspiration and uncle, Dr. Greg Steiner DDS, who told me back in the 1980s to do veterinary dentistry! A special note of gratitude to my old adventure buddy, Lynel Berryhill, whose support and technical help during my applications to the Dental College and Academy were invaluable. I couldn't have done it without you. I also owe a big thank you to Dr. Katie Kangas for her countless hours of editing. This has greatly improved your (the readers') experience.

And finally, this book is largely dedicated to my parents Jim and Toni. Without your emotional and financial support, my years of school, training, and practice would not have been possible. Thank you for going above and beyond as parents, friends, and business mentors. You're the best!

Thanks to all of you for the contributions you have made to my life, which in turn have led to the creation of this book.

Brook

CONTENTS

CONTENTS

CONTRIBUTORS

Chapter 1: Anatomy and Physiology
John R. Lewis, VMD, FAVD, DAVDC
Assistant Professor of Dentistry and Oral Surgery
Matthew J. Ryan Veterinary Hospital of the
University of Pennsylvania, Philadelphia, USA

Alexander M Reiter, Dipl Tzt, Dr med vet,
DAVDC, EVDC
Assistant Professor of Dentistry and Oral Surgery
Matthew J. Ryan Veterinary Hospital of the
University of Pennsylvania, Philadelphia, USA

Chapter 2: Oral Examination
Lee Jane Huffman, DVM, DAVDC
Pet Emergency Clinics and Specialty
Hospital, Ventura and Thousand Oaks, USA
This chapter is dedicated with all my love to
Rebeckah, Nonatime, and my wee 'Monsieur'.

Chapter 3: Veterinary Dental Radiology
Brook A. Niemiec DVM, DAVDC, FAVD
vetdentalrad.com

Chapter 4: Pathology in the Pediatric Patient
Brook A. Niemiec DVM, DAVDC, FAVD
Southern California Veterinary Dental Specialties,
San Diego, USA

Chapter 5: Pathologies of the Dental Hard Tissues
Gregg DuPont DVM, DAVDC
Shoreline Veterinary Dental Clinic, Seattle, USA

Chapter 6: Problems with the Gingiva
Linda DeBowes DVM, MS, DACVIM, DAVDC
Shoreline Veterinary Dental Clinic, Seattle, USA

Chapter 7: Pathologies of the Oral Mucosa
Brook A. Niemiec DVM, DAVDC, FAVD
Southern California Veterinary Dental Specialties,
San Diego, USA

Chapter 8: Problems with Muscles, Bones, and
Joints
Kendall G. Taney, DVM, DAVDC, FAVD
Center for Veterinary Dentistry and Oral Surgery,
Gaithersburg, MD, USA

Mark M. Smith, VMD, DACVS, DAVDC
Center for Veterinary Dentistry and Oral Surgery,
Gaithersburg, MD, USA

Chapter 9: Malignant Oral Neoplasia
Ravinder S. Dhaliwal DVM, MS, DACVIM,
DABVP
Pet Care Veterinary Hospital, Santa Rosa, CA, USA
This chapter is dedicated to my two little angels,
Siona and Nikita,
who have given a new perspective to my life.

Chapter 10: Pathologies of the Salivary System
Brook A. Niemiec DVM, DAVDC, FAVD
Southern California Veterinary Dental Specialties,
San Diego, USA

FOREWORD

Veterinary dentistry has exploded as a discipline within veterinary medicine over the past 20+ years, primarily due to the tireless efforts of those clinicians in the 1970s and early 1980s who took an often overlooked area of the patient, and turned it into a focus of major significance. Thanks to these pioneers in veterinary dentistry, many of us found our calling within veterinary medicine and provide a valuable service to animals throughout the world. In the early days of veterinary dentistry, those who had a special interest in dentistry would gather together and discuss conditions and treatments they had found to be particularly helpful or successful. Out of these meetings rose the organization of the American Veterinary Dental Society and the Veterinary Dental Forum. The Veterinary Dental Forum has grown to an annual meeting of nearly 1000 participants, a far cry from the early days of getting together around a cold beverage to talk about your most challenging/rewarding cases! Also blossoming out of the efforts of these pioneers has come the Journal of Veterinary Dentistry, a quarterly publication that is currently recognized internationally as the journal of record for veterinary dentistry. All these efforts were to help educate veterinarians about veterinary dentistry and to elevate the practice of veterinary medicine in general.

Though many aspects of veterinary dentistry are continuously evolving, one constant is the clinical practicality of veterinary dentistry. This is reflected in the organization and thought process throughout this book. Dr. Niemiec does an excellent job presenting many dental conditions from a very practical standpoint. Beginning with the initial oral examination, through the diagnostic procedures, such as dental radiography, Dr. Niemiec provides pragmatic tips along the way. Reading this text is similar to the way practitioners think through diagnostic challenges within their own practices. From the early chapters that focus on the normal oral/dental anatomy through the oral examination and diagnostics for all areas of the mouth, this text is a valuable reference for both the general practitioner and the seasoned veterinary dentist.

Those of us, like Dr. Niemiec, who have walked in the footsteps of those pioneers of the early days of veterinary dentistry, can only hope to carry on the tradition of educating others in our quest to relieve unnecessary patient suffering. This book is an excellent tribute to those practitioners.

With gratitude and thanks,

Michael Peak, DVM, DAVDC
Immediate Past-President, American Veterinary Dental College

This book is designed to be a quick reference for practitioners to identify the common oral pathologies in the dog and cat. All pathologies are demonstrated by typical photographic and, in some cases, radiographic examples. Along with the graphic examples is a concise but complete and current description of the pathology. The description includes etiology, pathogenesis, clinical features, differential diagnoses, diagnostic tests, and treatment/management. Each topic is then summarized in easy-to-read key points. This format will make identification and initial therapy of oral diseases much more efficient.

The first three chapters set a foundation for assessing and diagnosing oral pathology. Chapter one is a review of oral anatomy and physiology. In the style of the book, this is supported with numerous full color images. Chapter two presents a stepwise guide on how to perform a proper oral examination. These techniques will allow practitioners to find the subtle pathologies listed within the book. Finally, dental radiology is presented. The first part of chapter three discusses proper techniques for obtaining quality dental radiographs, and the latter part discusses proper diagnosis of dental radiographs with high-quality digital images.

Following this introduction, the book is presented by anatomic areas, to ease identification of unknown pathology. These areas include problems with the: teeth; gingiva; oral mucosa; bones, muscles, and joints; and salivary glands. Individual chapters have been created for pediatric oral/dental problems and malignant oral neoplasia. These unique topics are presented separately from the anatomical chapters to decrease time spent scanning the other chapters. Using this efficient format, if a patient under about 9 months is presented, the practitioner should only have to go beyond the pediatric chapter on rare occasions. Furthermore, if presented with a novel pathology, the practitioner may not know the name of the disease process, thereby making an index much less useful. By directly targeting the chapter which deals with that area of the mouth (for example the lesion is on the tooth), the practitioner can quickly scan just a few pathologies until he/she finds a picture that looks like the lesion in question. Then, in just a few minutes, the reader can learn all about the disease process, including what tests should be run to confirm the diagnosis as well as how best to manage it. Even experienced practitioners will benefit from the cutting edge information in this book.

In addition, the succinct and practical style of this volume lends itself to be a client-friendly education tool. The veterinarian can use this peer-reviewed book to back up their management recommendations. This is critically important in veterinary dentistry, as most pathologies do not have obvious clinical signs that owners recognize (fractured teeth for example). The prudent practitioner will encourage clients to read the brief description of their pet's particular pathology, thus improving client compliance with treatment recommendations. Since dental disease is present in almost all veterinary patients, I would consider having a copy in each exam room. This will aid all dental related discussions.

This book makes numerous treatment recommendations, but it is not a technical manual. For those practitioners interested in improving their technical skills, I recommend *Veterinary Dental Techniques*, 3rd edn, by Holmstrom SE, Frost P, and Eisner ER (eds), Saunders, 2004. However, these techniques (including dental radiology) are best learned through hands-on training at wetlabs. For a list of my wetlabs in San Diego, visit www.sdvdtc.com.

Brook A. Niemiec, DVM, DAVDC, FAVD

ABBREVIATIONS

AI	amelogenesis imperfecta
APD	air-polishing device
BPAB	black pigmented anaerobic bacteria
CBC	complete blood count
CEJ	cementoenamel junction
CI	calculus index
CK	creatine kinase
COC	calcifying odontogenic cyst
CT	computed tomography
CUPS	chronic ulcerative paradental stomatitis
DI	dentinogenesis imperfecta
DR	digital radiograph
EGC	eosinophilic granuloma complex
EMG	electromyography
FCV	feline calicivirus
FE	furcation exposure
FeLV	feline leukemia virus
FIV	feline immunodeficiency virus
FNA	fine-needle aspiration
FSA	fibrosarcoma
GI	gingival index
HIV	human immunodeficiency virus
IL-1	interleukin-1
IVIG	intravenous immunoglobulin
LEO	lesions of endodontic origin

MGM/ MGL	mucogingival margin/line
MM	masticatory myositis
MRI	magnetic resonance imaging
MTA	mineral trioxide aggregate
NSAID	nonsteroidal anti-inflammatory drug
OAF	oroantral fistula
OSA	osteosarcoma
PDL	periodontal ligament
PEG	percutaneous endoscopic gastrostomy
PI	plaque index
PTH	parathyroid hormone
RT-PCR	reverse transcriptase polymerase chain reaction
SCC	squamous cell carcinoma
SE	extrinsic staining
SI	intrinsic staining
SLE	systemic lupus erythematosus
SLOB	same-lingual/opposite-buccal
SRP	scaling and root planing
TEN	toxic epidermal necrolysis
TNF	tumor necrosis factor
TVT	transmissible venereal tumor
VOHC	Veterinary Oral Health Care Council

Anatomy and Physiology

John R. Lewis and Alexander M. Reiter

- **Canine dental anatomy**
- **Feline dental anatomy**
- **Rodent and lagomorph dental anatomy**
- **Dental terminology**
- **Tooth development**
- **Enamel, dentin, and pulp**
- **Periodontium**
- **Bones of the face and jaws**
- **Muscles, cheeks, and lips**
- **Neurovascular structures**
- **Joints of the head**
- **Hard and soft palates**
- **Tongue**
- **Salivary glands**
- **Lymph nodes and tonsils**

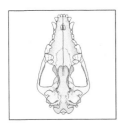 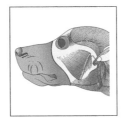 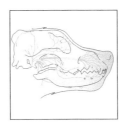 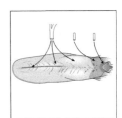

Canine dental anatomy

Accepted dental formulas for the deciduous and permanent dentition in the dog[1]:
- Deciduous teeth: (3 upper/3 lower incisors, 1 upper/1 lower canine, 3 upper/3 lower premolars) × 2 = 28 teeth.
- Permanent teeth: (3 upper/3 lower incisors, 1 upper/1 lower canine, 4 upper/4 lower premolars, 2 upper/3 lower molars) × 2 = 42 teeth.

The modified Triadan system is the most common numbering system in veterinary dentistry[2]. It provides a method of quick reference for verbal or written communication. Each quadrant is numbered as follows:
- Right upper quadrant = 100 (500 when referring to deciduous teeth).
- Left upper quadrant = 200 (600 when referring to deciduous teeth).
- Left lower quadrant = 300 (700 when referring to deciduous teeth).
- Right lower quadrant = 400 (800 when referring to deciduous teeth).

Each tooth is assigned a number within each quadrant. Beginning with 01 for the first incisor, teeth are consecutively numbered from mesial to distal. Since the dog has a full complement of permanent premolars, tooth numbering is consecutive from 01 to 10 on the maxilla and 01 to 11 on the mandible. Taking the quadrant and tooth number into consideration, three numbers are used to identify a specific tooth. For example, the permanent left upper canine tooth is referred to as tooth 204. The deciduous left upper canine is tooth 604 (**1A, B**).

CLINICAL RELEVANCE
- Knowledge of dental formulas and eruption times allows one to recognize abnormalities such as absent and supernumerary permanent teeth (*Table 1*). Identification of tooth type is also essential for accurate dental charting and record keeping.
- The permanent molars and first premolars are referred to as nonsuccessional teeth because they have no deciduous precursors.
- A deciduous tooth can be distinguished from a permanent tooth by its shape and diminutive size relative to permanent teeth. Deciduous premolars often mimic the shape of the adult tooth immediately distal to the deciduous tooth. For example, the deciduous upper fourth premolar has a crown shape similar to the permanent upper first molar.

Table 1 Eruption times of deciduous and permanent teeth in the dog[1]

	Deciduous teeth	Permanent teeth
Incisors	3–4 weeks	3–5 months
Canines	3 weeks	4–6 months
Premolars	4–12 weeks	4–6 months
Molars	No deciduous molars	5–7 months

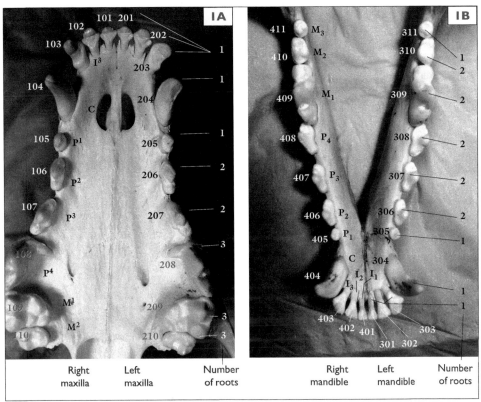

| | Right maxilla | Left maxilla | Number of roots | | Right mandible | Left mandible | Number of roots |

I Modified Triadan numbering system in the dog. **A:** Maxilla; **B:** Mandible. (Three-rooted teeth in red.)

Feline dental anatomy

Accepted dental formulas for the deciduous and permanent dentition in the cat[1]:

- Deciduous teeth: (3 upper/3 lower incisors, 1 upper/1 lower canine, 3 upper/2 lower premolars) × 2 = 26 teeth.
- Permanent teeth: (3 upper/3 lower incisors, 1 upper/1 lower canine, 3 upper/2 lower premolars, 1 upper/1 lower molar) × 2 = 30 teeth.

Several permanent premolars and molars have been evolutionarily lost in the domestic cat. Consequently, use of the Triadan numbering system in feline dental charting is slightly more complicated (**2A, B**). The 'rule of 04 and 09' refers to the fact that the canine (tooth 04) and the first molar (09) are present as reference teeth to allow counting forward or backward when numbering teeth[2]. For example, the lower first (05) and second (06) permanent premolars are absent in the cat, and thus the premolar closest to the canine tooth may mistakenly be numbered as the 05 tooth. Knowledge that the lower first molar (09 tooth) is the largest cheek tooth of the mandible allows one to count forward and identify the lower premolar closest to the canine as the 07 tooth (**2**). Quadrants are numbered as described under canine dental anatomy. As an example, the right mandibular third premolar is tooth 407. The left maxillary second premolar is tooth 206.

CLINICAL RELEVANCE

- The cat's dentition is different to the dog's in many ways. The total number of teeth is greatly decreased, and the crown shapes reflect the function of a true carnivore. Eruption times differ (*Table 2*).
- Since cats do not have occlusal table surfaces on their molars, they rarely develop true carious lesions.
- Cats are more commonly affected by tooth resorption than dogs.
- The groove on the buccal surface of the canine teeth of cats has been referred to as a 'bleeding groove', an adaptation of carnivore teeth which is thought to allow prey to bleed around the tooth while prehended by the cat.
- Variation in the number of roots exists in maxillary cheek teeth of cats, specifically the second and third premolar and first molar[3].

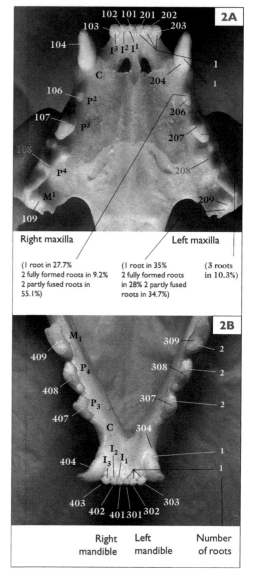

Right maxilla   **Left maxilla**

(1 root in 27.7% 2 fully formed roots in 9.2% 2 partly fused roots in 55.1%)

(1 root in 35% 2 fully formed roots in 28% 2 partly fused roots in 34.7%)

(3 roots in 10.3%)

Right mandible   **Left mandible**   **Number of roots**

2 Modified Triadan system in the cat.
A: Maxilla; **B:** Mandible. (Three-rooted teeth in red.)

Table 2 Eruption times of deciduous and permanent teeth in the cat[1]

	Deciduous teeth	Permanent teeth
Incisors	2–3 weeks	3–4 months
Canines	3–4 weeks	4–5 months
Premolars	3–6 weeks	4–6 months
Molars	No deciduous molars	4–5 months

Rodent and lagomorph dental anatomy

Rodents have a single set of teeth without precursors or successors. There is one large, chisel-shaped incisor tooth in each quadrant (i.e. two upper and two lower incisors). These teeth generally have yellow enamel (except in the guinea pig) and evolved for dorsoventral slicing action. Gnawing action wears away tooth substance that must be replaced, so incisors continue to grow throughout the rodent's life, never developing anatomical roots. Rats, mice, and hamsters typically consume high-energy foods (seeds, grain, and tubers) that require little chewing, and thus the cheek teeth are subject to little wear[4]. These rodents have three small molar teeth in each quadrant, with anatomical roots that stop growing once fully erupted[5,6]. In contrast, chinchillas and guinea pigs are true herbivores, consuming large quantities of low-energy foods (fibrous mountain vegetation), resulting in marked wear to the cheek teeth. They have one premolar and three molars in each quadrant, with large grinding surfaces (**3**). The chinchilla and guinea pig's cheek teeth also never form anatomical roots, growing continuously to compensate for constant wear[4].

Lagomorphs have two sets of teeth. The deciduous teeth are rarely seen since they are generally lost *in utero* or shortly after birth[7]. Rabbits have a second, smaller pair of maxillary incisor teeth ('peg' teeth) palatal to the first incisors. They are true herbivores and primarily use their incisors in a lateral slicing action. There are three maxillary and two mandibular premolar teeth on each side, with three molar teeth in all quadrants[5,6]. The enamel of all lagomorph teeth is unpigmented. As in true herbivorous rodents, the rabbit's incisors and cheek teeth lack anatomical roots and continue to grow throughout life[7].

CLINICAL RELEVANCE

- Herbivorous species are often fed concentrates in the form of grain or pellets (which are more suited to rats and mice), with only limited or no access to hay and natural vegetation. For many pet rodents and lagomorphs, the provided food does not match their natural diet. If the diet provides too little tooth wear to compensate for the natural growth of the teeth, tooth elongation may occur.
- Chinchillas and rabbits tend to have severe extension of the cheek tooth apices into adjacent tissues, causing palpable swellings on the ventral border of the mandible and orbital invasion with epiphora, proptosis of the eye, and conjunctivitis.
- Guinea pigs tend to have severe intraoral tooth overgrowth, leading to formation of sharp enamel points or spikes on the buccal and lingual surfaces of upper and lower cheek teeth, irritation and ulceration of the buccal and lingual mucosa, and 'trapping' of the tongue[4,7].

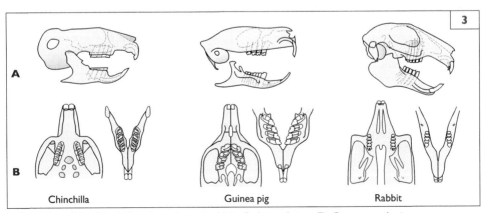

3 Dentition of the chinchilla, guinea pig, and rabbit. **A:** Lateral view; **B:** Open-mouth view.

Chinchilla   Guinea pig   Rabbit

Dental terminology

Dentistry has its own set of terms to describe accurately anatomical locations of the head and surfaces of individual teeth[6,8–11].

TERMS USED TO DESCRIBE A LOCATION OR DIRECTION IN REFERENCE TO THE ENTIRE HEAD

- Rostral – referring to a location toward the tip of the nose, analogous to the anatomical term 'cranial', but specifically used in describing locations on the head.
- Caudal – referring to a location towards the tail.
- Ventral – referring to a location towards the lower jaw.
- Dorsal – referring to a location towards the top of the head or muzzle.

TERMS USED TO DESCRIBE A LOCATION OR DIRECTION IN REFERENCE TO A TOOTH OR TEETH (4A, B)

- Mesial – the interproximal surface of the tooth that faces rostrally or towards the midline of the dental arch.
- Distal – the interproximal surface of the tooth that faces caudally or away from the midline of the dental arch.
- Vestibular – the surface of the tooth facing the lips: 'buccal' and 'labial' are acceptable alternatives.
- Facial – specifically refers to the surfaces of the rostral teeth visible from the front.
- Lingual – refers to the surfaces of the mandibular teeth that face the tongue.
- Palatal – refers to the surface of maxillary teeth that face the palate.
- Occlusal – refers to the surface of the tooth that faces the tooth of the opposing arcade.
- Proximal – referring to the mesial and distal surfaces of a tooth that come in close contact to an adjacent tooth.
- Interproximal – referring to the space between adjacent teeth.
- Coronal – referring to a location or direction toward the crown of the tooth.

- Apical – referring to a location or direction toward the tip of the tooth root.
- Line angle – line where two surfaces of the tooth converge (example: mesio-lingual).
- Point angle – point where three line angles converge (example: mesio-linguo-occlusal).

TERMS REFERRING TO ANATOMICAL STRUCTURES OF THE TOOTH

- Cusp – a pronounced point on the occlusal or most coronal portion of a tooth.
- Mamelon – one of the three rounded protuberances on the cutting edge of a newly erupted incisor tooth.
- Cingulum – rounded surface of the cervical third of the lingual or palatal surface of incisor teeth.
- Embrasure – the open spaces between the proximal surfaces of adjacent teeth that diverge from an area of contact.
- Dental bulge – expansion of crown at the gingival margin designed to deflect food particles away from the gingival sulcus.
- Enamel – highly mineralized inorganic hard tissue that covers the dentin of the crown, produced by ameloblasts.
- Dentin – hard tissue covered by enamel (crown) and cementum (root), produced by odontoblasts.
- Cementum – hard tissue covering the root surface, similar in composition to bone, produced by cementoblasts.
- Pulp – soft tissue within the tooth composed of odontoblasts, blood and lymph vessels, nerves, and layers of connective tissue.
- Pulp cavity – the entire space within the tooth, containing the pulp.
- Pulp chamber – the part of the pulp cavity contained within the crown of the tooth.
- Root canal – the part of the pulp cavity contained within the root of the tooth.
- Attached gingiva – gingival portion attached to underlying bone and tooth, extending from mucogingival junction to the gingival groove.

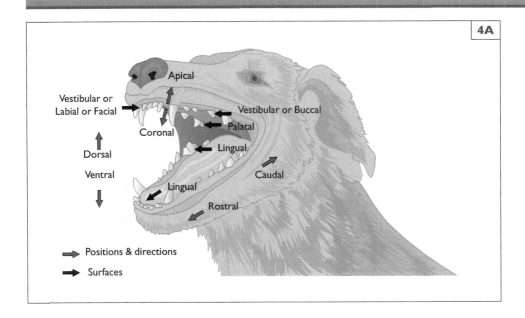

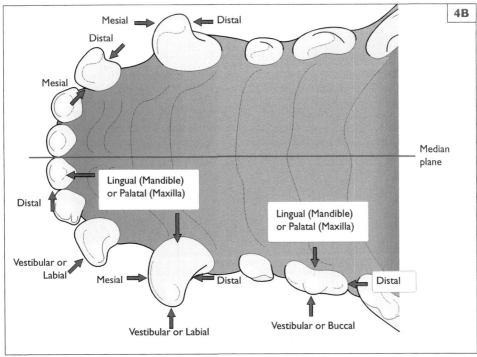

4 Dental anatomical terminology. **A:** Extraoral view; **B:** Intraoral view.

- Free gingiva – free gingival portion, extending from gingival groove to the gingival margin.
- Gingival margin – most coronal extension of the gingiva.
- Gingival sulcus (gingival crevice) – physiological space between free gingiva and tooth surface.
- Subgingival – referring to a structure or area that is apical to the gingival margin.
- Supragingival – referring to a structure or area that is coronal to the gingival margin.

OTHER TERMS

- Monophyodont – only one set of teeth will erupt and remains functional (e.g. dolphins and killer whales).
- Polyphyodont – many sets of teeth are continually replaced (e.g. sharks and crocodiles).
- Diphyodont – having two sets of teeth (e.g. humans and most domesticated mammals).
- Deciduous teeth – the first set of teeth which are shed and replaced by permanent teeth.
- Permanent teeth – the second set of teeth in diphyodont species.
- Successional teeth – permanent teeth which replace or succeed a deciduous counterpart.
- Nonsuccessional teeth – permanent teeth which do not have a deciduous counterpart.
- Homodont – dentition in which all teeth are uniform in shape.

- Heterodont – dentition with teeth of different shape and function (e.g. incisors, canines, premolars, and molars).
- Incisors – cutting teeth situated between the canine teeth.
- Canines – conical teeth situated between the third incisors and premolars, which function in protection, hunting, and prehension in carnivores.
- Premolars – cheek teeth distal to the canine teeth which serve to prehend and tear food in carnivores.
- Molars – cheek teeth distal to the premolars with occlusal surfaces responsible for grinding food (except in felines).
- Carnassial – referring to the upper fourth premolar and lower first molar teeth, which serve a shearing function in carnivores.
- Elodont – tooth that grows throughout life (e.g. chinchillas, guinea pigs, and rabbits; incisors of all other rodents; tusks of elephants and other animals; caudal teeth of aardvarks).
- Anelodont – tooth that has a limited period of growth.
- Hypsodont – tooth with long anatomical crown at tooth maturity; the tooth is continuously erupting as occlusal wear takes place (e.g. horses and ruminants).
- Brachyodont – tooth with shorter anatomical crown than root(s) at tooth maturity (e.g. cats and dogs).

Tooth development

Most domesticated animals undergo tooth development resulting in two sets of teeth, deciduous (also referred to as primary) and permanent dentition. Such animals are known as diphyodonts. The first signs of tooth development occur at approximately day 25 of gestation with thickening of embryonic oral epithelium, known as dental lamina. A series of invaginations of this epithelium results in the formation of the primordial tooth structure referred to as enamel organ, more appropriately called dental organ[12]. The dental organ progresses through a series of stages of bud, cap, and bell[13,14] (**5**). The bud stage is the initial coalescence of the dental lamina in locations corresponding to the future site of deciduous teeth. The cap stage begins when the bud develops a concavity on its deep surface. At this stage the dental organ is comprised of three parts including the outer enamel epithelium, the inner enamel epithelium, and the stellate reticulum. The addition of a fourth layer, the stratum intermedium, marks the beginning of the bell stage. The buds which form the deciduous dentition develop extensions called successional laminae. These form the permanent dentition after progressing through the bud, cap, and bell stages. Nonsuccessional teeth (permanent teeth without deciduous counterparts) develop directly from the dental lamina. The progressive growth of the roots results in tooth eruption, occurring at specific times for each tooth and species. Development of the teeth of dogs and cats results in four specific types of teeth, each serving a distinct purpose. The presence of different types of teeth with different functions is referred to as heterodont dentition[11].

CLINICAL RELEVANCE

- The incisors are designed to cut, prehend, and groom. Their concave lingual/palatal surface allows for scooping of food which facilitates transport into the oral cavity. The canines are used to penetrate and grasp prey or food and also function as defensive weapons in protection. In the carnivore they represent the teeth with the longest crown and root. The premolars assist in the ability to hold and carry, in addition to breaking food into smaller pieces. The occlusal surfaces of the molars grind food into smaller particles in preparation for digestion
- Abnormalities or disruptions of the normal sequence of tooth development may be an indication of past or ongoing disease.
- Disruption of ameloblasts during formation of enamel matrix protein may result in enamel hypoplasia and/or enamel hypocalcification. Common causes include infection with epitheliotropic viruses such as distemper, febrile episodes, metabolic or nutritional abnormalities, or trauma to a tooth during the formation of enamel prior to tooth eruption. Incomplete enamel coverage may cause tooth sensitivity, increased plaque retention, and development of carious lesions.
- Caries lesions, though rare in companion animals, are most commonly seen on the occlusal surface of the maxillary first molars due to developmental pits and fissures with incomplete enamel coverage of the occlusal surfaces.
- Ectodermal dysplasia is a genetic disease affecting structures of ectodermal origin including skin and teeth. Affected patients often exhibit oligodontia (multiple missing teeth), peg teeth (abnormally pointed crowns), and abnormally shaped or number of roots.

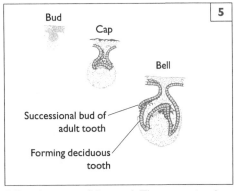

5 Development of the tooth. The successional bud of the permanent tooth can be seen forming from the dental lamina.

Enamel, dentin, and pulp

Enamel is the hardest tissue of the body due to its high mineral content, arranged in rods of densely packed calcium hydroxyapatite crystals. Hydroxyapatite accounts for 96% of enamel by weight (85% by volume). The remaining 4% is comprised of water, protein, and lipid. Although enamel is produced by cells called ameloblasts, mature enamel is acellular. Mineral exchange occurs between enamel and saliva. Demineralization of surface enamel by acids can be reversed by mineral exchange, but enamel cannot be repaired or regenerated due to the natural loss of ameloblasts after eruption of the tooth[12].

Dentin makes up the bulk of the adult tooth and is continually produced throughout life of a vital tooth. It is comprised of 70% mineral (calcium hydroxyapatite), 20% protein and lipid, and 10% water. Dentin is porous, with approximately 45,000 dentinal tubules per square millimeter in coronal dentin[12]. There are three main types of dentin. Primary dentin is the first dentin produced during development of the tooth. After development and eruption of the tooth, secondary dentin is produced throughout life of a vital tooth, causing the pulp cavity to become progressively narrower. Tertiary (reparative) dentin is produced in response to injury and irritation. Dentin is produced by cells called odontoblasts. Odontoblasts line the periphery of the pulp cavity, and their cytoplasmic processes extend into dentinal tubules. Each tubule also contains fluid, and some tubules contain nerves extending from the pulp. Tooth pain may result from fluid shifts and nerve stimulation due to changes in temperature, desiccation, or osmotic changes (e.g. foods with high sugar content) in the area of exposed tubules. If odontoblasts adjacent to exposed dentinal tubules survive the initial insult, they will produce tertiary dentin, which is

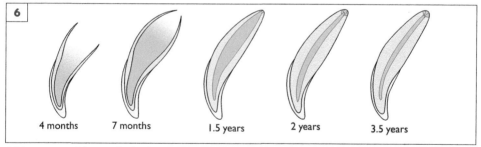

| 6 | | | | |
| 4 months | 7 months | 1.5 years | 2 years | 3.5 years |

6 Maturation of the tooth. As the tooth ages, the apical root forms a delta in dogs and cats, compared to a foramen in primates.

produced in a rapid, less organized fashion than primary or secondary dentin[11].

Pulp is comprised of four layers, beginning from the periphery[15]:

- Odontoblastic layer – responsible for production of secondary dentin throughout the life of the vital tooth and tertiary dentin in response to injury and irritation.
- Cell-free zone of Weil – acellular area which contains the subodontoblastic nerve plexus of Raschkow.
- Cell-rich zone – containing undifferentiated mesenchymal cells and fibroblasts.
- Pulp proper – containing major vessels, nerves, and connective tissue; direct stimulation of the pulp results in sharp, localizable pain associated with stimulation of myelinated A-delta fibers; dull throbbing pain is created by stimulation of unmyelinated C fibers.

CLINICAL RELEVANCE

- Fluoride has a beneficial effect upon enamel by substituting hydroxyl groups to form fluoroapatite, which is more resistant to acidic dissolution by cariogenic bacteria.
- The disorganization of tertiary dentin makes it prone to extrinsic staining, resulting in a brown color that may mimic pulp exposure. Determination of tertiary dentin versus pulp exposure can be made by running an explorer over the discolored area. If the discolored area feels smooth on exploration, it is likely to be tertiary dentin.
- Although enamel reaches its full thickness prior to eruption, dentin becomes continually thicker during the life of the tooth. Extracting immature teeth is sometimes difficult because these teeth are very fragile (**6, 7**[16]).
- Tooth enamel of dogs and cats is thin compared to that of human enamel[17].
- The 'dental bulge', a convexity of the cervical crown portion, is not due to an increased thickness of enamel, but rather a thickening of dentin in this area[17].

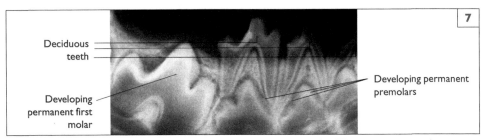

7 Radiograph of deciduous and developing permanent teeth in the dog. The permanent teeth are forming within the mandible. The first molar, being a nonsuccessional tooth, is more developed than the permanent premolars adjacent to it.

Periodontium

The periodontium consists of four components: the gingiva, periodontal ligament, cementum, and alveolar bone (**8, 9**).

The gingiva and adjacent connective tissue are durable, fibrous tissues that protect the subgingival attachment apparatus of the tooth. The gingiva is keratinized and consists of four layers: stratum corneum, stratum granulosum, stratum spinosum (prickle cell layer), and stratum basale. A space between the tooth and gingiva normally exists called the gingival sulcus. The normal sulcus depth is considered less than 3 mm in dogs and less than 1 mm in cats. The presence of rete pegs (epithelial ridges that interdigitate with underlying connective tissue) may cause a normal stippling of the gingival surface.

The periodontal ligament (PDL) acts as the shock absorber of the tooth. The principal fibers of the PDL, also known as Sharpey's fibers, travel transversely in the coronal portion of the root and more obliquely towards the apex. Some fibers connect adjacent teeth by traveling through or coronal to the alveolar septum. The periodontal space also contains vessels and cells. Epithelial cells within the periodontal space, called cell rests of Malassez, are remnants of the Hertwig's epithelial root sheath. These cells are thought to play a role in the maintenance and repair of the PDL. Radiographically, the PDL appears as a dark line surrounding the root.

The cementum is a hard tissue that covers the root and is produced by cementoblasts. Sharpey's fibers are embedded in cementum and traverse the periodontal space to anchor the tooth in alveolar bone. Cementum is similar in mineral composition and histologic appearance to bone. Cementum width increases with age. A variety of medical conditions can result in hypercementosis, an excessive production of cementum, most commonly seen in the apical portion of the root.

Alveolar bone surrounds the alveolar socket. Radiographically, an increased density of alveolar bone is visible adjacent to the periodontal space, referred to as the lamina dura. Bone is constantly remodeling in response to use and the forces placed upon it. Because of this, alveolar bone has the most rapid turnover of any bone in the body. Osteoclasts are responsible for resorption of bone, whereas osteoblasts produce new bone.

CLINICAL RELEVANCE

- Periodontal disease is the most common disease in companion animals. A thorough understanding of the normal attachment structures of the tooth allows for identification of pathological conditions and appropriate treatment.
- A periodontal probe is used to detect periodontal pockets of teeth affected by periodontal disease. The normal sulcus depth is considered less than 3 mm in dogs and less than 1 mm in cats. Deeper probing depths are evidence of a periodontal pocket.
- In cats, tooth resorption may be hidden by a focal area of granulation tissue or inflamed gingiva. Use of a fine dental explorer at the gingival margin allows for detection of lesions.
- Radiographically, the PDL appears as a dark line surrounding the root. An increased density of alveolar bone is visible adjacent to the periodontal space, referred to as the lamina dura.

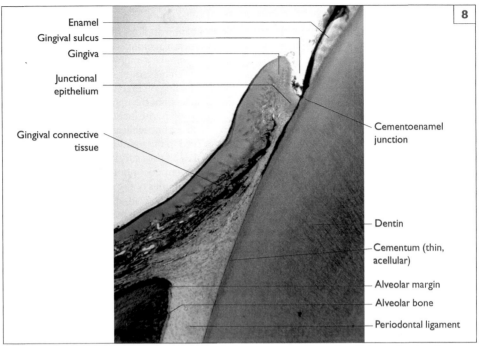

8 Photomicrograph of the periodontium. Cervical cementum is thin and acellular at the alveolar margin.

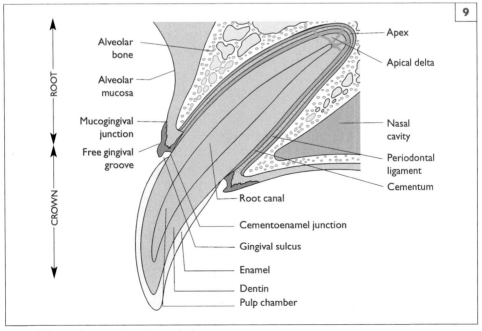

9 An adult maxillary tooth and its periodontium.

Bones of the face and jaws

Three terms are used to describe head shape. Mesaticephalic refers to a head of medium proportions, as seen in the majority of dogs and cats. Brachycephalic animals have short, wide heads such as Pekingese dogs and Persian cats. Dolichocephalic dogs and cats have long, narrow heads, such as the Collie and Siamese cat (**10**).

CLINICAL RELEVANCE

- Understanding the bony anatomy of the face and jaws is an important aspect in dentistry (surgical extractions, orthodontics) and oral surgery (mandibulectomy, maxillectomy, jaw fracture repair). The following diagrams depict some of the commonly encountered bones and structures of the face and jaws during surgical procedures(**11–15**)[18,19].

- Unlike humans, dogs and cats have right and left mandibles that are separated by a fibrocartilaginous synchondrosis (mandibular symphysis). This symphysis may exhibit various degrees of mobility depending on breed and age.
- The teeth of the upper jaw are confined to two bones: the incisors arise from the incisive bone while all other teeth are rooted in the maxilla. The palatine bone makes up the caudal portion of the hard palate but does not contain any teeth.
- The hamulus of the pterygoid bone is palpable bilaterally, dorsal to the soft palate and just lateral to midline. Inability to palpate these processes may suggest the presence of a nasopharyngeal/retrobulbar space occupying lesion.
- Brachycephalic dogs often exhibit crowding of teeth due to skull shape. As a result, rotation of teeth and periodontal disease are common.

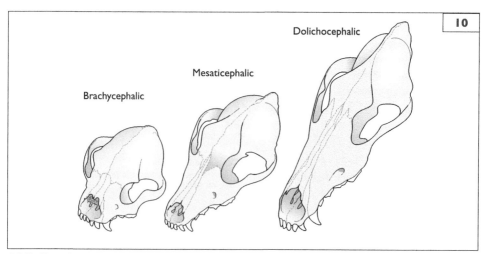

10 Skull conformation: brachycephalic, mesaticephalic, dolichocephalic.

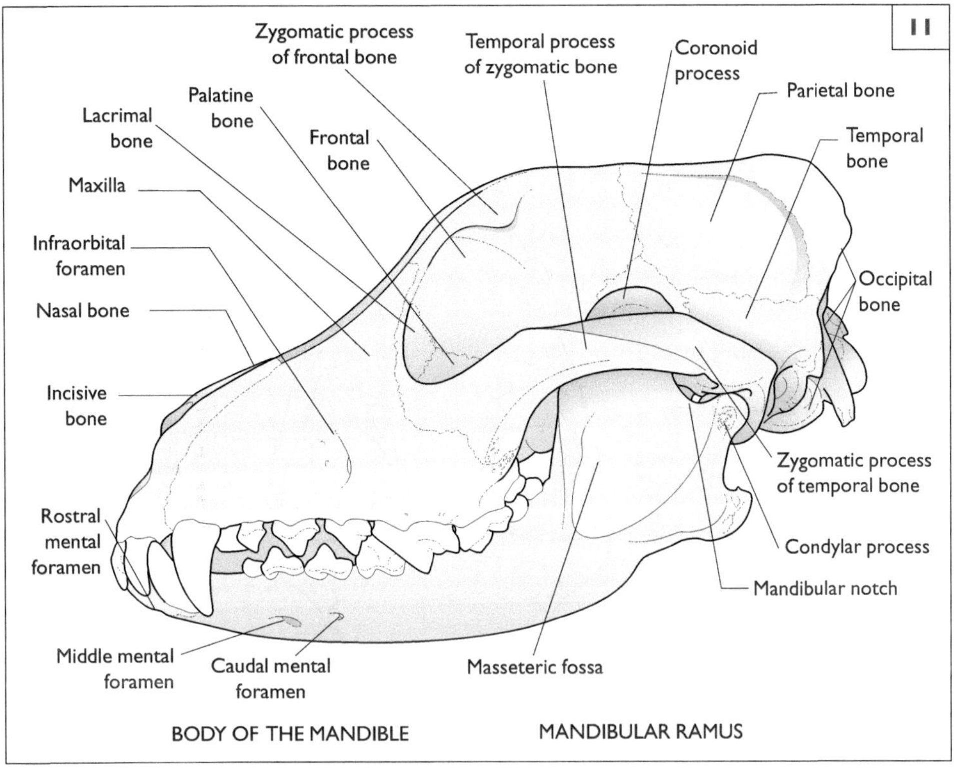
11
Zygomatic process of frontal bone
Temporal process of zygomatic bone
Coronoid process
Parietal bone
Temporal bone
Palatine bone
Lacrimal bone
Frontal bone
Maxilla
Infraorbital foramen
Nasal bone
Occipital bone
Incisive bone
Zygomatic process of temporal bone
Rostral mental foramen
Condylar process
Mandibular notch
Middle mental foramen
Caudal mental foramen
Masseteric fossa
BODY OF THE MANDIBLE
MANDIBULAR RAMUS

11 Bones of the face and jaws, lateral view.

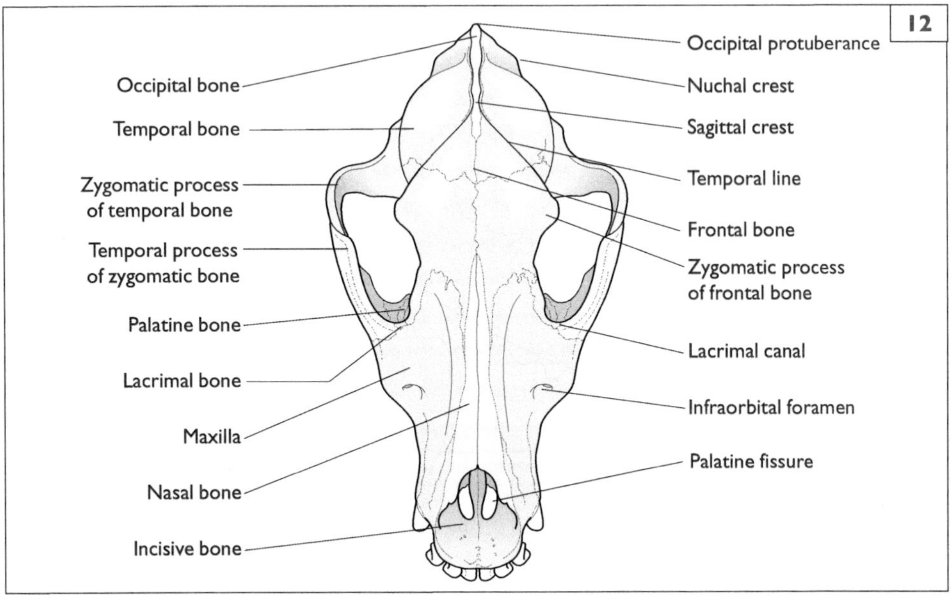
12
Occipital protuberance
Occipital bone
Nuchal crest
Temporal bone
Sagittal crest
Zygomatic process of temporal bone
Temporal line
Frontal bone
Temporal process of zygomatic bone
Zygomatic process of frontal bone
Palatine bone
Lacrimal canal
Lacrimal bone
Infraorbital foramen
Maxilla
Palatine fissure
Nasal bone
Incisive bone

12 Bones of the face and jaws, dorsal view.

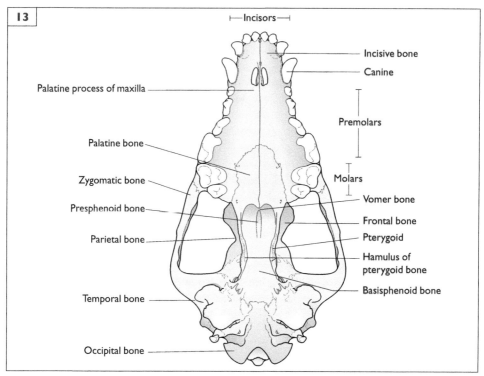

13 Bones of the skull, ventral view.

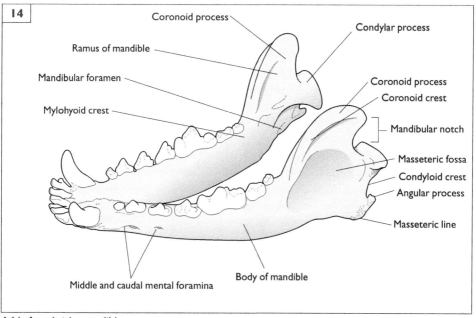

14 Left and right mandibles.

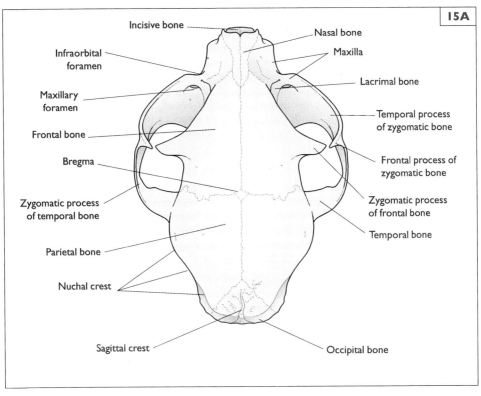

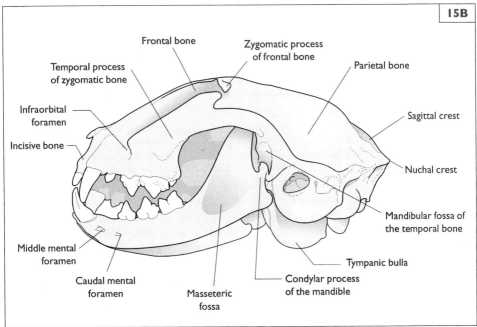

15 Bones of the face and jaws of the cat. **A:** Dorsal view; **B:** Lateral view.

Muscles, cheeks, and lips

MASTICATORY MUSCLES

The paired muscles of mastication include the masseter, temporal, pterygoid (medial and lateral), and the digastricus muscles. All function to close the mouth, with the exception of the digastricus muscle, which acts to open the mouth. Muscles of mastication, with the exception of the digastricus muscle, contain a special type of myofiber, referred to as Type 2M[20]. The masseter muscle originates ventral to the zygomatic arch and inserts to the ventrolateral mandibular ramus. The temporal muscle, the largest and strongest muscle of the head, occupies the temporal fossa and arises from the parietal, temporal frontal, and occipital bones. The muscle inserts at the coronoid process of the mandible and the dorsal portion of the zygomatic arch. The lateral pterygoid muscle arises from a bony ridge on the sphenoid bone and inserts on the medial surface of the condylar process. The larger medial pterygoid muscle arises from the lateral surface of the pterygoid, palatine, and sphenoid bones and inserts along the ventromedial border of the mandibular ramus and angular process. The digastricus muscle arises from the paracondylar process of the occiput and inserts on the caudal two-thirds of the ventral mandible. It consists of a rostral belly, innervated by the trigeminal nerve, and a caudal belly, innervated by the facial nerve[18] (**16,17**).

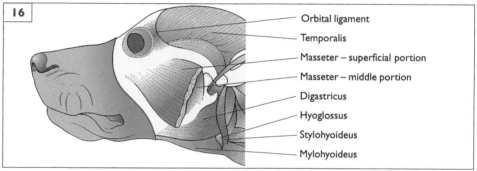

16 Muscles of mastication, lateral view.

Orbital ligament
Temporalis
Masseter – superficial portion
Masseter – middle portion
Digastricus
Hyoglossus
Stylohyoideus
Mylohyoideus

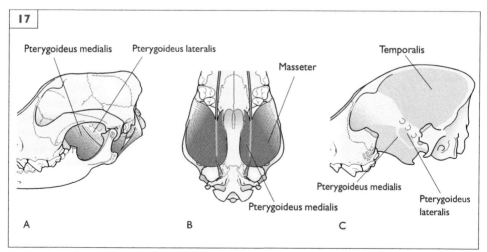

17 Muscles of mastication. **A:** Cutaway of mandible to show pterygoid muscles; **B:** Ventral view; **C:** Attachment sites of temporalis and pterygoids.

Pterygoideus medialis   Pterygoideus lateralis   Temporalis
Masseter
Pterygoideus medialis
Pterygoideus medialis
Pterygoideus lateralis
A   B   C

CHEEKS

The soft tissue of the cheeks of dogs and cats consists of four main layers: external skin, orbicularis oris and platysma muscles, buccinator muscle, and intraoral buccal mucosa. The portion of the cheek where the upper and lower lips converge is called the commissure. Three important structures contained beneath the soft tissues of the cheek run parallel in a rostrocaudal direction. The dorsal buccal branch of the facial nerve traverses in a horizontal plane just dorsal to the commissure. The parotid duct runs parallel to this structure at the level of the commissure. The most ventral of the three structures is the ventral buccal branch of the facial nerve. Rostrocaudal rather than dorsoventral incisions in this area will help to avoid inadvertent transection of these structures (**18**).

LIPS

The lips are not used as prehensile organs in dogs and cats, but they do function in communication and expression. Muscles that play a role in function of the cheeks and lips include the platysma, orbicularis oris, caninus, levator nasolabialis, incisivus superioris, incisivus inferioris, and levator labii muscles.

CLINICAL RELEVANCE

- The myofibers of the masseter, temporal, and pterygoid muscles contain a unique form of myosin which is sometimes targeted by immune-mediated mechanisms in dogs with masticatory myositis. Serum antibody titer determination and muscle biopsy are performed in dogs exhibiting pain on opening the mouth in order to rule out this disease.
- Some breeds (such as Sharpei dogs) exhibit 'tight lip syndrome', whereas other breeds (such as Newfoundlands) have a redundancy of lip tissue in the area of the lower premolars. Both conditions may result in lack of normal vestibule formation.
- When incising the soft tissues of the cheek, incisions should be made in a rostrocaudal rather than dorsoventral direction to avoid inadvertent transection of the parotid duct and branches of the facial nerve.
- When a unilateral mandibulectomy is performed, the tongue may protrude on this side. A commissurorrhaphy (movement of the commissure forward by incising and suturing) will minimize tongue deviation on the affected side.

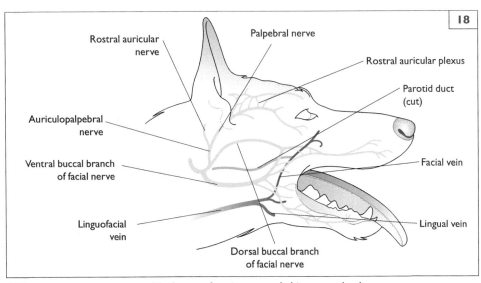

18 Important structures to avoid when performing a muscle biopsy or cheek surgery.

Neurovascular structures

Two cranial nerves are responsible for many of the afferent and efferent innervations of the structures of the head. The trigeminal nerve (cranial nerve V) divides into the ophthalmic, maxillary, and mandibular branches. All three branches are sensory, but the mandibular branch of the trigeminal nerve also supplies motor function to the muscles of mastication and other adjacent muscles. The lingual nerve, a branch of the mandibular nerve, contains afferent fibers that transmit tactile, pain, and thermal impulses from the rostral two-thirds of the tongue. The facial nerve (cranial nerve VII) provides motor function to many of the cutaneous facial muscles and the caudal belly of the digastricus muscle, and is responsible for taste in the rostral two-thirds of the tongue. The maxillary artery, a branch of the external carotid artery, provides blood supply to the upper jaw via infraorbital, palatine (major and minor), and sphenopalatine branches. The mandibular artery is a branch of the maxillary artery and provides blood supply to the lower jaw. Veins often exist concurrently with arteries and empty via the maxillary and linguofacial veins into the external jugular vein.

The following diagrams show important neurovascular structures of the face and mouth (**19–22**).

CLINICAL RELEVANCE

- Knowledge of nerves and vessels of the face, jaws, and tongue is essential when performing oral surgery.
- When performing mandibulectomies and maxillectomies, it is advisable to score the bone with a bur and then use leverage to break the remaining bony attachments; this technique allows for safe ligation of the mandibular and infraorbital vessels.
- When performing maxillectomies, surgical efficiency is critical. Bleeding may not be able to be controlled until the affected piece of jaw is removed. Have blood products available in case of severe bleeding.
- The infraorbital neurovascular bundle or its branches may be encountered when removing root tips from maxillary premolars and molars. This bundle runs between the mesiobuccal and mesiopalatal roots of the maxillary fourth premolar tooth. Avoid burring of bone or tooth in areas where

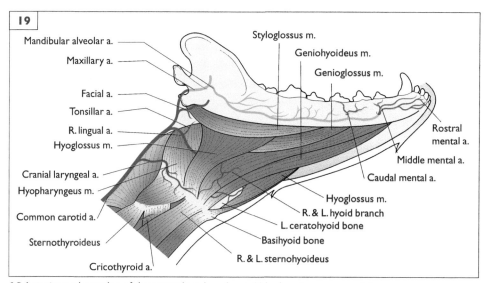

19 Arteries and muscles of the ventral neck and mandible. (a: artery; m: muscle)

visualization is difficult, and use the smallest bur possible (such as a 1/4 round bur) to minimize iatrogenic hemorrhage.

- The middle mental foramen is located lateral to the apex of the mandibular canine tooth. Be cognizant of this structure when creating a flap and window in the alveolar bone during extraction.
- The inferior alveolar artery is apical to the roots of the mandibular premolars and molars. Care must be taken when retrieving root tips from this area.

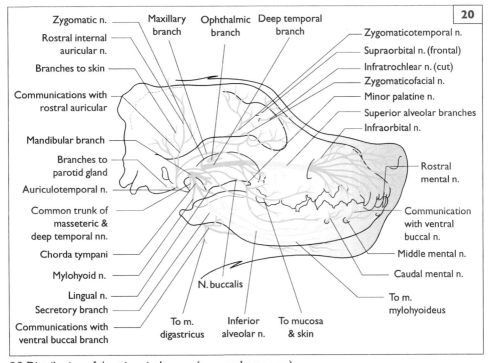

20 Distribution of the trigeminal nerve. (m: muscle; n: nerve)

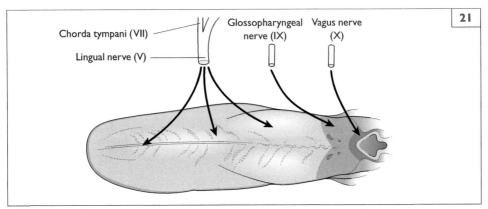

21 Sensory innervations of the tongue. The trigeminal (V) and facial nerve (VII) supply the rostral two-thirds, and the glossopharyngeal (IX) and vagus (X) nerves supply the caudal tongue.

22

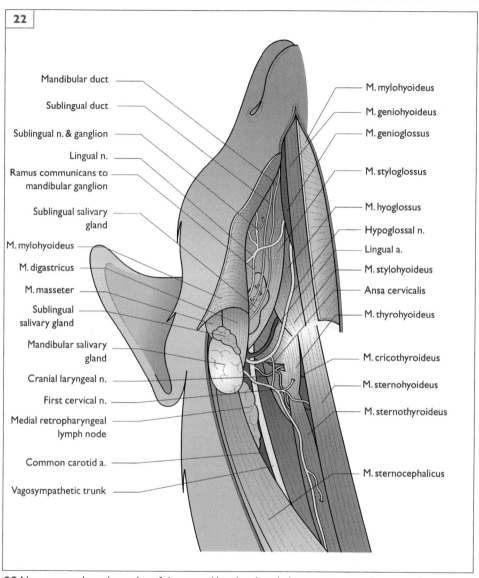

Mandibular duct

Sublingual duct

Sublingual n. & ganglion

Lingual n.

Ramus communicans to
mandibular ganglion

Sublingual salivary
gland

M. mylohyoideus

M. digastricus

M. masseter

Sublingual
salivary gland

Mandibular salivary
gland

Cranial laryngeal n.

First cervical n.

Medial retropharyngeal
lymph node

Common carotid a.

Vagosympathetic trunk

M. mylohyoideus

M. geniohyoideus

M. genioglossus

M. styloglossus

M. hyoglossus

Hypoglossal n.

Lingual a.

M. stylohyoideus

Ansa cervicalis

M. thyrohyoideus

M. cricothyroideus

M. sternohyoideus

M. sternothyroideus

M. sternocephalicus

22 Nerves, vessels, and muscles of the ventral head and neck. (a: artery; m: muscle; n: nerve)

Joints of the head

The temporomandibular joint (TMJ) is formed by the condylar process of the mandible and the mandibular fossa of the temporal bone[18]. A thin fibrocartilaginous disc lies between the hyaline cartilage-covered articular surfaces. The joint capsule attaches to the entire edge of the disc. Thus, the joint cavity is completely divided into a dorsal meniscotemporal compartment between the disc and the temporal bone, and a ventral meniscomandibular compartment between the disc and mandible. These two compartments do not communicate with each other. A thick band of fibrous tissue on the lateral aspect of the joint capsule forms the lateral ligament which tightens when the jaw opens[18,21]

The TMJ is a condylar joint that can move in flexion, extension, and translation. Translation refers to the mandible's ability to move rostrally and laterally. The degree of translational ability is related to the dietary habits of the animal. A strictly carnivorous animal will have less movement rostrally and laterally than an omnivore[21–23]. This difference in TMJ mobility is the result of the fit of the condylar process of the mandible within the mandibular fossa of the temporal bone. The strictly carnivorous cat has greater congruity of its mandibular condyle and fossa due to a more prominent retroarticular process and articular eminence; this results in decreased translational movement[21–23].

In conjunction with the rostral mandibular symphysis, subtle changes in angle and rotation of each mandible are possible and essential for normal function. The slight mobility in this fibrocartilaginous synchondrosis makes the two mandibles capable of limited independent movement. Simple opening and closing of the jaw does not require movement of the mandibular symphysis, but it may be necessary for chewing. Independent movement of each mandible may permit luxation of the TMJ to occur without fracture[21–23].

CLINICAL RELEVANCE

- Animals presenting with a TMJ problem may be reluctant or not be able to (fully) open (e.g. fractures, ankylosis, osteoarthritis) or close the mouth (e.g. fractures, luxation, open-mouth jaw locking)[22]. Clinical signs, palpation and diagnostic imaging help to rule out diseases of the eyes, ears, masticatory muscles, and other pathological conditions not related to the TMJ.
- The retroarticular process prevents caudal dislocation of the mandibular condyle; thus TMJ luxation usually occurs in a rostrodorsal direction.
- The more carnivorous an animal, the less translational TMJ movement is possible.
- Slight mobility in the mandibular symphysis allows limited independent movement of the two mandibles. The degree of symphysial mobility varies greatly depending on age, species and breed, which should not be incorrectly diagnosed as a symphysial separation (**23A,B**).

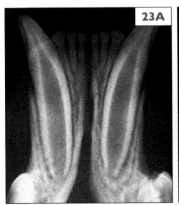
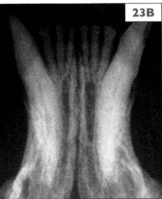

23 Radiograph of young (**A**) and geriatric (**B**) feline mandibular symphysis. As cats age, the symphysis normally becomes irregular and more poorly defined.

Hard and soft palates

The upper lip and rostral hard palate constitute the primary palate. The greater part of the hard palate and the soft palate constitute the secondary palate[18]. The nonelastic hard palate mucosa is developed into 6–10 transverse ridges, or rugae[9,18,24]. The incisive papilla is located on the midline rostral to the first ridge and just caudal to the maxillary first incisor teeth. On either side of this papilla are the incisive ducts that extend caudodorsally through the palatine fissures into the floor of the nasal fossae and communicate with the vomeronasal organ[9,18]. The free edge of the muscular but elastic soft palate curves laterocaudally to form the left and right palatopharyngeal arches, which merge with the walls of the pharynx. When the tongue is withdrawn from the mouth and moved to one side, a palatoglossal fold is developed on the opposite side, running from the body of the tongue to the initial part of the soft palate[18].

At its most caudal aspect, the maxillary bone has a pterygoid process that forms a notch or foramen together with the palatine bone, through which the minor palatine artery passes, providing the main blood supply to the soft palate. The major palatine artery (the main blood supply to the hard palate) passes through the palatine canal and emerges again at the major palatine foramen that is located near the transverse palatine suture, between the median palatine suture and the maxillary fourth premolar tooth. It runs rostrally in the palatine sulcus to the palatine fissures[18]. Within the palatine canal, the nerve and artery divide so that one or more accessory palatine arteries and nerves emerge on the horizontal process of the palatine bone through minor palatine foramina situated caudal to the major palatine foramen. A small rostral septal branch of the major palatine artery passes through the palatine fissure dorsomedially, and a small lateral branch passes through the interdental space between the canine and third incisor teeth[18] (**24, 25**).

CLINICAL RELEVANCE

- Whereas the hard palate forms a rigid partition between the oral and nasal cavities, the soft palate forms a valve. When elevated during swallowing, it closes off the nasopharynx, and when depressed during nose breathing, it closes off the oropharynx[18,25]. During swallowing, it works with the epiglottis, which closes off the distal airway, to allow a food bolus to cross the respiratory tract. Thus, the palate allows independent functioning of the respiratory and digestive systems and is especially important during the neonatal period, when sucking requires an airtight oral cavity. Palate defects can result in nasal discharge, sneezing, coughing, aspiration pneumonia, and failure to create negative pressure for nursing[18,25].
- The major palatine artery is the most important vascular structure of the palatal mucosa and needs to be preserved during surgical procedures.
- Hard palate mucosa lacks a submucosa; thus it remains nonelastic, and sufficient tissue needs to be elevated and freed for tension-free closure of palate defects.
- The incisive papilla is a normal anatomical structure and not a tumor.

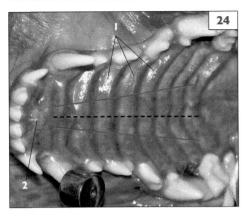

24 Hard palate, palatine rugae, and major palatine artery. Incisive papilla sits on the midline behind the incisors, and palatal mucosa forms a series of ridges and rugae that extend the entire length of the hard palate. The major palatine artery arises bilaterally from a foramen medial to the maxillary fourth premolar and travels rostrally under the palatal mucosa. (Black dotted line = palatal midline. Red line = course of major palatine artery. 1: Palatine rugae; 2: Incisive papilla)

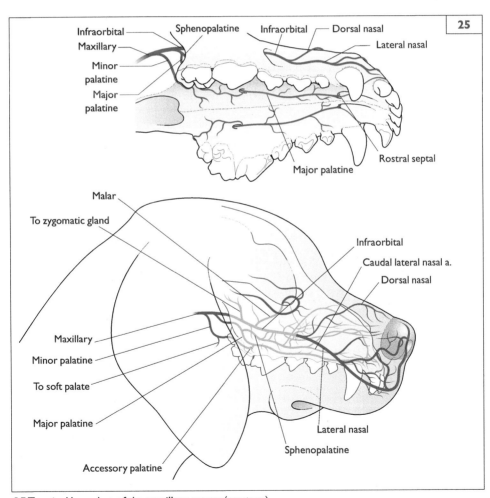

25 Terminal branches of the maxillary artery. (a: artery)

Tongue

The tongue is an elongated, mobile, muscular organ, extending from its attachment on the basihyoid bone to its free tip at the mandibular symphysis[18]. The rostral two-thirds compose the body, and the caudal one-third composes the root of the tongue. A dorsal median groove extends from the tip of the tongue to the level of the vallate papillae. Hairs arranged in a midline row or in two symmetric rows parallel to the midline are seen in an occasional dog[14].

The lateral margins of the tongue separate the dorsal and ventral surfaces. They meet rostrally in the formation of the thin and narrow tip. The free rostral end contains a ventral stiffening rod, the lyssa, formed of fat and muscle in a fibrous sheath. The tongue widens and gradually increases in thickness caudally. Its muscular structure is complex; the motor nerve supply is the hypoglossal nerve (XII). In newborn animals the lateral surfaces of the tongue are fimbriated. These marginal papillae function in suckling and disappear as neonates wean from liquid to solid diets[14].

The lingual mucosa is thick and heavily cornified dorsally but thin and less cornified ventrally. Although taste sensation is of little clinical significance in companion animals, the cornified stratified squamous epithelium forms papillae on the dorsum of the tongue: filiform, fungiform, vallate, foliate, and conical papillae[14,26] (**26, 27**). The sensory nerve supply is a combination of trigeminal (V), facial (VII), glossopharyngeal (IX), and vagus (X) nerves, combining special sensory responses from the taste buds with normal sensory function[18]. The dog's dorsal tongue surface is soft compared to the rather stiff and rough surface of the cat, which has firm papillae that point caudally. On the ventral surface there is an unpaired, median mucosal fold, the lingual frenulum, which connects the body of the tongue to the floor of the mouth. This frenulum is loose, allowing the tongue to extend a considerable distance[14]. A rounded and fimbriated fold of mucosa protrudes on each side of the lingual frenulum, which ends at the sublingual caruncle (area of orifices of mandibular and sublingual gland ducts). The sublingual vein is often located in the submucosa between the lingual frenulum and the lateral border of the fimbriated fold[18]. The lingual artery (a branch of the external carotid artery) provides blood supply to the tongue.

CLINICAL RELEVANCE

- The tongue is usually retained in the mouth except when the animal is panting. The major function of the tongue is to lap fluids and form food boluses that are propelled through the oropharynx during swallowing. Loss of approximately one-third of the tongue (half of the body of the tongue) may not necessarily be associated with clinical signs. Animals compensate for greater amounts of tongue loss by sucking in liquid food or tossing bolused food to the oropharynx[14].

- The sublingual area of cats is a common site for squamous cell carcinoma. During oral examination, the ventral tongue surface and sublingual tissues can be inspected by forcing the thumb of the hand that opens the lower jaw into the intermandibular area, thereby raising the tongue.

- Losing part of the tongue is more problematic in cats; even though they can eat and drink, they may be unable to groom effectively.

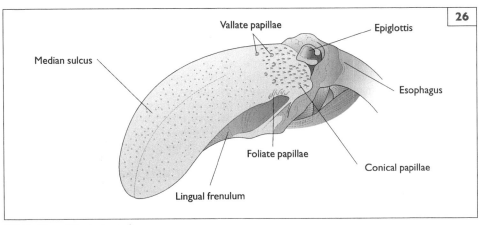

26 Papillae of the tongue, dog.

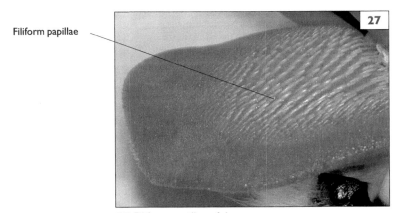

27 Filiform papillae of the tongue, cat.

Salivary glands

Scattered glandular tissue is present submucosally in the lips as the ventral and dorsal buccal glands[1]. The tongue, soft palate, and pharyngeal wall also contain acinar groups. The cat has a small circumscribed gland situated linguocaudally to each mandibular first molar tooth, which is called the lingual molar gland[27] (**28**). There are four pairs of major salivary glands in cats and dogs (**29**).

The parotid gland is a serous gland surrounding the horizontal ear canal. Its margins are indistinct because the gland lobules are held together loosely by connective tissue and blend with the subcutaneous fat and connective tissue of the muscles of the external ear. The parotid duct runs rostrally over the aponeurosis of the masseter muscle, and bends medially, opening into the mouth on a prominent papilla at the level of the maxillary fourth premolar tooth[1,18]. The mandibular gland is an ovoid structure caudoventral to the parotid gland. The maxillary vein covers the caudodorsal aspect of the gland. The mandibular lymph nodes lie on the dorsal and ventral surfaces of the linguofacial vein, which runs along the ventral aspect of the mandibular gland. The mandibular duct runs rostrally between the mandible and the root of the tongue and opens into the mouth at the sublingual caruncle (base of the frenulum of the tongue)[1,18]. The monostomatic part of the sublingual gland is intimately attached to the rostral surface of the mandibular gland. The polystomatic part is located more rostrally between the mandible and the tongue. The sublingual duct either opens as a separate passage on the sublingual caruncle, or joins with the mandibular duct, in which case there is only one opening. The mandibular and sublingual glands are both mixed (seromucous) glands[1,18]. The zygomatic gland is a mixed gland with an irregular ovoid shape that lies on the floor of the orbit ventrocaudal to the eye, immediately medial to the zygomatic arch and dorsal to the infraorbital nerve and vessels. Several ducts, of which the most rostral is the largest, run ventrally and open on a fold of mucosa lateral to the maxillary first molar tooth[1,18].

CLINICAL RELEVANCE

- There is minimal digestive enzyme activity in saliva of cats and dogs. The major function of saliva in cats and dogs is to lubricate the food and to protect the oropharyngeal mucosa. Saliva is rich in antimicrobial and buffering agents. Evaporative heat loss during panting is a secondary function in dogs. The mouth is richly endowed with serous and seromucous glands and mucus-secreting cells on the epithelial surface. Thus, removal of major salivary glands does not lead to xerostomia (dry mouth)[1].
- The intimate anatomical association of sublingual and mandibular gland-duct complexes requires resection of both structures if either of them is the cause of a mucocele.
- Because the mandibular gland is enclosed within a tight capsule, a rapid inflammatory increase in the size of the gland can lead to vascular compromise and necrosis.
- The prominent appearance of the cat's lingual molar gland may lead to an incorrect identification as an abnormal finding.

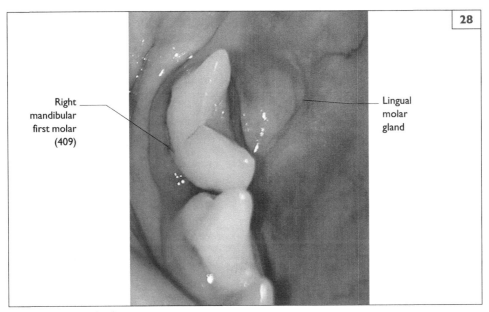

28 Lingual molar gland, cat.

Right mandibular first molar (409)

Lingual molar gland

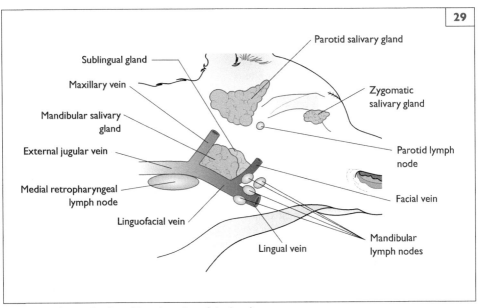

29 Major salivary glands and lymph nodes of the head.

Sublingual gland

Maxillary vein

Mandibular salivary gland

External jugular vein

Medial retropharyngeal lymph node

Linguofacial vein

Lingual vein

Parotid salivary gland

Zygomatic salivary gland

Parotid lymph node

Facial vein

Mandibular lymph nodes

Lymph nodes and tonsils

Lymph nodes act as filters of the lymph and germinal centers for lymphocytes and are surrounded by a capsule. The three lymph centers of the head are the parotid, mandibular, and retropharyngeal lymph centers[18,19]. One or two parotid lymph nodes are situated at the rostral base of the ear, under the rostrodorsal border of the parotid gland. Two or more mandibular lymph nodes lie ventral to the angle of the jaw, above and below the linguofacial vein. Buccal lymph nodes belonging to the mandibular lymph center can be found in less than 10% of dogs and are situated at the angle of the confluence of the facial and superficial labial veins, dorsal to the buccinator muscle[28,29]. The medial retropharyngeal lymph node is a large, elongated, transversely compressed node and lies along the craniodorsal wall of the pharynx. The mandibular gland and the brachiocephalic and sternocephalic muscles cover the node craniolaterally and caudolaterally, respectively. Several neurovascular structures course along the node's medial surface. In approximately one-third of cats and dogs, a lateral retropharyngeal lymph node is present, completely or partially covered by the caudal part of the parotid gland[18,19].

Some collections of lymphoid cells are not surrounded by a capsule, but rather by specialized epithelial cells that are capable of transporting antigen. These tissues do not filter lymph. Their main role is host defense at mucosal surfaces[19]. Dogs and cats possess several tonsil-like structures that are organized as a ring around the root of the tongue, palate, pharynx, and entrance to the larynx (**30**). However, only the palatine tonsils are conspicuous as large, ovoid, discrete bodies, each partly concealed in its own tonsillar fossa by a tonsillar fold derived from the soft palate caudal to the palatoglossal folds. This tonsil is attached by an elongated hilus to the lateral pharyngeal wall, through which it receives tonsillar arteries, and efferent lymphatics depart for the medial retropharyngeal lymph node. Like all tonsils, there are no afferent lymphatics[18].

CLINICAL RELEVANCE

- Regional lymph node enlargement indicates either tumor metastasis or reactivity related to oral inflammation. Enlarged lymph nodes should be evaluated by fine-needle aspiration or excisional biopsy. A single surgical approach has been developed to provide exposure for excisional biopsy of ipsilateral parotid, mandibular, and medial retropharyngeal lymph nodes through one incision[30].
- A negative lymph node aspirate or biopsy does not preclude the possibility of regional metastasis, which may occur along perineural or vascular routes, or metastasis to other lymph nodes.
- Lymph node staging of the primary neoplasm is an integral component of the multimodality treatment plan for the cancer patient.
- Evaluation of the mandibular lymph node alone in oral cancer patients may not provide a true indication of metastasis. Only 54.5% of cases with metastatic disease to regional lymph nodes have metastasis to the mandibular lymph node[31].

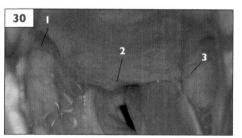

30 Tonsils and soft palate. The soft palate normally extends just beyond the caudal pole of the tonsils. Tonsils may normally be in or out of their tonsillar crypt. (1: Crypt of tonsil; 2: Soft palate; 3: Tonsil [out of crypt])

CHAPTER 2

Oral Examination

Lee Jane Huffman

- **Step 1: History**

- **Step 2: General physical examination**

- **Step 3: Orofacial examination**

- **Step 4: Conscious (awake) intraoral examination**

- **Step 5: The anesthetized orodental examination**

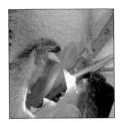
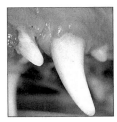
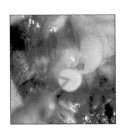
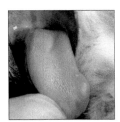

Step 1: History

Oral examination is prefaced by obtaining and verifying signalment and patient history while listening to the client, observing the patient, and performing the complete physical examination. Signalment-attributable risk factors are an important consideration when forming a differential diagnoses list.

Hands-off surveillance of the patient, owner, and additional pets (if present) allows identification of normal and maladaptive behaviors, as well as owner capability of providing restraint and homecare[1]. Have the owner describe what is wrong with their pet and write it down in the owner's words for objectivity and prioritization[2].

Initial questions should be open-ended and non-leading. Discussions should include details of the chief complaint, overall health status, use of the pet, and major past or current health problems (especially those compromising the immune or cardiopulmonary systems[2]). It is also important to discuss results of past tests and physical exams as interpreted by the owner, as well as previous or current treatments including the patient response as perceived by the owner. Thereafter, specific questions about the chief concern should include:

- Inception, frequency, and course.
- Perceived location.
- Associated signs, especially pain-related ones.
- Factors which aggravate, attenuate, or relieve the problem including response to prior treatment(s).

Important points of patient history include:
- Familial history of orofacial problems.
- Parafunctional behaviors such as: bruxism, increased or decreased chewing or grooming, pica, cage-chewing, decreased ability to open or close the mouth, yelping upon yawning, novel aversion to bite work or food, lateralized chewing, abnormal swallowing, novel preference for foods, quidding, rubbing the face against carpets or furniture.
- Ptyalism (increased saliva production).
- Pseudoptyalism (increased saliva escape from the oral cavity due to a conformational abnormality, for instance of the jaw or lips, or a swallowing disorder[3]).

- Halitosis.
- Orofacial swellings or draining tracts.
- Preferred chew objects and accessibility to foreign substances.
- Food and water bowl types.
- Sneezing, nasal discharge, or epistaxis.
- Fetid or blood tinged saliva[1].

Detailed history should be well documented as part of the legal medical record and include answers from client questionnaires written in their own words. It should also include previous test results (ideally graphed or charted for trend recognition), and past medical records. These records should be reviewed to elaborate further and verify the patient's history.

Client questionnaires can be pre-sent by mail or made available on the clinic website for thoroughness and saved appointment time. Thorough awareness of past history as relayed by the owner and past medical records allows:
- Recognition and appreciation of chronicity.
- Identification of relevant etiologic contributors or confounders, trends, and response to treatment(s).
- Evidence of the overall systemic health of the patient.
- Evaluation and trending of previous diagnostic results that need not be/should be repeated due to failure to provide an accurate picture of the acute situation or for trending purposes.

KEY POINTS
- Evaluation of signalment allows ranking of differential diagnoses according to intrinsic patient risk factors.
- Chief owner concern(s) should be written in the words of the owner for clinician objectivity and so that the concern(s) for which the patient presented is/are prioritized[2].
- A detailed patient history ensures attention to systemic health, allows determination of patterns and chronicity, and can be performed during initial survey of the pet, the owner, and their interactions. This will aid in diagnoses and future treatment recommendations.

Step 2: General physical examination

Complete physical examination should be performed in a comfortable and quiet environment with good lighting. Extra light for viewing inside the oral cavity may be provided by several methods including:

- Retracting surgery-type examination lights installed on the wall or ceiling.
- Inexpensive clip-on table lights.
- Hiking or head-loop lights.
- Ophthalmoscopic, otoscopic, or dental unit -attached (e.g. IM-3) transilluminators.
- Flashlights or pen lights.
- Videoscopy.

The physical examination should be as complete as possible and include:

- Body condition.
- Survey of the eyes and ears.
- Palpation of the neck including the thyroid gland.
- Palpation of all superficial lymph nodes[4].
- Thorough cardiothoracic evaluation.
- Abdominal/urogenital palpation.
- Appraisal of the haircoat, integument, and mucocutaneous junctions.
- Palpation and manipulation of joints and bones.
- Detailed neurologic assessment.

KEY POINTS

- Physical examination should be performed in a comfortable and quiet environment with good lighting. Poor lighting may obscure important findings.
- The complete physical examination should be as thorough as possible with special attention paid to body condition score and vital structures, given the need for general anesthesia for most veterinary dental diagnostics and therapeutics.

Step 3: Orofacial examination

Initially, do not open the mouth. Evaluate the head by utilizing visual and auditory observation as well as palpation. All senses are engaged and objective tests performed routinely or as indicated. During external orofacial survey examination, one should visually observe:

- Skull and jaw type (dolicocephalic, mesaticephalic, brachycephalic).
- Localized/generalized or increased/ decreased prominence of skeletal landmarks (e.g. muscle wasting or swelling; mass(es)).
- Partial or complete inability to open the mouth (trismus).
- Increased mouth opening (e.g.'dropped jaw' due to: mandibular neuropraxia; fractures; intraoral swellings or masses; nerve damage) (**31**).

- Soft tissue contracture (e.g. tetanus).
- Spasms or drooping (e.g. lower jaw; tongue; lips).
- Obvious lumps, swellings, or draining tracts (e.g. neoplasia; cellulitis; and/or abscesses).
- Facial asymmetries (e.g. dislocations; fractures; nerve damage; allergies or other inflammatory disorders; neoplasia) (**32**).
- Occlusion (e.g. genetic or environmental causes of malocclusion [e.g. fractures; TMJ luxations]).
- Jaw stability.
- Recurrent behaviors (e.g. licking or chewing at the skin; yelping upon yawning; bruxism).
- (Pseudo) ptyalism.
- Evaluation of air flow through the nostrils (slide test)[5] when indicated.
- Skin fold lesions (e.g. intertrigo).
- Puffiness of structures including eyelids, lips, jaws, and tongue (e.g. hypothyroidism; allergy).
- Weak maxillofacial bones 'rubber jaw' (e.g. hyperparathyroidism).

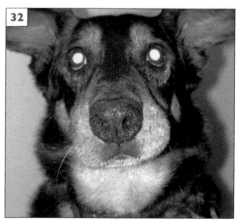

31 Lower jaw drooping (due to periodontal disease-induced bilateral pathological mandibular fractures) facilitating hands-off examination of the oral cavity. Gentle traction on the lip hairs enabled visualization of the fractures.

32 Facial asymmetry from baseball bat traumatism. Careful palpation of the lip and subsequent radiography revealed tooth fragments that were surgically extirpated from the mucosa of the dog's left upper lip at the time of standard endodontics on tooth 204.

During external orofacial survey examination, auditory observations during the examination should include the following:

- Clicking or popping noises before, during, and after anesthesia (e.g. TMJ disorder; malocclusions).
- Crying upon yawning (e.g. TMJ disorder; stomatitis; periodontal disease; oropharyngeal problem).
- Honking, reverse sneezing, sneezing, stertor or stridor (e.g. upper respiratory tract problems; oronasal fistulas; tumors).

Palpation of the head and neck should be performed as follows:

- Bimanually run your hands along the ventrum and sides of the mandibles, incisive, and maxillary bones, TMJs, zygomatic arches, and orbital rims (**33**).
- Run your thumbs or fingers dorsally to palpate the temporal line of the frontal bone (open fontanelles), the external sagittal crest, and external occipital protuberance[6].
- Palpate the muscles of mastication (temporal, masseter, medial pterygoid, digastric, and mylohyoid) and the neck muscles noting any pain or resentment, swelling, hypertrophy, or atrophy.
- While the animal's mouth is closed, place your index fingers in each of the external acoustic meatuses and gently pull rostrally, watching for a pain response[2].
- Palpate the TMJs while observing the animal's response.
- Assess the mandibular salivary glands and attempt palpation of the parotid salivary glands superficial portion just beneath the ear and behind the caudal border of mandible and TMJ[1]. Note swelling or pain (trauma; sialoliths).
- Palpate the mandibular and prescapular lymph nodes (e.g. reactive *vs.* infiltrative lymphadenopathy).
- Palpate the thyroid glands.
- Assess the position of the globes and ability to retropulse them.
- Detailed ophthalmoscopic and otoscopic examination are ideally performed given their proximity and possible shared or confounding conditions with the oral cavity (e.g. polyps; infections; extension of neoplasia).

- Particular attention should be paid to the skin of the head and neck, e.g. noting dander or keratin plugs, erythema, alopecia, lumps, or bumps.
- Examine for draining tracts. Any tracts should be sterilely swabbed (for cytology, culture-sensitivity) and gently pressed upon to assess pain, volume, and consistency of fluid.

KEY POINTS

- The first step of orofacial examination is external orofacial survey examination, which is performed without exogenous opening of the patient's mouth.
- Initial survey is performed by:
  1 Hands-off visual and auditory observation during history-taking.
  2 Physical examination.
  3 Palpation of the head and neck.
- Surface palpation of orofacial structures of the head and neck is performed in a systematic manner to avoid missed findings.

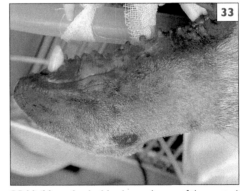

33 Visible and palpable shape change of the ventral mandibles with fistulation through the skin in the presence of abraded tips (C6) of the mandibular canines. Endodontic pathfinders failed to penetrate tertiary dentin in these areas. Radiography and histopathology confirmed chronic endodontic compromise of teeth 304 and 404.

Step 4: Conscious (awake) intraoral examination

Conscious oral examination should be as thorough as possible in order to recommend appropriate treatments, justify treatments in the presence of the owner, and arrive at representative estimates. An assistant photographer-restrainer-stenographer is helpful during conscious oral examination. Photographic documentation of findings objectifies them and allows them to be shared with colleagues, referring, or specialty veterinarians, and act as references for reassessment, study, and/or post-treatment results. For hygienic reasons and for owner peace of mind, one's hands should be washed and gloves ideally donned before placing them in the pet's mouth.

The intraoral examination should include four stages:
1 Evaluation of the lips.
2 Dental (hard tissue) evaluation.
3 Periodontal examination.
4 Oral cavity evaluation.

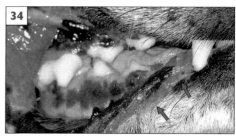

34 Mucosal, vermillion zone, right mandibular frenulum (arrows). Erythema and ulceration in a dog with systemic lupus erythematosus. Similar mucosal lesions would be expected with chronic ulcerative paradental stomatitis ('kissing lesions'). Odontic traumatism from tooth 104 might account for some of the erythema at the right mandibular frenulum. Note thickened saliva at the lip commissure likely secondary to subdued swallowing due to pain. Masticatory muscle atrophy was noted upon hands-off survey examination of this patient.

LIP AND MUCOSAL EVALUATION
Evaluate the integumentary component of the lips for:
• Clefts.
• Lacerations.
• Depigmentation (e.g. vitiligo), hyperpigmentation, or staining.
• Erythema, excoriation, or other inflammations (e.g.cheilitis; dermatitis, e.g. lip fold dermatitis).
• Puffiness (e.g. hypothyroidism[7]; allergy; injury; mass).
• Scaling (e.g. vitamin B deficiencies[1]; fungal infection[8]).
• Alopecia.
• Malodor.

Next, evaluate the vermillion zone (transitional zone between skin-covered facial component and mucosa-covered vestibular component of the lips) for:
• Depigmentations (autoimmune disease, e.g. lupus) (**34**).
• Raised red-brown ulcerations (e.g. eosinophilic granuloma complex; neoplasia).
• Other ulcerations (e.g. vitamin B deficiency)[1].

Gingerly lift up and down on the lips, paying attention to apparent looseness or tightness. Keep in mind that cheek and lip muscles counteract the tongue pressure on the teeth. Malocclusions or jaw length disparities may result with inappropriate lip tension[1,9]. Lip avulsion is usually obvious and is typically secondary to trauma. Limited lip commissure opening should be evaluated in light of signalment (e.g. microchelia of Schnauzers[1]), prior surgery (commisurroplasty), or scarring. Limited commissure opening is important to evaluate as it predisposes the patient to cheilitis due to food and saliva trapping in lip folds.

Evaluate the mucosa (**35**) for:
• Moistness (e.g. xerostomia).
• Color change.
• Masses.
• Fistulas.
• Ulcers (e.g. chronic ulcerative paradental stomatitis (CUPS).
• Other inflammation (e.g. cheek chewers) (**36**).
• Lacerations.
• Foreign bodies.

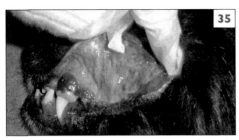

35 Unfolding of the mucolabial and mucobuccal folds to examine the mucosa vestibule for lesions.

The attached gingiva should be examined for changes such as color variations; enlargement; edema; or tendrelling up the tooth. Such findings may indicate neoplasia or resorptive lesions (TRs). Also check for bulbousness (especially at cat canines), gingival stippling (**38**), fistulation, recession, hyperemia, bleeding (spontaneous or examination-induced), or sulcal exudates. Soft tissue lesions are noted relative to teeth or normal soft tissue landmarks.

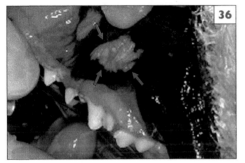

36 'Cheek chewers' lesion (arrows).

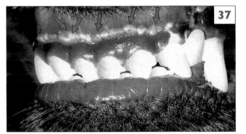

37 Suspected 'coccal bursitis' along the mucogingival margin above teeth 103 through 203 (arrows) due to soft tissue trauma and foreign body-type reaction to lodged bur or stiff hair fragments.

The salivary papillae represent the exit of the salivary ducts. These include the parotid papilla (which exits over the distal root of the maxillary fourth premolar), the zygomatic papilla (just caudal to it) and further caudal to this, the four zygomatic minor duct openings. Additionally, the buccal and labial salivary ducts are seen as small dots along the facial alveolar mucosa[1].

The mucogingival margin/line (MGM or MGL) demarcates the attached gingiva from the buccal mucosa. The MGM should be carefully examined for inflammation or fistulas, e.g. coccal bursitis (especially above the maxillary incisors), endodontic or periodontal fistulas (**37**).

The frenula are folds of alveolar mucosa forming a ridge of attachment between the lips and the gum. These include one maxillary frenulum (midline of the upper lip to the gingiva immediately above the two central incisors) and two mandibular frenula (lower lip distolabial to the mandibular canine). Evaluate the frenula for: 'tight lip'/loose attachment; debris collection; discoloration; and odontic traumatism.

38 Gingival stippling (epithelial (rete ridge/peg) interdigitation with underlying connective tissues) of the attached gingiva at tooth 308–309. It is less prominent in the cat than in the dog and can be present or absent in healthy or diseased gingiva. Its 'reduction or loss may be an indicator but does not automatically signify disease'[1].

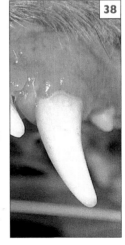

INITIAL DENTAL EVALUATION

Prior to performing a detailed dental evaluation, one should become fluent in tooth directional terms based upon the anatomical tooth surfaces (see *Table 3*).

G.V. Black's modified classification of tooth lesion location is helpful in more detailed localization of odontogenic pathoses or restoratives, and has recognized short-forms which are easy to chart (*Table 4*)[1].

The AVDC tooth fracture classification system defines fractures as follows:

Uncomplicated crown fracture (UCF): A fracture of the crown that does not expose the pulp.

Complicated crown fracture (CCF): A fracture of the crown that exposes the pulp.

Uncomplicated crown–root fracture (UCRF): A fracture of the crown and root that does not expose the pulp.

Complicated crown–root fracture (CCRF): A fracture of the crown and root that exposes the pulp.

Root fracture (RF): A fracture involving the root.

Table 3 Directional terms based upon anatomical tooth surfaces[1]

1 Proximal = surfaces of a tooth that come in close contact with an adjacent tooth

2 Coronal = direction/tooth surface/wall towards crown tip or occlusal surface

a Incisal = coronal @ incisors

b Occlusal = coronal @ premolars (PMs), molars (Ms)

3 Cervical = direction/tooth surface @ juncture of crown and root (neck)

4 Apical = direction/tooth surface towards root tip (*apex*), away from the coronal (incisal, occlusal) surface

5 Vestibular = direction/tooth surface facing lips or cheeks

a Labial = portion of incisors or canines facing lips

b Buccal = portion of PMs or Ms facing cheeks

6 Lingual = direction/tooth surface of maxillary or mandibular teeth facing tongue

7 Palatal = direction/tooth surface of maxillary teeth facing palate

8 Mesial = proximal surface of tooth closest to tooth ahead of it or facing towards rostral end of arch towards front midline

9 Rostral = proximal surface of tooth closest to tooth ahead of it or facing towards rostral end of arch

10 Distal = proximal surface of the tooth closest to the tooth behind it or surface facing in caudal direction of arch or laterally (away from midline)

11 Caudal = proximal surface of tooth (other than incisors) closest to tooth behind it or surface facing in caudal direction of quadrant/arch

12 Middle = middle third of the tooth

a between *coronal* and *cervical*

b between *cervical* and *apical*

c between mesial/rostral and distal/caudal

Table 4 G.V. Black's classification of tooth injuries[1]

Tooth injuries (caries, fracture, defect) are classified according to location (contiguous lesions or different classes may be exist) using Arabic or Roman numerals up to eight as follows:

Class 1 (C1) lesions occur in structural defects such as the cingulum of maxillary incisors, developmental grooves, and pit and fissures of Is, PMs, Ms

C2 = lesions of the proximal (+/− C1) surface of a PM or M

C3 = lesions of the proximal surface of an I or C but not including a ridge/incisal angle

C4 = lesion involving the incisal angle/ridge, proximal surface of an I or C

C5 = facial or lingual/palatal lesion involving cementoenamel junction (gingival 1/3rd) of any tooth but excluding pit or fissure lesions

C6 = lesion of an incisal edge or cusp of any tooth, including slab fractures

C7 = root lesion

C8 = root apex lesion

Table 5 Coronal line angles[1]

1 Mesiovestibular (MV)

a mesiolabial (ML) **b** mesiobuccal (MB)

2 Mesiolingual (ML) or mesiopalatal (MP)

3 Mesiocoronal (MC)

a mesioincisal (MI) **b** mesio-occlusal (MO)

4 Distovestibular (DV)

a distobuccal (DB) **b** distolabial (DL)

5 Distolingual (DL)/distopalatal (DP)

6 Distocoronal (DC)

a distoincisal (DI) **b** disto-occlusal (DO)

7 Linguoincisal (LI)/linguopalatal (LP)

a linguocoronal (LC) **b** linguo-occlusal (LO)

8 Vestibuloincisal (VI)

a faciocoronal (FC) **b** facio-occlusal (FO)

Table 6 Coronal point angles[1]

Mesiovestibuloincisal (mesiovestibulocoronal, mesiovestibulo-occlusal, mesiolabioincisal, mesiobuccocoronal, mesiobucco-occlusal)

Mesiolinguoincisal (mesiolinguocoronal, mesiolinguo-occlusal)

Distovestibuloincisal (distovestibulocoronal, distovestibulo-occlusal, distolabioincisal, distobuccocoronal, distobucco-occlusal)

Distolinguoincisal (distolinguocoronal, distolinguo-occlusal)

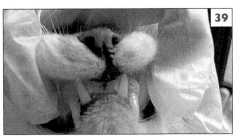

39 Assessing rostral occlusal relationships and comparing the visible periodontia of maxillary canines (teeth 104 and 204) for evidence of bulbousness. This cat exhibits an end-on incisor relationship, common to most cats. Note also the subtle inward arching of the line of maxillary incisors, another relatively common anecdotal finding in cats.

The eight (coronal) line angles are dividing lines formed between two of the five external tooth walls (vestibular, lingual/palatal, mesial, distal, and coronal). These are named for the walls forming them by substituting an o for the usual –al ending (*Table 5*)[1]. The four (coronal) point angles represent the point at which three of the line angles meet at a juncture, and so are named for the three surfaces that make the juncture or point (*Table 6*)[1].

The dentition should be evaluated thoroughly via the following steps:

1 Count teeth:
- Domestic canines have 42 permanent and 28 deciduous teeth.
- Domestic felines have 30 permanent and 26 deciduous teeth.

2 Evaluate occlusion (**39, 40**):
- Take photos to document (mal)occlusions.
- Determine whether teeth appear crowded, rotated, tipped (-version), or bodily moved (-occlusion)[1] (**41**).
- Determine whether a permanent dentition, mixed dentition, or deciduous dentition is present and compare this with expectations on the basis of patient signalment, nutrition, health (e.g. congenital hypothyroid dwarfism[10]), and the time of year[11].
- Evaluate occlusion based on accepted breed standards.

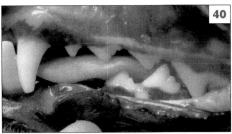

40 Evaluation of occlusal relationships of teeth from the left lateral aspect in a dog. Note slight relative mesiocclusion of the mandibular premolars in comparison to their maxillary counterparts. (Courtesy of Dr. Brook Niemiec.)

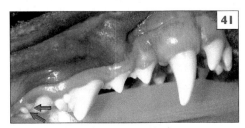

41 Upon external survey, this dog's nose appeared buckled. Note the denticles buccal to tooth 109 (erupted compound odontoma) (arrows), the buccal rotation of the mesial portions and crowding of teeth 106 and 107, and the apparent absence of tooth 105. Dental radiography confirmed compound odontomas at teeth 108 and 109.

In deciding if interceptive orthodontic extraction is required (and if so which tooth or teeth should be extracted), one should be familiar with the normal location of the permanent teeth. Except for the permanent maxillary canines (which erupt mesial to the deciduous), permanent teeth erupt lingual to their deciduous counterparts[1]. Besides relative positioning, other clues to differentiate deciduous teeth from permanent teeth include comparative whiteness, diminutive size, and degree of root development/resorption, eruption-exfoliation, and mobility.

If teeth or part of a tooth is apparently missing, evaluate both visually and manually for color change, fistulation, or bulging as possible sequelae of an unerupted or partially erupted tooth, or retained root tip. Since clinical signs are not always present, dental radiography is required to confirm that all parts of the tooth are truly absent and the tooth or area is not in need of treatment (e.g. excision of dentigerous cyst or extraction of retained root(s)). Note whether the hood of gingival tissue partially or completely covering an unerupted tooth (dental operculum)[12] appears tough, thickened, or fibrous, thus impeding eruption of the tooth[1] (**42**).

Determine if apparently extra teeth are present in the form of retained deciduous teeth or supernumerary teeth, as opposed to dilacerated or bigeminal/twinned crowns. If extra teeth or teeth-like structures (denticles) appear to be present, try to determine if these are truly extra or actually a single tooth. Radiographs will aid succinct diagnosis.

Note any other irregularities in the size and shape of teeth.

Dilaceration is an abrupt or extraordinary axial angulation, bend, or curve anywhere along the length of the tooth[13,14]. The position of the dilaceration depends upon the extent of tooth formation at the time of mechanical trauma, or hereditary developmental syndrome manifestation[13,15]. Crown (coronal) dilacerations[16] are visible clinically and may be esthetically displeasing and more plaque-retentive[17]. In contrast, root (radicular) dilacerations usually present incidentally on radiographs[15], and may pose endodontic, exodontic or orthodontic challenges[18], or inhibit tooth eruption[13,17].

Dens in dente/dens invaginatus[19] comprise one or more developmental invaginations/ intussusceptions. This means layers of inner 'tooth' are reversed such that enamel or cementum (if present) lay inside of the dentin +/− pulp tissues. Outer tooth enamel is not affected but inner tooth enamel/cementum +/− dentin may be missing, resulting in direct pulp exposure prior to calcification[20,21]. Dens in dente manifests clinically as exaggerated lingual pits +/− extra inter-radicular crown[1,14,19,20]. Histologically and radiographically it appears as tooth-like structure(s) within the affected tooth's pulp cavity[14,19]. Coronal dens in dente, not extending beyond the cementoenamel junction (type I) is much more common than radicular dens in dente which extends from the crown into (type II), or through (type III), the root[20,21]. Dens in dente has been reported in the dog but not in the cat[22].

42 Apparent absence of teeth 301 and 401 with hemorrhage and apparent fistulation over tooth 402, despite the presence of teeth 402 and 302. Operculectomy (excision of the thickened gingival covering) overlying the radiographically observable teeth 301 and 401 allowed for their subsequent eruption.

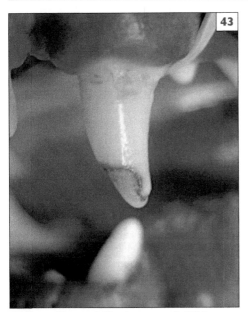

43 Enamel hypocalcification at tooth 402 in a dog, warranting dental radiography and treatment in the form of macroabrasion and restoration, endodontics, or exodontia as necessary. (Dog is in dorsal recumbency.)

Enamel pearl(s)/enameloma(ta) are usually singular but can be multiple, and manifest as small, spherical ectopic root deposit(s) with a predilection for molar furcations[23]. Primarily enamel, they usually contain a dentin core (rarely pulpal tissues), often obscured by a cemental covering[23]. In the absence of a cemental covering, long junctional epithelium (which allows extension of pathological periodontal pockets) occurs within the sulcus during the periodontal ligament's attempts to attach to the enamel[1,14]. Appearance of enamel pearls has been described in dogs[17].

Amelogenesis imperfecta and *dentinogenesis imperfecta* are collective terms for inherited formation or maturation disorders of enamel and dentin respectively, which occur in isolation or in syndromes in humans[24,25]. Models have only been reported in laboratory mice[25,26]. AI and DI may involve either primary and/or permanent dentitions more or less in a generalized pattern,

reflecting an inherited condition unrelated to temporal localized or generalized extrinsic aggressor agents[24,27].

Nonhereditary environmental enamel defects are relatively common in dogs and may occur during dental development due to local (trauma, infection) or systemic (infection, fluorosis, mineral deficiencies, or endocrinopathies) aggressor agents sufficient to affect enamel formation[14,24,25]. Hypoplastic types (enamel hypoplasia) exhibit quantitative enamel deficiencies[14]. Hypoplastic enamel is thin and/or has grooves and pits on its surface. Hypocalcified types exhibit qualitative enamel deficiencies manifested as pigmented, softened, and easily detached enamel (**43**). A so-far unused term in the veterinary literature, enamel hypomaturation, would be associated with qualitative enamel defects resulting in detachable, fine, porous, irregular opaque-white vertically banded pigmented teeth, whose enamel contrasts little with underlying dentin in radiographs[24]. The main clinical problems of enamel disorders are esthetics (discoloration), idiopathic resorption, delayed eruption or impaction, dental sensitivity, and loss of occlusal vertical dimensions[24]. Radiographs may reveal unerupted or resorbing teeth, and in hypomineralization cases, thin enamel contrasting little with the underlying dentin[24,25].

Erupted intraosseous compound or *complex odontoma*[28] (**41**) are slow-growing, benign and usually asymptomatic, nonaggressive odontogenic 'hamartomatous' tumors or true hamartomas[29,30]. Odontomas are composed of enamel, cementum, dentin, +/− pulp. They may develop before or after tooth eruption but rarely erupt into the oral cavity, so more are often discovered radiographically[29,30]. Compound odontomas are initially radiolucent and cystic. They eventually form a radiolucently-rimmed radiopaque mound of small, multiple, tooth-like components (denticles) or abortive teeth bearing only superficial similarity to rudimentary teeth[29-31]. Complex odontomas are irregular masses of amorphously calcified dental tissue composed mainly of mature tubular dentin[29-31]. Compound and complex odontomas are classified as intraosseous (if they occur inside bone) or extraosseus or peripheral (if they occur in the soft tissue covering the tooth-bearing portions of the jaws)[30].

Supernumerary/accessory roots or *supernumerary/accessory crowns/cusps* can occur in both dogs and cats (**44**). Extra cusps may develop independent of extra roots, but should alert the clinician to the possible presence of a supernumerary (SN) root. In feline maxillary third premolar teeth there is approximately a 10% incidence of SN roots[32,33]. The extra root and associated SN cusp tends to occur palatally mid-tooth. SN roots are relatively rare in dogs (2.87% incidence)[17]. In some dog breeds, SN roots are common enough to be viewed as a normal anatomical variation[17]. A study in greyhounds found a 36.4% incidence of SN roots[34]. In dogs, the teeth most commonly affected are the third premolars (44.44%) and first premolars (33.33%) (maxillary > mandibular)[34], followed by the fourth premolars (16.67%) and less commonly the second molars (5.55%)[17]. Thought to be caused by a developmental disturbance in Hertwig's epithelial root sheath, SN roots +/− associated SN cusps may present in both the deciduous and permanent dentition[35].

Fusion (developmentally conjoined teeth) appears clinically as a single tooth with a bifid crown or two teeth joined by enamel and/or dentin[14]. Concrescence is a form of fusion wherein already-formed teeth are conjoined by cementum only, before or after eruption[14]. This typically results in hypodontia (reduced number of teeth)[31]. Radiographically, these teeth may exhibit unusual pulp cavities[31].

Bigeminy/twinning (developmentally divided teeth) appears most commonly as a single tooth with bifid (cleft/branched) crown. Though occasionally complete bifurcation or twinning occurs, resulting in a normal-appearing tooth with adjacent SN teeth[12,14,31]. Radiographically, if incompletely bifurcated, these teeth exhibit enlarged or partially divided pulp chambers[31].

Macrodontia or *taurodontia* occurs when the crown appears abnormally large. Apparently small teeth may be microdontic (e.g. peg teeth) or deciduous.

In addition to calculus or plaque, look for exogenous material or surface texture abnormalities on teeth such as dental products, foreign bodies, or restorations. Note tooth staining and try to characterize it as extrinsic staining (SE) from plaque, metal, chlorhexidine, or fluoride; as opposed to intrinsic staining (SI) (**45**) from enamel opacities/hypocalcification, tetracycline staining, dental caries, pulp necrosis, tooth wear, hemorrhage, fluorosis, or root canal medicaments[1,36]. SI of part or the entire clinical crown is often easier to diagnose during the awake examination and can be pointed out to the owner as being problematic. SE can be evidence of chronic homecare with chlorhexidine, or maladaptive behaviors which can lead to more serious odontic pathoses or jeopardize proposed treatment(s).

Note dullness or opaqueness of teeth (**46**), which indicates endodontic compromise due to hemoglobin breakdown[1]. Transillumination

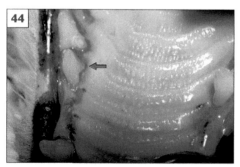

44 Supernumerary root of tooth 207 in a cat (arrow). Teeth 107 and 207 are most commonly affected with supernumerary roots in such a palatal location and can present a challenge during exodontia if not anticipated clinically and radiographically.

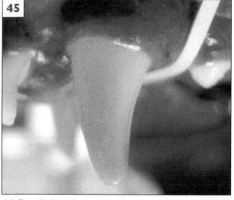

45 Purple-hued instrinsic staining of the apical portion of the crown of tooth 204. The tooth was radiographically confirmed to be suffering from irreversible pulpitis.

(use of light to examine the reflectivity of the internal tooth structures) (**47**) can be performed to help discern tooth opacities, coronal cracks, defects, and caries. Evaluate the surface of the teeth for:

- Abnormal lines which may indicate crazing or developmental aberrations and must be differentiated from normal anatomy (e.g. blood grooves on canines of cats).

- Loss of tooth substance (**48**) such as:
  - Enamel loss (enamel hypocalcification or chipping).
  - Wear = *attrition* (physiological/ masticatory) *vs. abrasion* (parafunctional habits).
  - Fracture.
  - Caries (**49**).

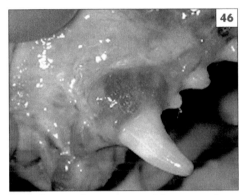

46 Dullness and opaqueness of the crown of tooth 204 suggesting probable endodontic compromise. Transillumination of the tooth contralateral (as in **47**) and adjacent teeth, in addition to dental radiography aided assessment of vitality.

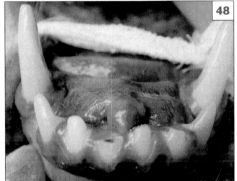

48 The rostral maxillary area of a dog suffering fracture +/− abrasion/attrition of teeth 102 and 201. Tooth 201 has cusp (C6), cingulum (C1), and incisal edge (C6) loss to the point of pulp exposure. Tertiary/reparative dentin will appear similar to the necrotic pulp observable at tooth 201, but will not be penetrable with an endodontic pathfinder (**50**). Note dullness and subtle pink-tinging of tooth 204 in comparison to tooth 104.

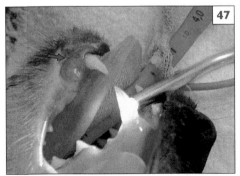

47 Transillumination of tooth 204 as an endodontic diagnostic aid to verify vitality. (Note apparently incidental prominence [color and size] of the left mandibular frenulum [arrow].)

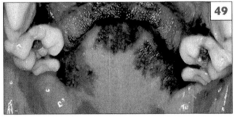

49 Obvious caries in the occlusal (C1) areas of teeth 109 and 209 observable during awake examination. Less conspicuous lesions, and all C1 areas of teeth should be explored to determine caries vs. tertiary dentin, calculus, or pits and fissures (normal areas which are deep or narrow and hence may be predisposed to debris-trapping with the risk of future caries).

Exposure of necrotic pulp can be hard to differentiate from tertiary dentin on concious exam. An endodontic pathfinder can be used to probe these areas in the awake animal given the nonsensitivity of such pulps (**50**). However, false negatives are expected due to technical difficulty in an awake animal, and should be attempted again once the animal is anesthetized. Even if these areas have tertiary dentin in place, as determined by probing, they should be radiographed and then re-radiographed every 6–12 months thereafter to ensure continued vitality. Pulp vitality testing is not currently reliable in veterinary medicine. If pulp-exposed, the tooth is defined as having a complicated tooth fracture.

Do not ignore injuries to the deciduous dentition. A fractured, pulp-exposed deciduous tooth is painful, readily inflamed and infected, and risks injury to the permanent tooth. Tooth injuries and pathoses should ideally be staged or graded. Many such grading and staging systems exist and the interested or advanced practitioner is encouraged to consult the recommended texts and websites.

INITIAL PERIODONTAL EVALUATION
During conscious oral examination, a preliminary generalized assessment of the periodontal health should be performed. This is only a generalized assessment at this time, encompassing the entire mouth. Dental scoring systems range from 0 to 3, with 0 being normal. Gingivitis scoring is known as gingival index (GI) and is defined as:
GI1 = Mild inflammation and color change, no bleeding on probing.
GI2 = Moderate inflammation and bleeding upon probing.
GI3 = Severe inflammation and spontaneous gingival hemorrhage.

There are several methods of measuring plaque indices (PI), the Silness and Loe is presented below:
PI1 = Plaque not visible by the unaided eye; however, it can be visualized on a probe after running along the tooth at the gingival margin.
PI2 = Gingival area covered by thin to moderately thick layer of plaque, plaque in sulcus.
PI3 = Significant abundance of plaque filling the sulcal area.

The calculus index (CI) is as follows:
CI1 = Calculus not exceeding 0.5 mm in width and/or thickness.
CI2 = Calculus not exceeding 1.0 mm in width and/or thickness, extending only slightly below the free gingival margin[1].
CI3 = Calculus exceeding 1.0 mm in width and/or thickness above and/or below the gum line.

Compare areas of the mouth. A heavier PI or CI on one side of the mouth may indicate lateralized chewing, with more build-up on the supposed painful side. In these cases, one should look more carefully for soft and hard tissue pathoses, and/or malocclusion(s). Higher CIs are expected on the caudal dentition, due to cheek trapping of debris and proximity to the zygomatic and parotid salivary ducts. If explainable by periodontal disease, higher GIs should directly correlate with higher PIs and CIs. Very few animals allow any periodontal probing upon awake examination, though this can be gently attempted to reinforce the need for treatment with apprehensive owners.

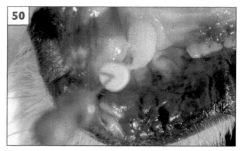

50 Endodontic pathfinder penetration of the pulp at tooth 204 in a cat. Note minimal cuspal tip (C6) loss. Any tooth substance loss from the canine of a cat is significant given the proximity of the pulp, warranting clinical probing and dental radiography.

TMJ EVALUATION

The TMJ examination should begin with hands-off observation of panting and mouth opening/closing behaviors. After the facial surfaces of the teeth are examined, open the mouth as wide as possible. Be especially careful in cases with severe periodontal disease or trauma due to the possibility of current or risk of jaw fracture. Note any behavioral or physical resistance to mouth opening (trismus) while listening for clicking or popping noises. Some breeds (terriers) or individuals are resistant to attempts to open their mouths, which may complicate diagnosis.

If noises are heard, the animal is resistant, or one is unable to open the mouth during awake examination, pathology should be suspected. Possible etiologies include:

- Neoplasia.
- Craniomandibular osteopathy.
- Masticatory muscle myositis.
- CUPS.
- Caudal mandibular fracture.
- Feline lymphoplasmacytic stomatitis.
- Tetanus.
- TMJ ankylosis/luxation/malfunction.

Complete TMJ evaluation, including ausculting the joint for subtle noises, will be facilitated by general anesthesia. At this time, additional diagnostics can be performed such as TMJ radiographs, CT, MRI, muscle biopsies, and measures of maximal mouth opening have not been quantified in the veterinary literature. Measurement of bite force in dogs has been studied but is not routinely performed[37].

TONGUE EVALUATION

Note the overall size and shape of the tongue (macroglossia or microglossia/bird tongue)[10,38]. Be careful not to overdiagnose macroglossia in brachycephalics who exhibit good function without traumatic exposure[39].

Evaluate the dorsum of the tongue starting at its root. In the cat, observe the membranous molar pads containing the lingual molar salivary gland between the tongue and the mandibular molar. Move rostrally along the tongue through its body and apex noting:

- Mobility.
- Flaccidity.
- Loss, prominence, or inflammation of papillae.

- Healed or active lacerations or punctures.
- Embedded foreign bodies (such as hair).
- Depressions.
- Apparent thickenings or masses.
- EGC (Huskies[40], cats[41]).
- Neoplasia.

KEY POINTS

- Thorough conscious oral examination allows appropriate treatments to be recommended and justified in the presence of the owner. This will help in the creation of more accurate estimates and improve compliance.
- An assistant photographer-restrainer-stenographer saves time, and prevents missed pathoses or notation thereof during conscious oral examination (**51**).
- The intraoral examination should include systematic evaluation of the lips, dental (hard) tissues, periodontium, and oral cavity. Abnormalities should be localized using adjacent anatomy and/or accepted classification schemes, and should be assigned appropriate dental indices and/or stages.

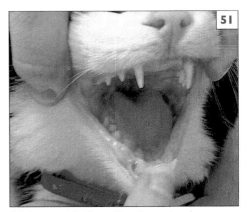

51 Assistant-facilitated hand-over head manipulation for open-mouthed examination in a cat.

Step 5: The anesthetized orodental examination

PREANESTHESIA AND INDUCTION

Perform the tests necessary to help diagnose systemic pathoses and determine safe anesthetic protocols according to the animal's age, history, and physical examination findings. Preanesthetic testing protocols can vary depending on the clinician and the owner's accepted and affordable standards of care. For instance, in some North American institutions, a complete preanesthetic senior (6–7 years and older) work-up might include blood pressure measurement, complete blood count (CBC), ECG, chemistry profile, electrolytes, coagulation, urinalysis, endocrine and infectious disease testing. Thyroid testing is important as hypothyroidism decreases healing ability and hyperthyroidism can lead to cardiac disease[42,43]. In addition, three-view thoracic radiographs +/- advanced imaging can be performed to discover occult intrathoracic pathoses such as primary or metastatic cancer[44]. The definition of a 'senior' patient may vary, and one must keep in mind that organ systems, species, and breeds of dogs age at different rates[44]. www.vasg.org is an excellent resource for preoperative testing recommendations.

Testing for immune-mediated, inflammatory (e.g. MM type 2M muscle fiber autoantibody testing[45]), and/or infectious diseases (e.g. FeLV, FIV, *Bartonella henselae*) may also be indicated. Based on preanesthetic evaluations, anesthetic protocols may be adjusted, anesthesia rescheduled until systemic disease is better managed or resolved, or anesthesia canceled entirely.

Preparations for anesthesia and surgery should include the following:
- Intravenous access.
- Fluid therapy.
- Anesthetic monitoring equipment.
- Parenteral medications including pre-emptive analgesia.
- External heat sources (which are extremely important in any dental procedure given the cold water irrigation of the oral cavity, especially in extended anesthetics).

Unconscious oral examination begins during anesthetic induction. Structures of the oropharynx not visualized upon conscious oral examination should be visualized at this point.

KEY POINTS
- Preanesthesia testing +/- imaging should be thorough to ensure a safe anesthetic event and to aid diagnosis of oromaxillofacial or systemic pathoses.
- Preparations for anesthesia and surgery should include placement of an intravenous catheter, initiation of fluid therapy, readying of anesthetic monitoring and support equipment (thermal support, ventilator), and the administration of pre-emptive analgesics and antibiotics if indicated.

PREPARATION FOR ANESTHETIZED EXAMINATION

The patient should be placed in dorsal recumbency as this allows one to view the entire oral cavity and its support structures during examination and charting. It also allows proper orientation of the periodontal probe. A roll or sand bag can be placed under the neck to promote drainage of irrigating fluids and saliva. Suction should always be used. Using a mouth gag will greatly facilitate the oral examination process by statically maintaining the open mouth position and deflecting the tongue and endotracheal tube. Select a properly sized mouth gag and remove it as often as possible to decrease TMJ strain.

A proper examination requires:
- Excellent general and spot lighting.
- Magnification.
- Explorer-periodontal probe.
- Dental mirrors (**52**).
- Wooden tongue depressor.
- Dry field (suction is helpful).

Examination may proceed in any order as long as it is consistent. Pathology and treatment should be noted using the AVDC approved abbreviations. These can be found in Appendix 1; however, for the most up to date list visit www.avdc.org. A key for the most common abbreviations should be provided on the front or back of the dental chart.

The dental chart should diagram the teeth and their proximal relations in some form. The most helpful charts show vestibular, occlusal, and lingual/palatal views of the teeth such that odontogenic or soft tissue lesions adjacent to these can be diagramed on or next to them, as seen from the appropriate viewpoint. Charts must allow room to mark pathological periodontal pockets in the areas at which they

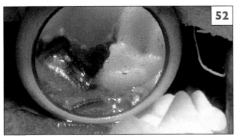

52 Use of a dental mirror to facilitate examination of the palatal and occlusal areas of tooth 109. Note apparent increased depth of the C I area of the tooth and slight discoloration. Use of a dental explorer aided diagnosis of an early carious lesion at this tooth. Dental X-ray was also performed on this and the contralateral tooth for comparison and to help stage endodontal and/or periodontal compromise.

Detailed oral examination and charting is best performed following the scaling/root planing/subgingival curettage procedure for two reasons. First, subgingival calculus may cause underestimation of a periodontal pocket. Second, evaluation and charting after cleaning may reveal areas of calculus, plaque, or other pathology in need of further treatment.

Some veterinary dentists prefer to scale their patients' teeth themselves for earlier recognition of problems. Alternatively, entrust this to an experienced staff member. The additional set of eyes and hands will decrease missed pathology, and will prevent fatigue of the primary clinician. After scaling/root planing/subgingival curettage, the oral cavity is assessed in detail. Blowing air perpendicularly against the teeth with a three-way irrigating syringe onto the teeth and into the sulci or pathological pockets will aid in the visualization of missed calculus (appears chalky-white), debris, or pathoses above and below the gum line. To avoid air emboli or subcutaneous emphysema, do not blow air into open pulp cavities or soft tissue cavernous areas.

occur from an occlusal vantage point. Dental charts should also provide areas adjacent to the teeth for common pathologies such as gingival recession or hyperplasia, furcation exposure, tooth mobility, and tooth substance loss. Finally, charts should leave room to note nonodontogenic findings. Example dental charts may be found in Appendix 2.

Prior to diffusion with rinsing agents (e.g. chlorhexidine), or scaling, reassess for:
- Previously restored teeth or appliances.
- Plaque, calculus, and gingival indices.
- SE, such as metal.
- Soft tissue masses.
- Inflammation.

Only hand instruments should be used in the area of restorations or appliances to prevent reverberation-induced loosening. Preprophylaxis photographs should be taken for documentation of pathology and for client education purposes. Halitosis should also be evaluated. Measurement of halitosis can be subjectively judged[46] and scaled from 0 to 3 or objectively measured using a sulfide monitor[47]. Causes of halitosis include:
- Periodontal disease, especially in the presence of dry mouth and/or stomatitis.
- Foreign body or tumor-induced necrosis and/or infection.
- Ketoacidosis.
- Uremia.

KEY POINTS
- In preparation for detailed anesthetized orodental examination and charting, the patient should be placed in dorsal recumbency as this allows one to view the entire oral cavity and its support structures, and allows proper orientation of the periodontal probe.
- In order to protect the patient's lungs from oral contamination, a properly sized and inflated endotracheal tube should be used. In addition, the neck should be slightly elevated to encourage drainage. Finally, suction should be utilized if available, and invested in if not.
- A properly-sized mouth gag prevents operator fatigue and allows better visualization by holding the mouth open and deflecting the endotracheal tube and tongue. Proper use prevents undue strain on the TMJs.
- Proper anesthetized examination requires excellent lighting, magnification, an explorer-periodontal probe, dental mirrors, a dry field (suction is helpful) and a consistent approach.

- Pathology and treatment should be noted on an appropriate dental chart using AVDC approved abbreviations.
- Prior to diffusion with rinsing agents or scaling, ensure notation of previously restored teeth or appliances, plaque, calculus, and gingival indices, SE, soft tissue masses, inflammation, and/or halitosis and obtain preprophylaxis photographs.
- Detailed oral examination and charting is best performed following the scaling/root planing/subgingival curettage procedure since subgingival calculus may cause underestimation of periodontal pockets. In addition, areas missed during cleaning can be detected and revisited.

DENTAL CHARTING AND PERIODONTAL EXAMINATION

Revisit all the structures assessed upon conscious oral examination, and any that were missed. Be systematic and thorough regarding the structures examined, process of examination, and the order of examination. Four-handed dental charting (periodontal probing and oral assessment by one person and notation of findings by another) on a specific dental chart is more efficient and ensures consistency.

Preface odontogenic findings by calling out the tooth number according to the modified Triadan tooth numbering system[48].

The modified Triadan system[48] is the accepted tooth identification system and allows one to communicate more efficiently. The teeth in respective quadrants are numbered clockwise starting with the right maxillary (100 series) and ending with the right mandibular (400 series) for permanents, and 500 through 800 for the deciduous. Teeth are numbered for the primitive carnivore which had a full complement of premolars (four) and molars (three) in each quadrant[49]. Kittens have 26 teeth, puppies 28, cats 30, and dogs 42. Despite debate, accepted scientific anatomical nomenclature dictates that there are no molars in the deciduous dentition. In addition, the most rostral premolar(s) and most caudal molars are absent in normal feline dental formulae[1]. Canines are always numbered as 04s and first molars are always 09s. Hence the permanent maxillary right canine is tooth 104. Adult cats lack all 05s and mandibular 06s (second premolars), and do not have teeth numbering higher than the 09s (first molars).

Kittens lack all molars (09s) in addition to the teeth missing in adults. Puppies lack all molars (maxillary 09s and 10s, mandibular 09s, 10s, and 11s), in addition to all 05s (first premolars). Even seasoned clinicians must remind themselves of the numbering system when dealing with puppies and kittens as their fourth premolars look and function like permanent first molars.

Notify the stenographer of retained, SN, or missing teeth. Radiographs are required to confirm that missing teeth are truly absent. Visually inspect and palpate areas of missing teeth for fistulation, inflammation, or hyperplasia. When charting the teeth, be specific. Localize the lesion according to tooth landmarks such as cusps, developmental grooves, line and point angles. Lesions may also be localized by G.V. Black's modified classification (*Table 4*). Furthermore, deficits should be staged according to accepted indices. Size and shape changes of teeth should be noted, photographed and/or diagrammed. SI or SE, dullness, physiological or pathological grooves, crazing, or tooth substance loss should be recorded. These areas require examination with an explorer or endodontic pathfinder for smoothness, ledging, or deficits. All tooth deficits or areas of discoloration should be explored for carious lesions or pulp exposure. If the probe locates areas of stickiness, or sinks at all into the tooth, this is indicative of a carious lesion or pulp exposure. Hemorrhage or audible differences (duller pitch) could also suggest the presence of these lesions. Areas of pulp exposure can be vital (pink and bleeding) or nonvital (dark and necrotic). Discolored areas that are tan in color (*vs.* dark) and which do not allow any sinking of the probe (i.e. no stickiness) are likely to be covered with reparative dentin and do not require treatment or attention in the absence of radiographic evidence of endodontic disease. Clinical and radiographic recheck of discolored areas previously deemed healthy is indicated at future prophylaxes to detect progression of endodontic disease not currently evident. Transillumination should be performed in all cases of questionable tooth vitality.

Note any tooth changes:
- Positioning,-version, -occlusion, extrusion, infraclusion (**53**).
- Rotation and by what degree.
- Crowding.

Finally, an explorer is pointed perpendicular to the teeth and gently run along them at the gingival margin to determine areas of possible resorption. Resorption will feel rough, and can be delineated from the furcation of multirooted teeth, which will feel smooth.

Before beginning detailed periodontal examination, be familiar with the markings on the provided periodontal probe. There are numerous periodontal probes, and each has specific measurement markings. Probe the sulcus around the tooth by 'sounding' (walking the probe around the tooth while gently pressing on the sulcal floor)[2]. Each tooth should be evaluated at a minimum of 8 locations (line angles, see *Table 5*). Be careful not to skirt the teeth without gently probing the sulcus at line angles, as pockets can be missed this way. Normal sulcal depth in dogs is 0–3 mm and in cats is 0–0.5 mm[1]. Thus, a probe that cannot measure ≤1 mm increments is essentially useless in a cat. Above normal sulcal depth values, depths are considered pathological and should be noted on the dental chart by their millimeter depth and location. For example a P4 MB 107 denotes a pathological periodontal pocket of 4 mm at the mesiobuccal aspect of the permanent maxillary right third premolar tooth[1]. Normal measurements for an animal differ between individuals and regions of the mouth. Of concern are aberrant measurements (e.g. a 3 mm sulcal depth when 1 mm depths are consistently found) or a 3 mm depth found at an incisor as well as a canine. If the periodontal probe drops into an area beyond its marked measurements, then oronasal fistulation (ONF)(**54**) or oroantral fistulation (OAF) should be suspected. Such fistulations can be confirmed clinically by blood or irrigating fluids emanating from the ipsilateral external nare during probing or alveolar irrigation[11,50]. The summation of trabecular bone and maxillary sinuses preclude radiographic confirmation of an oronasal fistula (ONF)[31,51].

Note gingival hypertrophy (GH) with associated pseudopocketing and record gain in millimeters. Likewise, note gingival recession or pseudorecession (supraeruption), and record loss in millimeters. For example GR4 DL 104

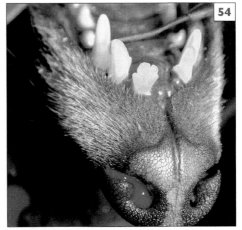

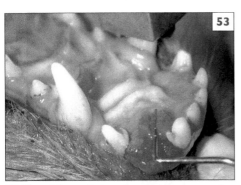

53 Use of the periodontal probe to measure the diameter of a tooth-displacing epulis. (Note distoversion of tooth 203 and slight labioversion of tooth 202.) The probe can also be used to manipulate the tumor away from the teeth to discern potential origins.

54 Clinical diagnosis of an oronasal fistula in a dolicocephalic breed. Bleeding upon probing of the periodontium distopalatal to tooth 204 resulted in rhinorrhagia from the ipsilateral nare. Note insertion of the probe beyond its anodized markings. The chief concern upon presentation was chronic sneezing. (Also note mildly bulging gingiva at radiologically-confirmed missing teeth 101, 201, and dilaceration of the cusp of tooth 202 which was diagnosed as fused with tooth 201.)

represents 4 mm gingival recession at the distolabial aspect of the permanent maxillary right canine. Record furcation exposure (FE) in multirooted teeth, noting the orientation of their entrance (line or point angles) and FE index (**55**)[52].

Stage 1 (F1, furcation involvement) exists when a periodontal probe extends less than half way under the crown in any direction of a multi-rooted tooth with attachment loss.

Stage 2 (F2, furcation involvement) exists when a periodontal probe extends greater than half way under the crown of a multirooted tooth with attachment loss but not through and through.

Stage 3 (F3, furcation exposure) exists when a periodontal probe extends under the crown of a multirooted tooth, through and through from one side of the furcation out the other.

When moving to the adjacent teeth, note blunting or absence of the interdental papillae, which represents interproximal gingival recession. In addition to pockets and furcations, sinus tracts can also be probed. Introduction of gutta percha can help radiographically delineate the morphology and course of these defects[2].

Assess mobility of the tooth by attempting to move it horizontally or depressing it vertically. A periodontal probe turned perpendicular in relation to the tooth is useful in assessing mobility of the bunodont maxillary molars. Using the butts of two mouth-mirror handles is more useful in assessing the mobility of secodont teeth (i.e. canines). Assign a mobility index to each tooth as follows[2]:

M0 = Normal physiological movement.
M1 = Slightly more than physiological movement.
M2 = <1 mm of horizontal movement.
M3 = >1 mm of horizontal movement and/or ability to depress/infraclude the tooth apically (vertically).

Always compare contralateral and adjacent teeth when assessing mobility. Take care not to mistake physiological tooth movement (e.g. due to positioning in the mandibular symphyseal fibrocartilage) for pathological movement. Be wary of teeth that exhibit novel version or occulsion, have greater mobility than expected, or permanent teeth that self-exfoliate. In these cases, further work-up (radiography, biopsy) is recommended. Causes of increased mobility include:

• Periodontal disease.
• Neoplasia.
• Acute periradicular abscess (e.g. carnassial).
• Root fracture.
• Trauma.
• Chronic bruxism.
• Orthodontic tooth movement.
• Hyperparathyroidism.

A generalized GI is best assigned after individual tooth assessment with periodontal probing. Soft tissue inflammation in the absence of inciting debris should make one suspicious of tooth resorption, immune-mediated disease, tooth retention, or neoplasia.

55 Undermining of the furcation areas at teeth 408 and 409. Periodontal probe exploration confirmed an F1F (furcation undermining, facial entry at tooth 408), and an F2F (non through-and-through furcation exposure, facial entry) at tooth 409.

KEY POINTS

- During anesthetized oral examination, systematically revisit all the structures assessed upon conscious oral examination, and any that were missed.
- Use four-handed dental charting and the modified Triadan tooth numbering system.
- Odontogenic pathoses should be localized according to tooth landmarks such as cusps, developmental grooves, line and point angles and/or G.V. Black's modified classification, and staged according to accepted indices.
- During probing, pathological periodontal pocketing, GH with pseudopocket or (pseudo)recession, FE, tooth mobility, and generalized GI are noted and charted.
- Be familiar with how to maximize the usefulness of the explorer-probe and verify probe markings before charting these measurements

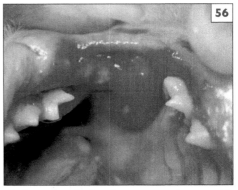

56 Open-mouthed oral examination in a cat with inflammation lateral to the palatoglossal folds. This area is typically inflamed in pets with stomatitis. (Note views of the soft palate, hard palate, mucosa, tongue, and sublingual areas afforded on this open-mouth view.) (Courtesy of Dr. Brook Niemiec.)

ORAL CAVITY EVALUATION

Examine the remainder of the oral cavity systematically as during awake examination, but in more detail. During intubation and the oral examination, look towards the oropharyngeal area. Use your finger, a tongue depressor, or laryngoscope to depress the root of the tongue to enhance visualization. Examine the epiglottis, soft palate, arytenoid cartilages, vocal folds, laryngeal saccules if everted, tonsillar crypts, palatine tonsils, and the palatoglossal folds. It is important to evert the palatine tonsils by gently pulling forward on the rostral aspect of the tonsillar crypts with the blunt periodontal probe. This allows for evaluation of tonsillar presence, size, lobulation, pigmentation, mottling, and crypt foreign bodies. Abnormalities are best investigated by biopsying both tonsils since bilateral synchronous tonsillar lesions (e.g. squamous cell carcinoma) have been reported[53]. Evaluate the continuation of the soft palate ventral to its caudal pillars or palatoglossal folds (**56**)[54].

Evaluate the soft palate for elongation, prominent palatal gland ducts, ulcerations, abrasions, burns, color changes, foreign bodies, redundant midline tissues (especially in brachycephalics), and clefting. Move rostrally to the hard palate and evaluate for clefting, asymmetric rugae, debris-trapping between the rugae (especially in brachycephalic breeds) (**57**), rugal flattening, ulcerations, swellings, masses, and foreign bodies (**58**). Finally, examine the incisive papilla and its lateral incisive ducts for size and debris (usually hair) entrapment.

Using a gloved finger, palpate the soft and hard palates as well as the underlying bones. Pay attention to asymmetry. Asymmetric junctures of the rugae at the raphe may be an indication of tendency toward (secondary) cleft palate formation. It is not uncommon to find this asymmetric rugal pattern in parents of cleft palate puppies[1]. Check the rugal folds for food or hairs trapped between them and any resultant excoriations or ulcerations. A cotton swab can be used to tease such debris gently from the area before definitive treatment. If appliances have been removed, note any areas of contact irritation and medicate or treat these as necessary.

While examining the palates, re-evaluate the occlusal and lingual surfaces of the teeth. Common problem areas include:
- The occlusal surfaces of teeth 109 and 209: caries in dogs.
- Attached gingiva palatal to teeth 108 and 208: gingival recession, FE, foreign bodies, OAFs.
- Attached gingiva at 104 and 204: vertical pocketing +/− ONFs (especially in Dachshunds).

Patency of salivary ducts can be assessed by pressing lightly caudal to the papilla and rolling the finger towards the duct, or by passing a catheter[1].

Carefully examine the tongue's dorsal, lateral, and ventral surfaces as well as underlying structures (**59**). Evaluate the tongue and any suspicious areas for thickness and texture. The tongue should be strong and mobile. Observe the margin of the tongue for ulcerations from CUPS or immune-mediated disease. In suckling puppies, marginal papillae are normal. Look at the ventrum of the tongue and structures in the floor of the mouth for pathologies such as edematous swelling, 'tongue chewer lesions', masses, lacerations, ulcerations, and foreign

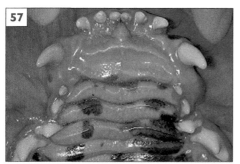

57 A treatable problem[1] of hair-trapping between closely approximated rugal folds and between the incisive papilla and teeth 101 and 201 in a brachycephalic breed. Note symmetry of the rugal folds at the median raphe of the hard palate, and symmetrical 90° rotation of teeth 107 and 207.

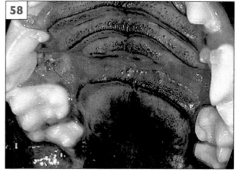

58 Hard palatal trauma due to a chronically wedged stick between teeth 108 and 208. Note grass trapped palatal to tooth 108. Recession to the point of furcation exposure was discerned upon detailed periodontal probing during unconscious oral examination.

bodies. The lingual frenulum attaches the body of the tongue to the floor of the oral cavity.

Examine the tongue and sublingual structures from the rostrum. Note especially the lingual frenulum and the area below the tongue tip, including the paired sublingual caruncles which mark the exit of the sublingual and mandibular salivary ducts[1]. Pressing a thumb in the intermandibular space to elevate the tongue will allow better visualization (**60**). Measure any masses found in the oral cavity and describe pertinent landmarks.

Check for mobility at the mandibular symphysis, but do not over interpret mobility or rush to treat a case orthopedically that exhibits good function, occlusion, and TMJ comfort. These cases may benefit more from periodontal work-up and treatment. Evaluate mouth opening, lateral movement of the mandibles, and movement of the TMJs for palpable/audible clicks or crepitus, or excessive movement felt by the non-manipulating hand. Clicks and crepitus are best heard by holding the bell of a stethoscope over one TMJ before testing the other side. Re-evaluate the lymph nodes, salivary glands, muscles, thyroid glands, and neck. Re-examine the skin for evidence of wounds or dermatologic conditions. Take photographs to document major findings and those in need of treatment.

KEY POINTS

- During unconscious oral examination, all components of the oral cavity must be systematically examined as during awake examination, but in more detail.
- Based on the findings of the conscious and anesthetized examination, create a dental plan for the patient. Rework the estimate and obtain owner consent for further diagnostics (such as dental radiographs, biopsies, fine-needle aspiration) and/or treatments.

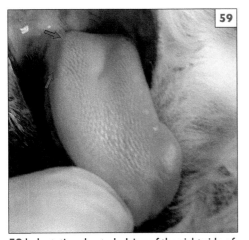

59 Indentation due to bulging of the right side of the dorsum of the body of the tongue in a cat (arrows). The right lateral sublingual area (visualized using the technique in **60**) had been invaded by a squamous cell carcinoma.

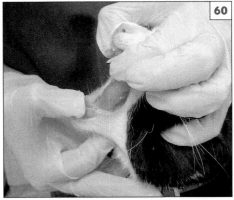

60 Technique for visualizing the rostral and lateral sublingual areas on a cat, by placing a forefinger in the intermandibular space. Alternatively, the thumb may be placed here and the middle finger placed on the mandibular incisors to displace the mandible ventrally, leaving the index finger free to manipulate the apex of the tongue.

CHAPTER 3

Veterinary Dental Radiology

Brook A. Niemiec

- **Step 1: Patient positioning**

- **Step 2: Film placement within the patient's mouth**

- **Step 3: Positioning the beam head**

- **Step 4: Setting the exposure**

- **Step 5: Exposing the radiograph**

- **Step 6: Developing the radiograph**

- **Step 7: Techniques for various individual teeth**

- **Step 8: Interpreting dental radiographs**

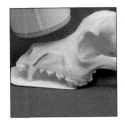 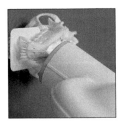 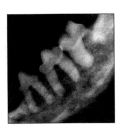 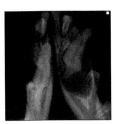

Step 1: Patient positioning

The first step in creating quality dental images involves positioning of the patient. Utilize sand bags, v-trays and other implements to improve stability and placement of the patient.

TECHNIQUE[1-5]

Position the patient so that the area of interest is convenient to the radiographic beam. Except in rare instances, the object or tooth to be radiographed is positioned 'up'. For ease of determining angles, the patient should be positioned as follows:

- Maxillary teeth = ventral recumbency.
- Mandibular canine and incisor teeth = dorsal recumbency.
- Mandibular premolar and molar teeth = lateral recumbency with the affected side 'up'.

When the operator is proficient in visualizing the correct angle, many maxillary images can be obtained with the patient in lateral recumbency, which avoids rolling the patient numerous times during procedures.

KEY POINTS

- The angles required for veterinary dental radiology are easier to visualize when the teeth are perpendicular or parallel to the table.
- For the vast majority of images, the patient should be positioned with the object tooth nearest the X-ray tube head.

Step 2: Film placement within the patient's mouth

Film placement in veterinary dentistry is challenging due to the inability to visualize the roots. Correct placement of the film will minimize retakes.

TECHNIQUE[1-5]

When utilizing standard film, there is an embossed dot (or dimple) on the corner of the film (**61**). The side of the film with the palpable dot should be placed towards the X-ray beam, and this side of the film is white for most film types. The opposite or 'back' side of the film will usually be colored. Place the film in the mouth so that the entire tooth (including the root) will be imaged (if possible). The roots of all teeth are much longer than the crown in veterinary patients. This is especially true of canine teeth which have roots that are at least twice as long as the visible crown. Always err on the side of having the film further into the mouth to ensure imaging the entire root structure. The film should be placed as close as possible to the object (generally touching the tooth and gingiva) to minimize distortion (**62**). Finally, ensure that the embossed dot is not over the area of interest.

KEY POINTS

- The white side of the film is placed toward the tube head and the colored side away.
- The film is placed *within* the mouth to avoid superimposition of the opposite arcade.
- Roots are much longer than most people realize.

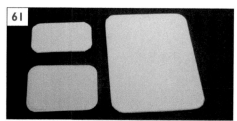

61 Standard dental film, clockwise from top left: Size 1, 4, 2. Embossed dot is best seen in bottom left of size 4 film.

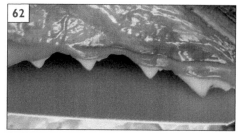

62 Proper positioning of film for a maxillary premolar radiograph.

Step 3: Positioning the beam head

Correct placement of the tube head, in relation to the patient and the film, is important to create the most accurate image. This is the most difficult and frustrating part of veterinary dental radiology. Once the steep learning curve is mastered, dental radiology becomes much easier and efficient.

TECHNIQUE[1-5]

There are two major techniques for positioning the beam head in dental radiology, both of which are used daily in veterinary practice.

Parallel technique[2]: By the strict definition, this technique is used only on the mandibular premolar and molar teeth. All other teeth have anatomical structures (palate or mandibular symphysis) that preclude parallel film placement. Place the film parallel to the tooth and perpendicular to the X-ray beam (**63**). This technique is similar to standard radiographic techniques of skeletal bone (e.g. spine) or body cavity (e.g. thorax). This technique provides the most accurate image (**64**).

Bisecting angle technique[2]: This is by far the most common positioning technique used in veterinary patients (as the parallel technique cannot be physically achieved for the majority of teeth). The bisecting angle technique uses the theory of equilateral triangles to create an image that most accurately represents the tooth being radiographed. Place the film as parallel as possible to the tooth root. Then measure or approximate the angle between the tooth root and film. This angle is divided in half (bisected) and the X-ray beam placed perpendicular to this imaginary angle (**65**).

By utilizing this technique, the operator will create the most accurate representation of the tooth root length (**66**). If the calculated angle is incorrect, the radiographic image will be distorted, creating an image that is longer or shorter than the object being radiographed.

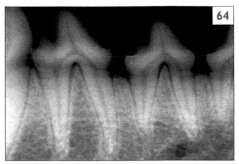

64 Resultant radiograph of the technique in **63**.

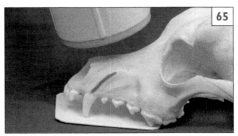

65 Bisecting angle radiograph for the maxillary canine in a dog. The purple line is the angle of the tooth root and the green line is the bisecting angle between it and the film. Note that the beam is aimed perpendicular to the green line, not the film.

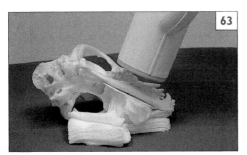

63 Parallel technique for mandibular premolar/molar teeth in a dog.

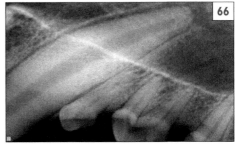

66 Proper bisecting angle of the maxillary canine from **65**.

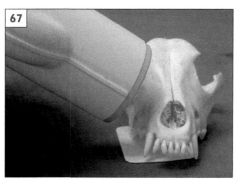

67 Improper angulation of the radiographic beam. The angle of beam to film is too small.

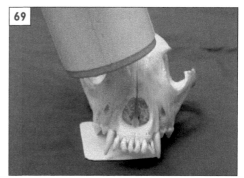

69 Improper angulation of the radiographic beam. The angle of beam to film is too great.

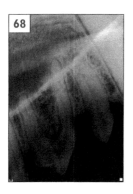

68 Resultant radiograph of the technique used in **67**. Note the elongation of the roots.

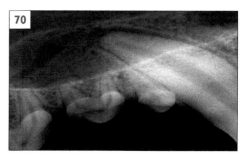

70 Resultant radiograph of the technique in **69**. Note the foreshortening of the premolar roots.

The best way to visualize this concept is to think of a building creating a shadow from the sun. The building (tooth root) is at a 90° (right) angle to the ground (film). In this case, the bisecting angle would be 45°. Early and late in the day, the sun is at an acute angle to the building and casts a long shadow. In dental radiology, this occurs when the angle of the X-ray beam to the tooth is too small (or more perpendicular to the tooth root) (**67**). This improper angle will result in 'elongation' of the image (**68**). At some point in the late morning and early afternoon, the sun is at a 45° angle to the building, which is the bisecting angle. The shadow that is cast is an accurate representation of building height. As the sun continues travelling up in the sky, the shadow shortens. In dental radiology, this occurs when the angle of the X-ray beam to the object is too great, and is known as 'foreshortening' (**69, 70**). This error usually occurs when the X-ray beam is relatively perpendicular to the film.

KEY POINTS
- Parallel technique is only used for mandibular premolars and molars.
- The maxillary cheek teeth are at an approximately 90° angle to the film.
- The incisors and canines have crowns with approximately 90° angles to the film; however, the root angles are close to 40°.

Step 4: Setting the exposure

This involves setting the amount of radiation that will be used to expose the image. It differs from standard radiology in that the kVp and Ma are held constant in dental radiology. Only the time is adjusted.

TECHNIQUE[1-5]

If you are using a machine that requires manual setting of the exposure (**71A**), you will need to create a technique chart for your system. This is similar to the one used for a standard radiology machine, except only one variable needs to be adjusted (time). Start with the sample charts provided, and adjust to your individual machine (*Table 7*). Note that the digital settings are much lower than those for standard film (*Table 8*). If you are utilizing the computer controlled system, set the controls for the species, size of the patient, and tooth to be imaged (**71B**). If the setting is proper and the exposure is incorrect, the easiest way to make corrections is to change the f setting. By pressing this button, the numbers will go up on both sides. The one on the left is the f number and the one on the right is the exposure time. If you continue to press the button, it will continue to increase the exposure time until it reaches f number 9, when it will markedly decrease and the f number will go back to 1. If the radiograph is overexposed (too dark), decrease the f number by 1. If it is underexposed (too light), increase the number by 1. Continue this process until you have correct film exposure. Generally, the f number will be the same for all radiographs on a given machine.

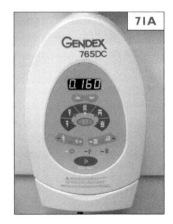

71A; Manual controlled radiograph machine.

Table 7 Dental radiology technique chart for standard film

	Mandible^	Maxilla^	Extraoral maxilla^
Cat	8–12	10–14	14–18
Dog (toy)	9–12	10–16	
Dog (small)	12–16	14–18	
Dog (medium)	18–22	20–28	
Dog (large)	22–28	28–36	
Dog (giant)	26–34	32–42	

^in **pulses** for D speed films. For E speed films decrease the exposure to half.

	Mandible*	Maxilla*	Extraoral maxilla*
Cat	0.13–0.2	0.17–0.23	0.23–0.30
Dog (toy)	0.15–0.22	0.17–0.27	
Dog (small)	0.2–0.26	0.23–0.30	
Dog (medium)	0.30–0.37	0.33–0.47	
Dog (large)	0.37–0.47	0.47–0.6	
Dog (giant)	0.43–0.57	0.53–0.70	

*in **seconds** for D speed films. For E speed films decrease the exposure to half.

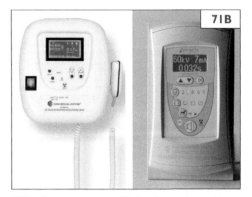

71B; Computer controlled radiograph machine. Note settings for size of patient, tooth, and f setting.

The exposure for direct digital radiographs (DRs) is far less than that for conventional film, so be sure the computer is on the digital setting prior to exposure. Some older machines may not have the ability to create such a short exposure time and must be replaced prior to utilizing digital systems.

KEY POINTS

- Manual adjust machines will require a basic technique chart, with only one variable (time).
- Computer controlled versions are set according to the computer and adjusted with the f number.
- Digital sensors require much less exposure than conventional film.
- Time is the only variable in dental radiology.

Table 8 Dental radiology technique chart for digital sensors[a,b]

	Mandible^	Maxilla^	Extraoral maxilla^
Cat	0.032–0.04	0.04–0.05	0.05–0.063
Dog (toy)	0.04–0.05	0.04–0.063	
Dog (small)	0.04–0.05	0.04–0.063	
Dog (medium)	0.04–0.063	0.05–0.063	
Dog (large)	0.05–0.08	0.063–0.08	
Dog (giant)	0.05–0.08	0.063–0.10	

^in seconds.

[a]Note these numbers are a guide only, since dental machines and digital systems are highly variable.

[b]Phospor sensor plates have a very wide range of acceptable exposure; use the lowest possible setting.

Step 5: Exposing the radiograph

This is the act of actually creating the image by exposing the film to radiation.

TECHNIQUE[1–4]

It is strongly recommended that everyone leave the room prior to exposing the radiograph, to reduce staff X-ray exposure. If this is not possible, stand at least 6 feet (2 meters) away at a 90–130° angle to the primary beam (to the side of the tube head, not in front or behind). Most dental radiograph generators have a hand held switch. These switches are 'dead man's' style, which means if you release finger pressure during the exposure, the production of X-rays will stop. On a manually adjusted dental radiology unit, this will result in an underexposed or light radiograph, while on a computer controlled dental radiology unit, an error message will illuminate and you must restart the process. Make sure to press the button until the machine stops beeping. When using a digital system, this will be a very short time.

KEY POINTS

- Leave the room when possible during X-ray exposure.
- Make sure that the button is depressed until it stops beeping to ensure proper exposure.
- Digital exposure time is very short.

Step 6: Developing the radiograph

Dental radiographs can be developed via hand developing, automatic dental film processors, or standard radiograph processors. Hand developing will be described further in this chapter. For automatic dental processing, refer to the operating manual for that piece of equipment. This author does not recommend standard radiograph automatic processors for developing dental films.

REMOVAL OF FILM FROM THE PACKET

Removal of the film from the packet is the first step in developing dental radiographs, regardless of the method chosen. Carefully open the package by grasping the tag. Once opened, three components will be encountered: the film, a piece of black paper, and a lead sheet (**72**)[4,6]. The paper will either be in front of the film (towards the tube head) or wrapped around the film entirely. The lead sheet is behind the film. These all feel very different. Remove these contents and separate the film from the other pieces. Grasp only the very corner of the film to avoid finger print artifacts[2]. For hand development, placing the film clip on the edge of the film prior to separation will help to avoid touching the film (**73**).

KEY POINTS
- Make sure to separate all three components prior to developing.
- Avoid touching the film with fingers as this will create artifacts.

DEVELOPING DENTAL RADIOGRAPHS BY HAND

This is by far the most common and least expensive method of developing dental radiographs. It involves developing the film with chemicals by hand, without the use of an automatic processor[2–4,6]. This method is similar to dip tank developing that was previously used for standard films.

Technique

Hand developing can be performed in a dark room using household cups or bowls, or in the operatory room utilizing a chair-side developer. A chair-side developer unit holds the chemicals for developing and fixing the film, which are visualized through a colored filter (**74**). Advantages of chair-side developing include time efficiency and allowing for continual patient monitoring by the technician during the development process[2,3,6].

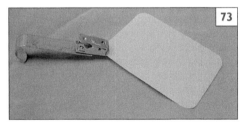

73 Proper positioning of film clip on the corner of the film.

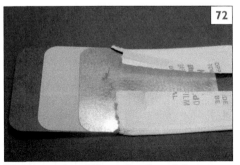

72 Opened dental film packet. From left: paper, film, lead.

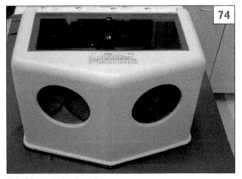

74 Chair-side developer.

Hand developing methods may utilize two different techniques to produce an image correctly on the film. The techniques employ the use of either time/temperature or observation by the person developing the film (sight developing)[6]. Both methods employ a two-step rapid development solution. The solutions designed for standard radiographs are a poor substitute since time of development will be greatly increased, and the quality of development and fixation will be inferior[6].

Time/temperature development is performed by continually monitoring the temperature of the developing solution, and utilizing this information to determine the required development time by consulting the manufacturer's recommendation[6]. This is the most scientifically correct method of development, but can be cumbersome[4].

Sight development is accomplished by dipping the film in the developer for a short time, removing it, and then critically examining the film with the safe light or through the filter[4,6]. This process is repeated until the first hint of an image appears, indicating the film is properly developed. Sight development has significant advantages over the time/temperature technique. First, continuous temperature monitoring is not necessary. Note that the solution temperatures typically rise during the day (especially if there are numerous films being developed), which affects (hastens) development time. This can result in overdeveloped films unless the technician performs frequent temperature readings. The biggest advantage of sight developing, however, is that an experienced technician can adjust for minor technique errors by relatively over- or under-developing the film[6]. This will not compensate for major errors, but will avoid some retakes.

Once the film is carefully removed from the packet, it is placed into the developer solution. To ensure full development, take care to submerge the entire film for the allotted time, or until developed. Following proper development, the film is rinsed by agitating in distilled water for 1 minute, and then placed in the fixer. The film may be evaluated for a short period after complete submersion in the fixer for 1 full minute. However, in order to archive the film for later viewing, it should be replaced in the fixer for a minimum of 10–30 minutes depending on the condition of the fixer[3,6]. If the film stays in the fixer for a prolonged period, it will not be adversely affected.

The film must be thoroughly rinsed after completing the fixation process. Proper rinsing requires the film to be placed in the water rinse for a minimum of 10 minutes. However, if true archival quality is desired, a 30 minute rinse is recommended[3,6]. In order to avoid fixer solution dripping down from the clip and ruining the image, the film should be transferred to a clean clip and quickly rinsed again before drying[6].

The radiograph must be dried completely prior to storage, or the films will stick together resulting in significant film damage[2,3,6]. Drying can be accomplished with a dental film dryer or hair dryer. Alternatively, the radiographs may be hung to air dry. However, a full 24 hours should be allowed for complete drying if the air drying method is used. When drying multiple radiographs, they can be transferred to a multifilm clip.

Chemicals used in hand developing must be replaced frequently when using small cups. Six ounces of developer will generally develop 10–15 size # 4 films, or a larger number of smaller # 2 films, before replenishment is necessary[3]. Regardless of the quality of development or fixing and rinsing, some degradation of the film quality is expected over time. Therefore, it is recommended to take high quality digital photos of the radiographs and store them in a folder on a computer which is routinely backed-up (**75**). This, in essence, is a permanent copy of the film and will also facilitate telemedicine with specialists or other veterinarians. For instructions on how to take quality digital images of dental films, visit www.vetdentalrad.com and click on how to prepare files, and then digital camera.

KEY POINTS
- Make sure film is completely covered by developing and fixing solutions to avoid undeveloped areas.
- Films can be viewed after 1 minute of fixing, but then need to be returned to the fixer.
- Fix for a minimum of 10–30 minutes.
- Rinse for a minimum of 10 minutes, but preferably 30 minutes.
- Dry completely prior to storage.
- Take a digital photograph of the images, especially important ones.

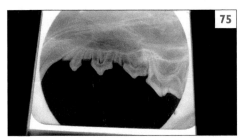

75 Digital picture of a standard film for archival and telemedicine.

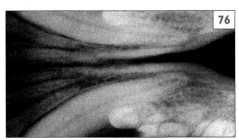

76 Underexposed or underdeveloped film. Note how 'light' the image is.

ERRORS OF EXPOSURE AND DEVELOPMENT

There are numerous opportunities for errors in the creation of dental radiographs which are directly related to developing or exposure. These differ from errors of angulation (covered earlier in this chapter).

Errors in exposure or development will result in poor quality or unreadable films. Common errors include underexposure/ developing, overexposure/developing, under-fixing, and under-rinsing[2–4,6,7].

Underexposed or underdeveloped radiographs will appear washed out or 'light' (**76**). This can result from insufficient exposure or developing time as well as exhausted developer. This problem can be corrected by increasing development time or exposure. If the problem persists, replace the solutions.

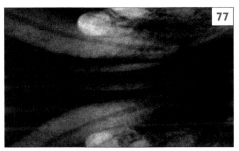

77 Overexposed or overdeveloped film. Note how 'dark' the film is.

Overexposed or overdeveloped film will result in a radiograph that is 'dark' (**77**). This problem is usually corrected by decreasing exposure time, but occasionally decreasing the development time may be preferred.

Extreme underfixing will cause the film to blacken prior to viewing. Slight under fixing will cause the radiograph to yellow over time. Immediate film blackening can be avoided by leaving the film in the fixer for a minimum of 1 minute before viewing. Long-term viewing ability (years) will be achieved by fixing for a total of 30 minutes[6].

Initially, the radiograph will not be adversely affected by insufficient rinsing. However, the fixer that remains on the film will turn it brown over time, resulting in unreadable films (**78**). The biggest problem with this error is that it is not discovered at the time of the procedure,

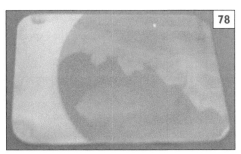

78 Under-rinsed film 1 year post exposure. Note the browning and poor film quality.

only later on review. Therefore, the films can not be re-exposed. This problem can be avoided by rinsing the film thoroughly. Current recommendations for proper rinsing are 30 minutes in a container, or several minutes under running tap water[3,6].

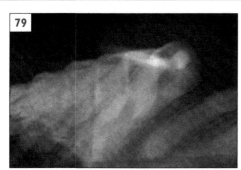

79 Washed out or fogged film.

Fogged or unclear radiographs (**79**) can occur secondary to a variety of problems and these may be frustrating to identify and correct. The most common causes are: old or exhausted solutions, old film, poor radiographic technique, light exposure, and improper light filter or developer type[2]. Troubleshoot through this list, and the cause will usually be elucidated. Light fogging (due to leakage) in a darkroom can be confirmed by placing a coin on an opened film for a few minutes and then developing the film. If the coin is visible, there is a light leak.

KEY POINTS
- If the film is too dark, decrease the exposure or development time.
- If the film is too light, increase the exposure or development time.
- Completely immerse the film in the solutions to ensure complete development.
- Fix the film for 30 minutes for archival quality.
- Make sure to evaluate the *entire* film.
- Rinse the film completely to avoid browning artifacts.

Step 7: Techniques for various individual teeth

It should be noted that the techniques listed below are for mesaticephalic dogs and cats. Dolichocephalic and especially brachycephalic breeds may have significantly different angles.

Mandibular premolars and molars
Views of the mandibular premolars and molars involve the most basic veterinary dental radiographic technique. This is because these views are generally accomplished via the parallel technique[4]. An exception to this may be the first and second premolars in dogs and third premolars in cats. The interference of the mandibular symphysis makes exposing the apices of these teeth impossible with parallel technique in certain breeds[8]. The alternate technique for these teeth is discussed in the next section.

Technique[2,8,9]
The patient is placed in lateral recumbency with the arcade to be imaged facing up. The film is placed parallel to the teeth on the lingual surface of the teeth/mandible, and the tube head positioned perpendicular to both the teeth and the film (**80**).

Key points
- These are the most basic radiographic views as parallel technique is used.
- Alternate imaging may be necessary for apices of mesial premolars.

Mesial mandibular premolar teeth
As stated previously, most mandibular teeth can be imaged using the parallel technique[2]. However, in some patients there is a problem with imaging the apices of the mesial premolars[2,8]. Typically, this is the third premolar (especially the mesial root) in cats, and the first and second premolars in dogs. The challenge with imaging these teeth is the interference of the mandibular symphysis. A standard parallel view will not image these apices.

To image the entire arcade, the bisecting angle technique is often necessary[2]. This technique can be utilized to image the entire arcade or just the mesial premolars, with a second film utilizing standard parallel technique (which is more accurate) for the molars and distal premolars.

Technique[2,8]

The film is placed in the patient's mouth at approximately a 90° angle to the tooth roots, so that the lingual edge of the film is touching the opposite mandible. The beam is then placed perpendicular to the angle between the tooth roots and the film, which is approximately 45° (81). Note that there may be slight elongation, which is a fair tradeoff for viewing the apices.

Key points

- This technique is challenging, but often necessary to image the apices of the mesial premolars.
- Two views are ideal in these cases as: 1) the molars and distal premolars are most accurately depicted with the standard parallel view, and 2) the mesial premolars are fully imaged (if slightly elongated) using this bisecting angle technique.

Mandibular incisors and canines

All six mandibular incisors and both mandibular canines can be exposed on the same film in cats and small to medium breed dogs[8,9]. In some cases, the exposure may need to be decreased for the incisors, although the angle is the same. Large breed dogs (and medium breeds if using digital sensors) will generally require one film for each of the canines, and one for the incisors[9]. The technique is a slight modification of the parallel technique.

An important point to consider when imaging the canines and incisors is that the roots curve backward to near a 45° angle in many cases. Consequently, the roots and crowns have significantly different angles. Since the roots are typically the area of interest, use the angle of the *root* (not the crown) for your bisecting angle calculation[8,9]. This technique is much closer to parallel than an image of the crown.

Another important point to consider when imaging canine teeth is their (often underestimated) length. The apex of the canine roots end over the mesial root of the second premolar. It is very common for the novice to miss the root tip apices. Place the distal edge of the film *behind* the second premolar to ensure imaging of the entire tooth[8,9].

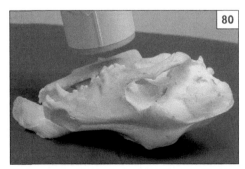

80 Proper parallel technique for the mandibular premolars and molars.

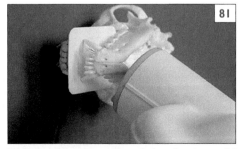

81 Proper bisecting angle technique for the mesial mandibular premolars. This will image the entire root system without distorting the image unduly.

Technique[2,8,9]

Place the patient in dorsal recumbency with the head fully extended. Place the film square with the mandible, so that the film covers the entire intended area. The tube head is placed in parallel alignment with the patient's head in a rostro-caudal plane, perpendicular to the film. Then rotate the tube head down to an angle that is approximately 75° to the film, keeping in line with the patient's head (**82**). This is now the bisecting angle for the roots.

In large canine breeds, the small size of the film may require that the incisors be exposed separately from the canines. In this case, the first view is taken with the leading edge of the film sticking out just in front of the incisors. This film will image the incisors. To image the entire canine root, place the film so that the edge is back beyond the level of the second premolar. In larger breeds, this view will typically not image the coronal area of the incisors.

Key points
- This is very close to parallel technique.
- Calculate the angle based on the backward sweeping roots, not the crown.
- In cats and small breed dogs, only one film is necessary for all eight teeth in most cases.
- In large breeds, the angle is the same but the film placement is slightly different.

Maxillary incisors

The bisecting angle technique is used when taking radiographs of the maxillary incisors[2]. In cats and most small breed dogs, all six incisors can be exposed on one film. In large breed dogs, left and right side views may need to be exposed separately (especially if utilizing digital sensors). In certain canine breeds (especially dolichocephalics), the lateral incisors may need to be imaged separately since they will be superimposed on the canines[9]. In this case, the tube head will need to be moved in the horizontal plane to image the lateral incisors properly.

As with the mandibular canines and incisors, the maxillary incisor roots also curve backward to near a 45° angle in many cases[8,9]. This results in the roots and crowns having significantly different angles. Since the roots are typically the area of interest, remember to use the angle of the *root* and not the angle of the crown for your bisecting angle calculation.

Technique[2,8,9]

The patient is placed in sternal recumbency with the head level with the table. The film is placed in the mouth so that the upper canines are resting on it and a small amount of the film is in front of the incisors. The tube head is positioned parallel with the patient's head in the horizontal plane and angled approximately 80° to the film in the rostro-caudal plane, which is the approximate bisecting angle for the distally curved roots (**83**).

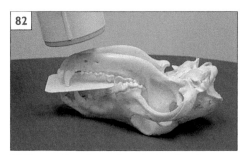

82 Proper bisecting angle technique for the mandibular canines and incisors.

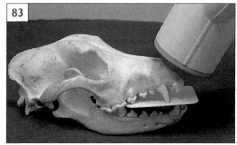

83 Proper bisecting angle technique for the maxillary incisors.

In some cases, the lateral incisor will be imaged over the canine. If overlap occurs (or is suspected to occur), this can be corrected by rotating the tube head in the lateral plane, thus allowing visualization of the tooth without interference. To perform this rotation, keep the tube head at the same angle in the rostro-caudal plane and rotate it approximately 30° laterally in the horizontal plane.

Key points
- Use the angle of the root (not the crown) for the bisecting angle technique.
- The proper rostro-caudal angle is 80° in most cases.
- All six incisors may be imaged on one film in most cases.

Maxillary canines
The technique for maxillary canines uses the bisecting angle principle: remember to consider the root rather than the tooth. Each maxillary canine must be imaged on a separate film[8,9]. Separate views are necessary because the root of the maxillary canines lie over the maxillary first and second premolars (P2 in the cat). If the canines are imaged straight on (i.e. one rostral view is taken), they will overlap with the premolars on the image (**84**)[8,9]. Additionally, it is important to remember that the apex of the canine root is at approximately the mesial root of the second premolar. Therefore, the film needs to be placed distal to the P2 in order to image the entire root.

Technique[2,8,9]
The patient is positioned in sternal recumbency with head fully extended. The film is placed in the mouth between the maxillary canines, with the front of the film behind the incisors but just in front of the canines. Be sure to have the back edge of the film at least to the level of P2. Start with the tube head positioned straight on with the nose. The ideal angle for this radiograph in the cat is 80° rostro-caudal and 20° in the lateral plane[10] (**85**). Likewise for the dog, 80° rostro-caudal is the ideal angle[11]. The lateral angle is less clear-cut, but an angle between 20° and 30° degrees appears to give the best image[11] (**86**). The 80° rostro-caudal angle compensates for the backward sweep of the canines, and the 20° lateral angle removes the premolar interference while minimizing distortion.

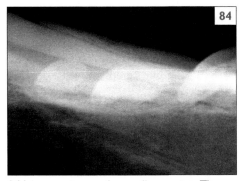

84 Improper image of a maxillary canine. The interference of the premolars makes evaluation impossible.

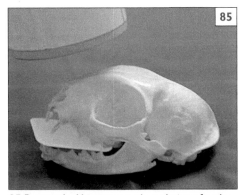

85 Proper dual bisecting angle technique for the maxillary canine in a cat.

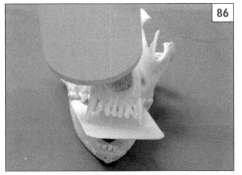

86 Proper dual bisecting angle technique for the maxillary canine in a dog.

Key points
- Both maxillary canines *cannot* be imaged on the same film.
- The beam head requires angling in both planes to create a proper image.
- For both dogs and cats, an 80° angle rostrocaudal is ideal. The entire tooth cannot be imaged in medium and large breed dogs when using a digital sensor.

Maxillary molars and premolars
These views are the most challenging to obtain of the veterinary dental radiographs. This is especially true of the maxillary fourth premolars which will be covered in the next section. A precise bisecting angle technique[2] is needed to achieve a quality radiograph of the maxillary molars and premolars.

Technique[2,8,9]
The patient is positioned in sternal recumbency with head extended. The cusp tips of the teeth to be imaged should be resting on the film, which is relatively flat against the palate. The tube head is centered over the desired tooth to be imaged and placed at an approximate 45° angle to the film (**87**). In dogs, proper technique will produce an excellent image of the premolars and an acceptable image of the molars, but cause superimposition of the mesial and palatal roots of the fourth premolar. In cats, this will give an excellent view of the second premolar and part of the third premolar, but the zygomatic arch interferes with the maxillary fourth premolar, third premolar, and first molar (**88**).

Key points
- This is a difficult technique due to the angle required.
- This will create good images of the mesial premolars, but not the P4 in either species.
- Alternate techniques are required for the P4 in dogs and P3–M1 in cats.

Maxillary fourth premolar in dogs
In order to image the mesial roots of the maxillary fourth premolar separately, the tube head must be rotated around the dog's head in the horizontal plane. This is the most difficult technique in the dog as two precise angles are necessary to create a proper image. Proper positioning will separate the mesial roots so they can be visualized independently.

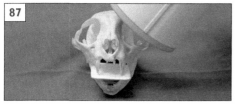

87 Proper bisecting angle technique for the maxillary premolars and molars in a dog.

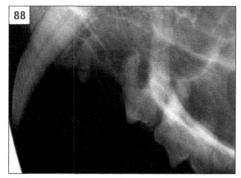

88 Zygomatic arch interference makes the standard bisecting angle technique less than ideal in the cat.

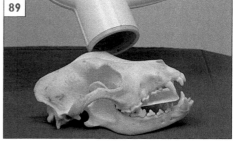

89 Proper distal tube shift technique for the maxillary fourth premolar in a dog.

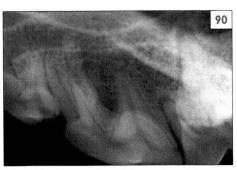

90 Resultant image from **89** revealing all three roots. From left: mesio-buccal, mesio-palatine, and distal.

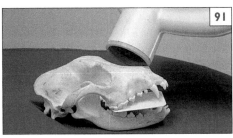

91 Proper mesial tube shift technique for the maxillary fourth premolar in a dog.

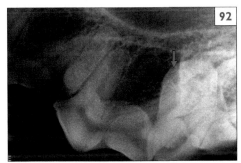

92 Resultant image from **91** revealing only the mesial roots. From left: mesio-palatine, mesio-buccal. The distal root is superimposed on the first molar (arrow).

This technique utilizes the SLOB rule, which stands for same-lingual/opposite-buccal[3,4]. The more buccal (or labial) object will move in the opposite direction as the tube shift, where as the more lingual (or palatal) object will move in the same direction relative to the tube shift. This is also known as the 'tube shift technique'[2].

Technique[2,9]

Option 1: Distal tube shift technique: the tube head is rotated around the patient's cranium distally so that it is pointing more toward the front of cranium, at approximately a 30° angle (**89**). The resultant radiograph will reveal the mesial roots separately (**90**). In this case, the mesio-buccal root is imaged most mesial and the mesio-palatine will be between the mesial-buccal and distal roots. This is typically the preferred option because the entire tooth can be imaged on one film in most cases.

Option 2: Mesial tube shift technique: to utilize this technique, the tube is shifted approximately 30° mesially, so that the tube head is pointed towards the back of the patient (**91**). The resultant view reveals the mesio-palatine root imaged mesial to the mesio-buccal root (**92**). The major deficiency with this technique is that the distal root is now superimposed over the first molar. Thus, an additional exposure will be required to evaluate the distal root.

Key points
- Proper imaging of this tooth requires precise horizontal and vertical beam angulations.
- If evaluating only for periodontal disease or retained roots, this may not be necessary as the straight lateral view may suffice in these cases.
- Distal tube shift is more commonly performed since all three roots can be evaluated in the same image.

Maxillary fourth premolar in cats

In veterinary dental radiology, the major difference between canine and feline patients is the techniques used for the maxillary cheek teeth. In dogs, quality radiographs of these teeth can be exposed with the standard bisecting angle technique. However, in cats the position of the zygomatic arch does not allow a clear view of the third and fourth premolars since it will be superimposed over these roots[2,8]. Due to this limitation, two additional techniques are now currently utilized to get a clear image of these tooth roots in cats.

Technique[2]

Extraoral technique[2]: This method is difficult to master, but it allows these teeth to be visualized without interference of the zygomatic arch or elongation of the roots. Place the film on the table with the embossed dot facing up and the patient in lateral recumbency, with the teeth to be imaged *down* on the film. The film should be placed so that the ventral aspect is just visible below the cusp tips of the teeth to be imaged. This will ensure that the majority of the film is available to image the roots. Make sure that the film covers the entire arcade (second premolar to first molar) in the rostral-caudal direction. For this view, a size 4 film is preferred (if available) to reduce placement errors.

Place a radiolucent gag between ipsilateral canines to open the mouth fairly wide. The patient's head should be slightly rotated so that the mandible is about 20° above the maxilla. The tube head is then positioned so that it points into the oral cavity, such that the cusp tips of the opposite arcade will be imaged approximately 3 mm below the root apices of the intended arcade to be imaged. The angle produced is approximately 25° from perpendicular, which then creates the approximate 45° angle necessary to depict the root length accurately (**93**). Variation on the angle depends on the anatomy of the particular patient. Note that the zygomatic arch (arrow) is now visualized apical to the tooth roots, giving a clear picture of the entire root system (**94**). Splitting of the tooth roots (SLOB rule) is very difficult to achieve in this view. If this is critical, use the acute angle technique described below.

An important point to remember when utilizing the extraoral technique is that the film needs to be marked in some way to distinguish right *vs*. left. This is due to the fact that the embossed dot is now facing into the mouth, as opposed to out of the mouth as in the intraoral techniques. Therefore, when the films are viewed they will be interpreted as the contralateral arcade. In our practice, the embossed dots on dried films are filled in with a

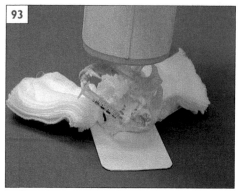

93 Proper extraoral technique for the maxillary premolars in a cat.

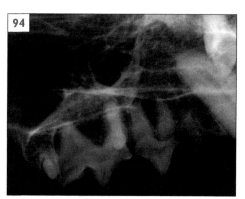

94 Resultant image from **93** revealing the roots with minimal zygomatic arch interference.

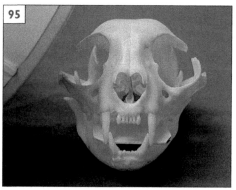

95 Proper acute angle technique for the maxillary premolars in a cat.

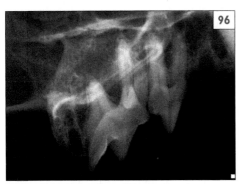

96 Resultant image from **95** revealing the roots with minimal zygomatic arch interference, but with slight elongation of the roots.

Step 8: Interpreting dental radiographs

Interpreting dental radiographs is similar to interpreting a standard bony radiograph. However, dental radiographic changes can be much more subtle than those observed with standard radiographs. In addition, there are numerous pathologies which are unique to dental radiology. Finally, there are many normal anatomical structures that may mimic pathological changes.

Differential diagnoses
- Normal anatomy.
- Artifacts.

KEY POINTS
- Be careful not to over interpret pathology.

DETERMINING WHICH TEETH HAVE BEEN IMAGED
This is the first step in interpreting the radiograph, and is more difficult than most people think. It requires knowledge of anatomy as well as dental films.

Technique[2,3,12,13]
The key to identifying the film correctly is the embossed dot, which is on one corner of the film. When the film is properly positioned for exposure, the convex surface will point at the radiographic tube head, and the concave side into the patient's mouth. There is no way to expose a diagnostic radiograph with the film in backwards, due to the lead sheet on the back side of the film. Therefore, when interpreting the film, the embossed dot is facing out of the mouth. Determining which tooth or teeth is imaged requires three steps.

The first step is to place the convex (raised) side of the dot toward you. This orients the film as if you were looking at the patient from a few feet away. Imagine that your eyes are in the same position that the X-ray tube was in when the film was taken. *Once the dot is toward your eye, do not flip the film over*. This step is automatically done for you when using digital dental film systems. This is labial film mounting, which is the accepted standard of the AVDC for film viewing.

Next, determine if the image is maxillary or mandibular. Then, rotate the film so maxillary

red permanent marker to denote that the extraoral technique was utilized. Other practices will mark an L or R on the film with a permanent marker or use small paper clip markers prior to exposure.

Acute angle technique[2]: This technique is similar to the standard bisecting angle; however, the teeth are purposefully elongated to remove the zygomatic arch interference. This technique lends itself to splitting the mesial roots of the upper fourth premolar better than the extraoral technique. The mesial tube shift is preferred in feline patients due to the close proximity of the third premolar mesially, and the smaller first molar distally. Perform a standard bisecting angle technique, but angling the beam at 30° as opposed to 45° (**95**)[2]. This will remove the zygomatic arch interference; however, it results in a slightly elongated image (**96**).

Key points
- Due to the interference of the zygomatic arch, alternate imaging is recommended for the maxillary premolars and molars in cats.
- The extraoral technique is more difficult, but gives the most accurate image.
- The acute angle technique is easier and preferred in cases where splitting the mesial roots is necessary.
- Remember to mark the films if the extraoral technique is used.

teeth have the roots pointing up, as if you were outside the patient's mouth looking in. Mandibular quadrants are rotated so that the roots point down.

Finally, determine if the film is from the right or left side. The simplest method is to identify which end of the radiograph is towards the front of the patient and which is toward the back. Imagine the patient standing in front of you with the nose in one direction and the back of the head in the other direction. Then, simply imagine the whole patient standing in front of you facing that direction. If the patient's nose is pointed to the right, you are looking at the right side of the patient. If the patient's nose is pointed left, you are looking at the left side of the patient's mouth. When positioned as described above, views of incisors and canines have right and left swapped, similar to looking at AP abdominal films. For example, the left side of the correctly positioned film is actually the right side of the patient.

Key points
- The embossed dot will point out of the mouth.
- Orient the film as it would be in the patient's mouth.
- Use the embossed dot to determine right from left.
- Remember, if the extraoral technique was used, the film will be opposite of what is expected.
- Incisors and canines are swapped left and right.

Normal dental radiographic anatomy[2,12,14–16]
There are a number of structures within the oral cavity that can mimic disease. Knowledge of normal radiographic anatomy will help avoid over interpretation.

Radiographic features
Normal alveolar bone will appear gray and relatively uniform throughout the arcade. It is slightly more radiopaque than tooth roots, and appears slightly but regularly mottled. Bone should completely fill the area between the roots (furcation) and end at the 'neck' or cementoenamel junction (CEJ) of the teeth. The root canals should all be the same width, allowing for differences in the diameters of the

roots. There should be no radiolucent areas in teeth or bone. A thin dark line (periodontal ligament) should be discerned around the roots of the teeth (**97**).

Differential diagnoses
There are several normal anatomical findings that are commonly misinterpreted in dental images as pathological. In views of:
- Mandibular cheek teeth: a horizontal radiolucent line will be seen near the ventral cortex, which is the mandibular canal. There are two circular radiolucent areas seen in the area of the apices of the first three premolars. These are the mental foramina (middle and caudal) (**98**).

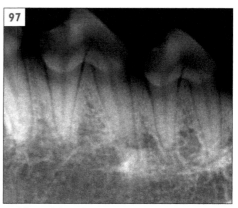

97 Normal dental radiograph of the mandibular premolars of a dog. This shows normal bone which completely fills the furcation and regular periodontal ligaments.

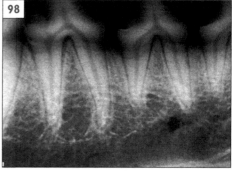

98 Mesial mandibular premolars of a dog. Note the radiolucent circle apical to the mesial root of P2. This is a mental foramen.

- Mandibular incisal area: a radiolucent line will be observed between the first incisors which is the fibrocartilaginous mandibular symphysis (**99**).
- Rostral maxillary area: there are paired radiolucent areas distal to the second incisors. These are the palatine fissures (**100**).
- At the apex of the canine teeth: there is commonly a significant widening of the periodontal ligament. This may appear to be a periapical lesion, but is differentiated from pathology because it is very regular and v-shaped, as opposed to irregular and round (**101**). These 'chevron effect' is a normal finding. If any doubts persist as to a lesion being pathological, obtain radiographs of the contralateral tooth for comparison.

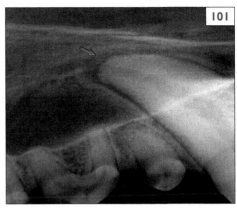

101 'Chevron effect' at the apex of a maxillary canine (arrow).

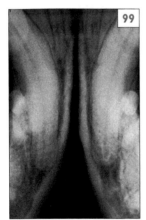

99 Mandibular canine/incisor radiograph of a dog. The black line in the center is the mandibular symphysis.

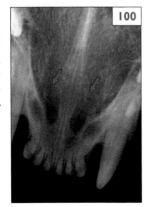

100 Maxillary incisor area of a cat. Note the paired radiolucent areas, these are the palatine fissures (arrows).

Diagnostic tests

Any questionable areas should be evaluated by exposing a second, comparative view.

A suspect periapical lucency (especially in the area of the mandibular premolars) should be evaluated with an additional film. Expose a radiograph with a slightly different angle in the horizontal or vertical plane. If the lucency is still centered on the apex, it is likely to be real. If the lesion moves off the apex or disappears, it is an artifact. Suspect changes in the diameter of a tooth should be compared against surrounding and contralateral teeth. Surrounding teeth can be seen on the same film with the 'lesion'. The contralateral view should be taken at the same angle as the original. It is important to note that root canals are not exact cylinders (especially canines). A lateral view may have a very different canal width than a V/D view[17].

Key points

- Knowledge of normal oral anatomy and skeletal landmarks will aid in radiographic evaluation and help avoid over interpretation.
- Imaging the contralateral tooth will help in determining normal from pathology.
- Periapical disease almost never affects only one root of a multirooted tooth.
- Pathological lesions are rarely smooth and regular.

Periodontal disease

Definition
Periodontal disease is defined as inflammation of the gingiva or periodontium, their active recession, or their altered state with or without current disease[4].

Etiology and pathogenesis[4]
The combination of bacterial induced inflammation and host response will result in osteoclastic resorption of bone. This proceeds in a nonlinear pattern as long as the inflammation persists. Removal of the inflammation (prophylaxis, homecare) will stop the progression. However, the bone loss is irreversible without advanced periodontal therapies which may or may not be effective. For a more detailed discussion of periodontal disease, see Chapter 6.

Radiographic features[12,18,19]
Bone resorption results in crestal bone loss to a level below the CEJ. This decrease in bone height may also result in furcational exposure. The most common pattern of bone loss in veterinary patients is horizontal[4]. Horizontal bone loss occurs when there is generalized loss of a similar level across all or part of an arcade[2] (**102**). The other pattern is called angular (vertical) bone loss. Angular bone loss occurs when there is one area of recession below the surrounding bone[2] (**103**).

An important point to remember is that bone loss does not become radiographically evident until 30–50% of the mineralization is lost in a bony region[2]. Therefore, radiographic findings will always underestimate bone loss. In addition, bone loss on only the lingual/palatal or facial surface may be hidden by superimposition of bone or tooth, thus resulting in a nondiagnosed bony pocket. Always interpret radiographs with the above information as well as the oral examination findings in mind.

Differential diagnoses
- Neoplasia.
- Trauma.
- Foreign body.
- Fungal infection.
- Metabolic disease (secondary hyperparathyroidism).

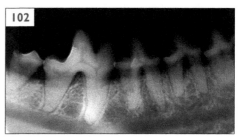

102 Horizontal bone loss in the mandibular premolars.

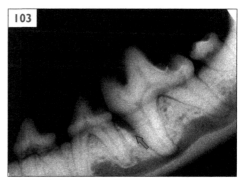

103 Vertical or angular bone loss on the mandibular first molar (arrow).

Diagnostic tests
Biopsy and/or blood panel in questionable cases.

Management
See periodontal disease, Chapter 6.

Key points
- Dental radiographs will underestimate the amount of bone loss from periodontal disease, and should not be relied on as the sole tool in diagnosis and treatment planning.
- Full mouth radiographs are mandated in cases of periodontal disease affecting more than one or two teeth.

Endodontic disease

Definition[4,12]

The endodontic system is a collection of connective tissue, blood vessels, and nerves which serve to defend the tooth[20]. This is also commonly referred to as the pulp or root canal system. Endodontic disease is defined either as tooth nonvitality or any inflammation to the pulp of the tooth[21]. If the tooth is vital, the inflammation can be either reversible (meaning the tooth will live) or irreversible (leading to tooth death and infection)[21].

Etiology and pathogenesis

Radiographic signs in endodontic disease are most commonly created by tooth death and secondary infection. As a tooth matures, secondary dentin is produced causing a decrease in canal width[20]. When a tooth becomes nonvital, this development generally stops secondary to the death of the odontoblasts. Consequently, a nonvital tooth will have a wider root canal than the surrounding vital teeth[20]. Conversely, on rare occasions, the inflammation associated with tooth death can also induce hypercalcifcation resulting in a smaller canal. This is especially common in teeth that are periodontally diseased[20]. In addition, pulpal inflammation may result in an area of internal resorption[2]. Periapical changes occur when the inflammatory/infectious agents extend through the apical delta of the tooth, resulting in osteoclastic bone resorption[4]. See Chapter 5 for a detailed discussion on endodontic disease.

Radiographic features[2,12,16,22,23]

The vast majority of teeth radiographically diagnosed with endodontic disease are nonvital and infected. Vital teeth (regardless of the level of inflammation) will rarely show obvious radiographic signs of the disease process. Endodontic disease may be demonstrated radiographically in several ways, and an individual tooth may have one, some, or all of the different changes listed below. Note however, that only one of the changes needs to be present to establish a presumptive diagnosis of endodontic disease. These radiographic changes can be grouped into two major categories: 1) changes in the bone, or 2) changes in the tooth.

Bony changes: The classic and most obvious finding is periradicular rarefaction (**104**). More subtle changes may include a widened periodontal ligament, a thickened or discontinuous lamina dura, or periradicular opacities. It is important to be aware of superimposed lucencies which are artefactual. These structures (i.e. mental foramina) can be imaged over an apex and falsely appear as osseous rarefaction secondary to endodontic disease. There are several clues that these and other superimposed lucencies are artefactual. First, superimposed artifacts are typically seen on only one root, whereas it is very rare to find a true periapical lesion on only one root of a multirooted tooth. In addition, artifacts tend to be regular in appearance, whereas true periapical lesions appear more ragged. If any area is in question, it is best to expose an additional film with a slightly different angle. If a periradicular lucency is still centered over the apex, it is likely real and not an artifact.

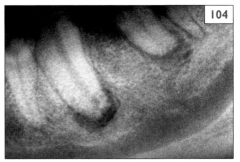

104 Periapical rarefaction on the mandibular first molar, indicating infection of the tooth.

Tooth changes. The classic appearance of a tooth with endodontic disease is a root canal with a different diameter (typically wider) than of surrounding teeth (**105**). This width discrepancy can be compared to any tooth (taking the size of tooth into consideration), but it is most accurate to compare with the contralateral tooth. It is important to expose the comparison view at the same angle, as root canals (especially in canine teeth) are not perfect cylinders. A change in the beam angle may affect the apparent canal diameter[2]. Pulpitis can occasionally result in increased dentin production, thus resulting in an endodontically diseased tooth with a smaller root canal than the contralateral tooth. This could lead to a misdiagnosis of the endodontically diseased tooth as healthy and *vice versa* with the healthy tooth. Hence it is important to evaluate the adjacent teeth as well as the contralateral.

Endodontic disease may also be manifested radiographically as internal resorption. This results from osteoclastic activity within the root canal system due to pulpitis. These changes create an irregular, enlarged region within an area of the root canal system. Finally, external root resorption can be seen with endodontic disease. It will appear as a defect of the external surface of the root, generally accompanied by a loss of bone in the area (see periradicular lucency above). External resorption most commonly occurs at the apex in companion animals (due to the lack of nonapical ramifications) and is quite common in cats with chronic periapical disease.

Differential diagnoses
- Cyst.
- Neoplasia.
- Normal anatomy.
- Superimposed structures.

Diagnostic tests
Dental radiographs are generally diagnostic, and contralateral views should be exposed in questionable cases. Transillumination (see Chapter 2) can be used to help determine vitality in intact teeth. Finally, consider histopathology in nonclassic appearing or nonresponsive lesions.

Management
Treatment of nonvital teeth is directed at removal of the infected root canal system[17,24]. This is ideally performed via standard root canal therapy. The other option for treating endodontically diseased teeth is complete extraction of the tooth. However, many owners are committed to optimum care as well as function and aesthetics and should be offered referral for endodontic therapy[4]. See Chapter 5 for a detailed discussion on endodontic therapy.

Key points
- The 'classic' radiographic sign of endodontic disease is periapical rarefaction. other signs include increased (or decreased) canal diameter, internal and external resorption, and as periapical opacities.
- Although there are numerous radiographic signs of endodontic disease, only one needs to be present to establish a diagnosis.
- True periapical lucencies are rarely present around only one root of a multirooted tooth.
- Root canal therapy or extraction is mandated for all nonvital teeth regardless of cause.
- Occasionally, cystic structures or neoplasia can mimic endodontic disease.

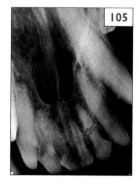

105 Widened pulp chamber on a maxillary left first incisor (arrow), indicating tooth nonvitality.

Feline tooth resorption (TR)
Definition[25,26]
TRs are defined as odontoclastic destruction of feline teeth, and are classified as either type 1 or type 2. In type 1 there is no replacement by bone, whereas in type 2 there is replacement of the lost root structure by bone.

Etiology and pathogenesis[4,26]
TRs are very common in our feline patients. The etiology at this point is unknown. TRs are not bacterial in nature, although bacteria can create the inflammation which activates the odontoclasts. There are numerous studies producing different theories but none have been proven at this time. Osteoclastic resorption will generally begin at the cervical line of the tooth and progress at varying rates, until in some cases no identifiable tooth remains. The reader is directed to Chapter 5 for a full discussion on this disease process.

Clinical features[4,26]
Type 1 TRs are typically associated with inflammation such as gingivostomatitis or periodontal disease. In these cases, it is thought that the soft tissue inflammation has activated the odontoclasts. This type will have significant resorption of the teeth and tooth roots that is *not* replaced by bone.

Type 2 TRs are usually associated with only localized gingivitis on oral examination, in contrast to the more severe inflammation due to periodontal disease or gingivostomatitis seen with type 1. The other key difference is that with type 2, the lost root structure will be replaced by bone.

Radiographic lesions[2,12,19,25,27]
Type 1 lesions will have normal root density in some areas (as compared with surrounding teeth) and a well defined periodontal space (**106**). These teeth often have a definable root canal in the intact part of the tooth. Additionally, type 1 lesions are generally associated with periodontal bone loss (either horizontal or vertical).

The radiographic appearance of type 2 lesions is that of teeth which have a different radiographic density as compared to normal teeth, as they have undergone significant replacement resorption (**107**). Findings will include areas with no discernable periodontal ligament space (dentoalveolar ankylosis) or root canal, and in late stages there will be little discernable root structure (ghost roots).

Differential diagnoses
- Caries.
- Neoplasia.
- Metabolic disease (hyper parathyroid hormone).
- Trauma.
- External resorption.

Diagnostic tests
Dental radiographs are generally diagnostic. In questionable cases other diagnostics should be considered such as: histopathological testing, culture and sensitivity, and blood work.

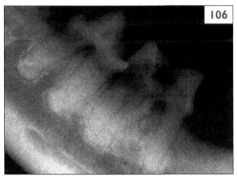

106 Type 1 TR. Note the normal periodontal ligament and root canal. This indicates the need for complete extraction.

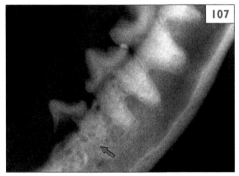

107 Type 2 TR. Note the significant resorption (arrow), indicating that crown amputation may be an acceptable method of therapy.

Management[27]

The importance of dental radiography in TR cases cannot be overstated. Type 1 lesions typically retain a viable root canal system, and will result in pain and endodontic infection if the roots are not completely extracted. However, the concurrent presence of a normal periodontal ligament makes these extractions routine. With type 2 lesions, there are areas lacking a normal periodontal ligament (ankylosis) that also commonly demonstrate varying degrees of root resorption, which makes extraction by conventional elevation difficult to impossible. The continued resorption in type 2 teeth is the basis for crown amputation therapy[28]. The reader is directed to Chapter 5 for a full discussion on TRs.

Key points
- Dental radiographs are critical in treatment planning for TRs.
- Type 1 TRs will typically have an intact root canal system and therefore require *complete extraction.*
- Type 2 TRs have often undergone significant replacement resorption and MAY be treated with crown amputation if resorption is severe enough.
- Restoration is rarely indicated due to the progressive nature of these lesions.

Neoplasia
Definition
Neoplasia is defined as the abnormal growth of cells that is not responsive to normal growth control[29]. Neoplasms can be further classified by their biologic behavior as benign or malignant.

Etiology and pathogenesis
Benign oral soft tissue neoplasms do not invade bone. They do grow, however, and the increasing size will place pressure on the alveolar bone. This expansive pressure will result in osteoclastic resorption on the leading edge of the tumor. In this way, the bone is slowly remodeled to accommodate the enlarging growth[2]. Cystic structures will tend to follow this same pattern of growth, with cystic fluid rather than tumor cells, filling the created void.

Malignant oral neoplasms generally directly invade and replace adjacent bone early in the course of disease[4]. This progresses from a small invasive branch and slowly expands in the area, thus eventually replacing virtually all of the natural bone with tumor cells.

Radiographic features[12,30]
If bone involvement occurs with a benign growth it is expansive, since benign oral soft tissue neoplasms do not invade bone. This pattern of growth will result in the bone 'pulling away' from the advancing tumor leaving a decalcified soft tissue filled space in the tumor site. Bony margins are usually distinct due to the homogeneous periosteal reaction. Finally, this expansive growth will result in tooth movement (**108**).

Cystic structures will appear as a radiolucent area with smooth bony edges. Similar to other benign growths, they grow by expansion and thus displace the other structures (e.g. teeth). Dentigerous cysts are typically seen as a radiolucent structure centered on the crown of an unerupted tooth (**109**).

Malignant oral neoplasms generally invade bone and result in irregular, ragged bone destruction (**110**). Initially, the bone will have a mottled 'moth eaten' appearance, but radiographs late in the disease course will reveal a complete loss of bone in the area. At this time, the teeth will appear to float in space. If the cortex is involved, an irregular periosteal reaction will be seen. In advanced cases, the root apices may develop a spiked appearance.

Differential diagnoses
- Osteomyelitis (bacterial or fungal).
- Periodontal disease.
- Endodontic disease.
- Metabolic bone disease.

Diagnostic tests
Histopathological testing is always necessary for proper diagnosis since a variety of benign or malignant tumors will look similar radiographically. In addition, osteomyelitis can result in similar radiographic findings to malignant tumors. Finally, aggressive tumors will show no bone involvement early in the course of

disease. The prudent practitioner will note the type and extent of bony involvement (if any) on the histopathology request form, and may even include copies of the radiographs and pictures, to aid the pathologist's interpretation of the lesion. Always make sure to get a representative sample for histopathology. All too often a malignancy is misdiagnosed as inflammation due to a sample being taken too superficially.

It is key to interpret the histopathology result in light of the radiographic findings. A diagnosis of a malignancy without bony involvement should be questioned prior to initiating definitive therapy such as aggressive surgery, radiation therapy, or chemotherapy. Conversely, a benign tumor diagnosis with significant bony reaction should be further investigated prior to assuming that the patient is safe.

Additional diagnostic tests in questionable cases include complete blood panel, urinalysis, bacterial and/or fungal culture, as well as fungal serology.

Management

Treat the tumor based on the histopathological diagnosis. For more detailed information on treatment of oral neoplasia, see Chapter 9.

Key points

- Benign tumors do not invade bone but will grow by expansion, creating smooth bony margins and moving other tissues such as bone and teeth.
- Cysts generally appear as distinct, rounded, radiolucent areas with smooth bony edges.
- Malignancies create a 'moth eaten' appearance in the bone.
- Histopathology is necessary to establish neoplasia from non-neoplastic processes, and to determine the type of neoplasia.
- Be sure to obtain a histopathology sample of diagnostic quality.

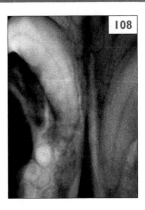

108 Acanthomatous ameloblastoma around the mandibular canine of a dog. Note that the tooth is being moved.

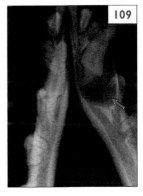

109 Large dentigerous cyst (arrow) from a mandibular canine in a dog.

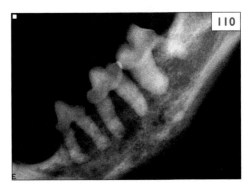

110 Squamous cell carcinoma in the mandible of a cat. There is significant bone loss and a mottled appearance to the mandible, especially the ventral cortex. Note also that the teeth have been moved by the disease.

Pathology in the Pediatric Patient

Brook A. Niemiec

- **Persistent deciduous teeth**
- **Fractured deciduous teeth**
- **Malocclusions (general)**
- **Deciduous malocclusions**
- **Class I malocclusions**
- **Mesioversed maxillary canines (lance effect)**
- **Base narrow canines**
- **Class II malocclusion (overshot, mandibular brachygnathism)**
- **Class III malocclusion (undershot)**
- **Class IV malocclusion (wry bite)**
- **Cleft palate**
- **Cleft lip (harelip)**
- **Tight lip**
- **Hypodontia/oligodontia and anodontia (congenitally missing teeth)**
- **Impacted or embedded (unerupted) teeth**
- **Dentigerous cyst (follicular cyst)**
- **Odontoma**
- **Hairy tongue**
- **Enamel hypocalcification (hypoplasia)**
- **Feline juvenile (puberty) gingivitis/periodontitis**
- **Oral papillomatosis**

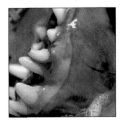
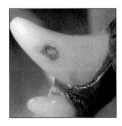
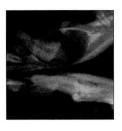
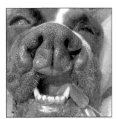

Persistent deciduous teeth

DEFINITION
A deciduous tooth is considered persistent as soon as the permanent tooth erupts into the mouth[1]. The permanent tooth does not need to be fully erupted for the deciduous to be considered persistent.

ETIOLOGY AND PATHOGENESIS
The most common cause for a deciduous tooth to be persistent is an incorrect eruption path of the permanent tooth[1,2]. When the permanent tooth erupts along its natural path, it places pressure on the apex of the deciduous tooth resulting in root end resorption in the deciduous tooth[3,4]. The steady coronal advancement of the permanent tooth will result in continued resorption. This progresses until the deciduous root is sufficiently resorbed, at which point it exfoliates, and the permanent tooth assumes its normal position in the mouth.

When the permanent follows an unnatural path, there will be no impetus for the root of the deciduous tooth to be resorbed. This will result in the deciduous tooth persisting and the permanent tooth erupting alongside. This is contrary to the classic but mistaken belief that a persistent (retained) deciduous tooth *causes* the permanent tooth to erupt in an unnatural position. This malpositioning of the permanent teeth may or may not be genetically dictated. However, due to the pattern of occurrence within breeds and head types, it is currently viewed as of genetic origin[2].

Another possible cause of persistent deciduous dentition is primary impaction or ankylosis of the deciduous tooth[4]. If these conditions occur (which are exceedingly rare), the result will either be impaction of the permanent, or improper eruption creating a persistent deciduous tooth[4].

The lack of a permanent successor as well as nutritional or hormonal imbalances are also potential causes of persistent deciduous teeth[4]. These cases however, will not have a permanent tooth in place.

CLINICAL FEATURES
This is most common in toy and small breed dogs, but can occur in any breed as well as cats[1]. Persistent deciduous dentition is often bilateral,

and the most common teeth affected are the canines (**111**), followed by the incisors, and finally premolars (**112**)[2]. Clinical examination will reveal additional teeth in the arcades, which often appear crowded. In addition, the adult dentition may be deflected into an abnormal position (**113**)[1]. This unnatural position may cause tooth, gingival, or palatine trauma leading

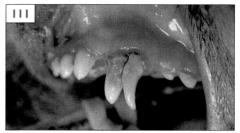

111 Persistent maxillary canine in a dog. Note mesial displacement of permanent tooth.

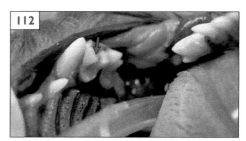

112 Persistent maxillary fourth premolar (arrow) in a dog. Note labial displacement of permanent teeth.

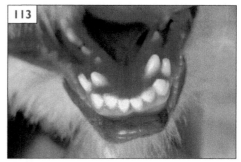

113 Persistent mandibular canines in a dog. Note lingual displacement of permanent teeth.

to damage to these structures (**114**)[1,2]. This may also result in traumatic pulpitis in the permanent dentition[5]. Studies have shown these orthodontic problems can occur within 2 weeks after the first sign of adult dentition eruption[2].

In addition to orthodontic consequences, periodontal problems also occur with persistent deciduous dentition (**115**). This results from the deciduous and permanent teeth sharing the same gingival collar. The abnormal anatomy results in a weakened periodontal attachment and increased susceptibility to future periodontal disease[1,2]. This is even more concerning given the fact that the patients who tend to retain teeth (toy and small breeds) are also prone to significant periodontal disease. Remember, the permanent tooth does not need to be completely erupted for these problems to occur. In fact, problems begin as soon as the permanent tooth starts to erupt.

DIFFERENTIAL DIAGNOSES
- Supernumerary teeth.
- Persistent deciduous without a corresponding permanent.
- Malformed crown (twinning/gemini teeth).

DIAGNOSTIC TESTS
Dental radiographs are critical to diagnosis and therapy. Dental radiographs will help the practitioner to determine:
- Deciduous from permanent dentition.
- Location of the developing permanent tooth/teeth.
- Integrity of the deciduous root structure.

MANAGEMENT
There should never be two teeth of the same type in the same place at the same time[1,2,4]. Therefore, any persistent deciduous teeth should be extracted *as early as possible* to lessen the untoward effects[1,2,4]. *Do not wait* until 6 months of age to perform the extractions along with neutering[5]. The time of permanent dentition eruption (except for molars which have no deciduous counterpart) is between 3 and 6 months[4]. This occurs at approximately the same time of the last booster vaccination. Therefore, it is strongly recommended that an oral evaluation accompanies this visit. In addition, owners should be instructed to examine their pet's mouth on at least a weekly basis to ensure the prompt removal of these teeth[5].

The extraction procedure can be very difficult owing to the considerable length and thin walls of the deciduous tooth (**116**)[2,5]. Additionally, there is often resorption and ankylosis of the retained deciduous tooth.

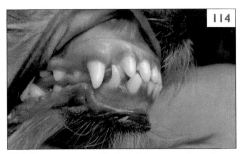

114 Persistent mandibular right canine in a dog. Note lingual displacement of permanent canine and secondary occlusal trauma.

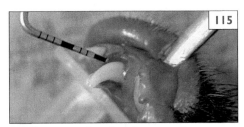

115 Deep periodontal pocket secondary to a persistent mandibular canine in a dog.

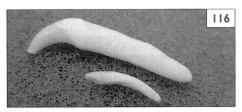

116 An extracted deciduous maxillary canine and incisor. Note that the roots are approximately four times the length of the crown.

Deciduous tooth extraction must be performed carefully and gently with a great amount of patience, to avoid damaging the developing permanent tooth[2,4,5,6]. Some veterinary dentists perform surgical extractions for deciduous canines to decrease the possibility of causing iatrogenic damage[1,6]. However, others (including this author) prefer simple (closed) extractions for the majority of deciduous extraction cases due to decreased surgical time and trauma[2]. Current literature recommends closed extractions in cases with significant root resorption and a surgical approach when the tooth appears intact[1,6].

Root fracture is a common occurrence during extraction attempts. If this occurs, every effort should be made to remove the remaining piece[1,4]. A retained root tip may become infected, or more commonly act as a foreign body and create significant inflammation[4,6]. There are rarely any clinical signs associated with this, but the patient suffers regardless. Complete root tip removal is critical in these cases, as the root tip alone is sufficient to deflect the adult tooth from its normal eruptive path[4]. Retained roots are best extracted utilizing a surgical approach[1,2].

Dental radiographs should be exposed following extraction to confirm complete removal of the deciduous tooth as well as document the continued presence and proper condition of the permanent teeth.

KEY POINTS

- Persistent deciduous dentition is typically due to malpositioning of the permanent dentition and is therefore of genetic origin.
- Persistent deciduous teeth will cause orthodontic as well as periodontal complications very quickly (within days) following eruption of the permanent teeth.
- Extractions should be performed promptly and very carefully.
- Fractured root tips must be extracted (using a surgical approach if necessary).

Fractured deciduous teeth

DEFINITION
Fracture of a deciduous tooth which exposes the pulp chamber.

ETIOLOGY AND PATHOGENESIS
These fractures are almost always traumatic in origin. Typical traumatic incidents include being hit by a ball/bat/car, a fall, or by abnormal chewing behavior. Deciduous teeth are longer and thinner walled than their adult counterparts, and are therefore more prone to fracture[5]. In addition, the relatively large size of the pulp chamber compared to permanent dentition ensures that almost any fracture will result in pulp exposure (especially in felines)[4,6].

CLINICAL FEATURES
Some patients may present with a history of trauma, but fractured teeth are more often found on routine examination. Veterinary patients rarely show any signs of pain due to the stoic nature of these species[7]. However, we do know that these teeth injuries are very painful for the patient[8]. Oral pain in pets with pulp-exposed teeth was substantiated in a veterinary study which demonstrated that pain upon chewing was significantly increased in dogs with pulp exposure *vs.* those without[9].

The most common deciduous teeth to fracture are the canines, but any tooth can be affected[6]. The fractured tooth can be identified as shorter than the contralateral tooth, and the pulp will be evident. If the fracture is fresh, it may be pink and/or bleeding (**117**). In addition, probing the tooth under general anesthesia will confirm pulp exposure and result in hemorrhage.

If the fracture is not recent and the pulp exposure is chronic, the pulp appears dark brown or black (**118**). Pulp infection and abscessation occur relatively quickly in deciduous teeth[5,6], which is most likely due to the large diameter of the pulp chamber. If tooth death and abscessation have occurred, clinical signs may include swelling or a draining tract at or near the root apex (**119**, **120**)[6]. The abscess drains directly onto the crown of the developing permanent tooth, which may result in damage to the permanent tooth, such as enamel hypoplasia[5,6,10,11].

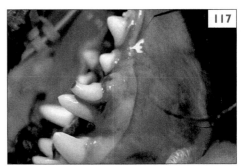

117 Fresh fracture of a deciduous maxillary right canine (504). Note the pink pulp chamber.

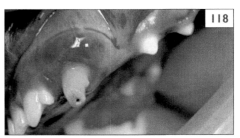

118 Chronic fracture of a deciduous mandibular right canine (804). Note the black pulp chamber.

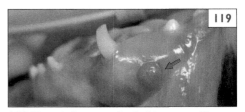

119 Chronic fracture of a deciduous maxillary right canine (504). Note the black pulp chamber and draining abscess (arrow).

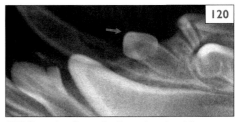

120 Dental radiograph of a patient in with a fractured deciduous mandibular left canine (704). Note the root resorption and abscessation is occurring near the crowns of developing teeth (arrow).

DIFFERENTIAL DIAGNOSES
- Tooth malformation.
- Fractured adult tooth.

DIAGNOSTIC TESTS
Visual examination is diagnostic. Dental radiographs *must* be exposed to confirm that the affected tooth is deciduous, as well as to determine root integrity and proximity of the permanent dentition[1,5].

MANAGEMENT
Regardless of the lack of clinical signs, and the fact that the tooth will exfoliate naturally in the relatively near future, *therapy is mandated.* Extraction of the fractured tooth is the treatment of choice[2,4,6]. This will alleviate the pain and (potential) infection from the exposed dental pulp[4,6]. Extractions of deciduous dentition are challenging, as the roots are longer and thinner than those of permanent dentition[2,5]. On occasion, the roots may be resorbed which makes routine extraction impossible.

Deciduous tooth extractions must be performed carefully and gently with a great amount of patience. This will help avoid fracturing the deciduous root as well damaging the developing permanent tooth[1,2,6]. Some veterinary dentists perform surgical extractions for deciduous canines to decrease the possibility of causing iatrogenic damage[1,6]. However, others (including this author) prefer simple (closed) extractions for the majority of deciduous extraction cases due to decreased surgical time and trauma[2]. Current literature recommends closed extractions in cases with significant root resorption and a surgical approach when the tooth appears intact[1,6].

Root fracture is a common occurrence during extraction attempts. If this occurs, every effort should be made to remove the remaining piece[1,4]. A retained root tip may become infected, or more commonly act as a foreign body and create significant inflammation[4,6]. There are rarely any clinical signs associated with this, but the patient suffers regardless. Retained root pieces are best extracted utilizing a surgical approach[1,2].

Dental radiographs should be exposed following extraction to confirm complete removal of the deciduous tooth as well as document the continued presence and proper condition of the unerupted permanent teeth. If extraction will result in the loss of a valued dental interlock, vital pulp therapy or root canal therapy may be performed[4,6]. An additional benefit of endodontic (*vs.* exodontic) therapy is the avoidance of scar tissue formation (operculum) which could result in an impacted permanent tooth.

KEY POINTS
- Fractured deciduous teeth are very painful and will quickly become necrotic and result in a draining abscess.
- Untreated deciduous fractures may lead to damage of the permanent tooth.
- Expedient treatment (generally extraction) is mandated.
- Extractions must be performed carefully to avoid damaging the developing permanent tooth.

Malocclusions (general)

DEFINITION
This is an occlusion that is not standard for the breed. It may be purely cosmetic or result in occlusal trauma. For descriptions of each class and a more detailed discussion on their respective etiology, clinical signs, and treatment options, see the individually classified malocclusions which are covered on the following pages.

ETIOLOGY AND PATHOGENESIS
There are several different potential etiologies for orthodontic problems, which are broken into two categories, genetic and nongenetic in origin. The most common cause of malocclusions is hereditary[4]. This often results from the line breeding of domestic animals (pets) for a certain size or type of head, or other desired characteristics[2]. In addition, malocclusions can result from the mating of parents with dissimilar jaw sizes causing an imbalance of maxilla and mandible[2]. Stockard explained that malocclusions also result from the degree of expression of the *achrondoplasia* gene within a patient[12]. This gene is carried by most small and toy breed dogs. Additional genetic causes include tongue size, lip and cheek tension (or lack thereof), and presence of a cleft palate[10].

In general, jaw length malocclusions (class II, III, IV) are considered genetic and tooth discrepancies (class I) are considered nongenetic[4,13]. A notable exception to this is mesiocclusion of the maxillary canines (lance effect) seen in Shelties and Persians, which is considered genetic[2,13].

Nongenetic causes of malocclusions include local and systemic influences which may occur before or after birth[4]. Local disturbances include trauma, early or delayed loss of primary teeth, cystic formation, or behavioral issues such as bruxism or abnormal chewing. Systemic disturbances include issues such as severe illness, nutritional disturbances, or endocrine diseases.

CLINICAL FEATURES
These patients often do not show any overt clinical signs other than the jaws or teeth being out of alignment. Depending on the class and severity of the problem, oral trauma may be present and can result in bleeding, oral pain, periodontal disease, traumatic pulpitis, and possibly an ONF[5,14]. A jaw length discrepancy will reveal an incorrect alignment of the mandible and maxilla. Other presentations can have a normal jaw length with a tooth or teeth out of alignment.

DIFFERENTIAL DIAGNOSES
- Normal bite for the breed (i.e. normal class III in a bracheocephalic breed).
- Temporomandibular joint (TMJ) dislocation.
- Mandibular fracture.

DIAGNOSTIC TESTS
Visual examination is diagnostic; however, dental radiographs should be exposed prior to definitive therapy.

MANAGEMENT
Therapy for malocclusions is relative to type and severity of the disease process. Options include[5]:
- No therapy (if purely cosmetic).
- Extraction of the offending tooth or teeth.
- Orthodontic correction using appliances.
- Coronal amputation and vital pulp therapy.

Remember that many orthodontic problems are hereditary and therefore the owner must receive genetic counseling prior to any orthodontic correction procedure[2,4,5]. In addition, strictly cosmetic correction is not in the patient's best interest. The pain associated with orthodontic adjustment, and the numerous anesthetics required, makes orthodontic therapy a disservice to the otherwise healthy patient. The practitioner should obtain a signed consent form for any orthodontic correction case in a non-neutered patient[4].

KEY POINTS
- Many, but not all, malocclusions are genetic in nature.
- Perform genetic counseling for all owners.
- Orthodontic correction is a long and uncomfortable process for the patient, and results are unpredictable.

Deciduous malocclusions

DEFINITION

This is an occlusion that is not standard for the breed during the deciduous dentition[4]. It can be any class of malocclusion, and may be temporary or develop into a permanent problem.

ETIOLOGY AND PATHOGENESIS

Orthodontic problems arise from several different sources. These can be genetic or nongenetic. In general, jaw length discrepancies (class II, III, IV) are considered genetic and tooth discrepancies (class I) (**121**) are considered nongenetic[4,13,15]. The jaw length discrepancies are most commonly seen in the deciduous dentition, whereas tooth alignment issues are usually normal in the deciduous and only present as a malocclusion in the permanent dentition.

In some cases, the patient may be genetically programmed for a normal bite and only temporarily maloccluded. In these cases, the alignment problem is typically mild. These temporary malocclusions occur when the maxilla and mandible grow at varying rates during development due to an independent jaw growth surge[4]. In contrast, severe malocclusions within the deciduous dentition should be considered permanent.

In many cases, the deciduous dentition is trapped by a tooth or the soft tissues on the opposite arcade, which interferes with programmed jaw growth and subsequent self correction[5]. This is called an *adverse dental interlock*[4].

CLINICAL FEATURES

These patients most often come from breeders, as these clients are likely to perform oral examinations on young animals. Oral examination will reveal that the mandible and maxilla do not rest in the correct occlusion. Any orthodontic presentation is possible; however, class II (overshot) (**122**), III (undershot) (**123**), and base narrow (**124**) are the most common presentations (see individual classes for full description of the malocclusions).

Depending on the class of malocclusion (especially class II and base narrow) palatine/gingival/lip/tooth trauma may occur[5]. One major difference between adult and deciduous malocclusions is the anatomy of the teeth involved. The deciduous teeth (especially canines) are much sharper than the corresponding permanent tooth. Therefore, trauma and pain are more intense initially, so are

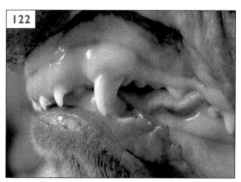

122 Significant deciduous class II malocclusion in a dog. Note the palatine trauma.

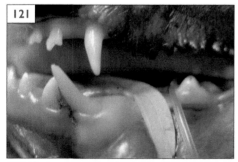

121 Mesiocclused deciduous maxillary right canine (504) in a dog.

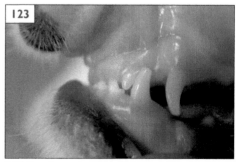

123 Significant deciduous class III malocclusion in a dog.

more likely to be clinically evident early in the course of disease (**125, 126**). This may result in pain or bleeding as the presenting complaint. Patients will commonly show no outward signs

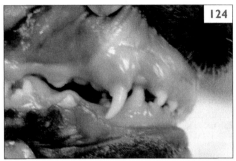

124 Base narrow malocclusion in a dog with secondary palatal trauma.

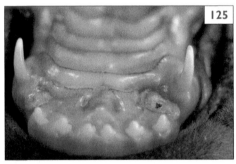

125 Palatine trauma associated with the base narrow malocclusion in **124**. Note the purulent exudate in the defects

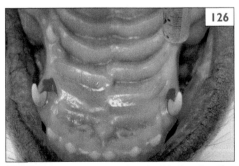

126 Palatine trauma associated with the class II malocclusion in **122**.

of distress. However, occlusal trauma is painful and may cause local infection, regardless of the lack of clinical signs, therefore expedient therapy is mandated[5].

An additional problem that may occur with a deciduous malocclusion which results in an adverse dental interlock, is the hindrance of normal skeletal growth. In cases of deciduous class II malocclusions, this has resulted in downward bowing of the mandible[2,4].

DIFFERENTIAL DIAGNOSES
Normal bite for the breed (i.e. class 0 type III in a bracheocephalic breed)[16].

DIAGNOSTIC TESTS
Visual examination is diagnostic; however, dental radiographs of the surgical area are required prior to extraction[5]. These radiographs are critical to document the presence (or absence), location, and integrity of the permanent dentition. Furthermore, the root structure of the deciduous teeth will be elucidated.

MANAGEMENT
If occlusal trauma is present, extraction of the offending deciduous teeth should be performed as quickly as possible to minimize the trauma and relieve the patient's discomfort[5]. Even if there is no current occlusal trauma, selective extraction of the deciduous teeth should be performed to remove the adverse dental interlock and allow jaw movement. This is termed *interceptive orthodontics*[4,5,13].

Deciduous extractions should be performed as soon as the problem is noted (ideally at 4–8 weeks)[4,5,13]. This will allow the maximum amount of growth as well as relieve pain as expediently as possible[4,5]. Deciding which teeth to extract can be difficult. Obviously, any tooth that is creating trauma should be extracted. When performing pure interceptive orthodontics, the simple rule is to extract the teeth on the jaw that needs to grow. However, recent texts recommend extracting any deciduous tooth that is or *is likely to become* a hindrance to movement, while not extracting teeth that may be creating a *favorable dental interlock*[2,4,5]. Favorable dental interlocks most commonly occur with class III malocclusions where the mandibular canines are close but still distal to the maxillary lateral incisors[4].

Extractions of deciduous dentition are challenging as the roots are proportionally longer and thinner than those of permanent dentition[2,5]. Deciduous tooth extraction must be performed very carefully and gently, with a great amount of patience[1,2].

Another reason to take great care during deciduous extractions is to avoid damaging the developing permanent tooth[2,6]. Some veterinary dentists perform surgical extractions for deciduous canines to decrease the possibility of causing iatrogenic damage[1,6]. However, others (including this author) prefer simple (closed) extractions for the majority of deciduous extraction cases due to decreased surgical time and trauma[2]. Current literature recommends closed extractions in cases with significant root resorption and a surgical approach when the tooth appears intact[1,6].

Root fracture is a common occurrence during extraction attempts. If this occurs, every effort should be made to remove the remaining piece(s)[1]. A retained root tip may become infected, or more commonly act as a foreign body and create significant inflammation[4,6]. There are rarely any clinical signs associated with this, but the patient suffers regardless. Complete root tip removal is even more critical in the case of a malocclusion, as the root tip alone is sufficient to deflect the adult tooth from its normal eruptive path[4]. Retained roots are best extracted utilizing a surgical approach[1,2].

Dental radiographs should be exposed following extraction, to confirm complete removal of the deciduous tooth as well as document the continued presence and proper condition of the unerupted permanent teeth.

KEY POINTS
- If occlusal trauma is occurring, it is painful (regardless of the lack of clinical signs).
- Extractions should be performed as early as possible to alleviate pain and allow for maximum jaw growth.
- Be careful during extraction to avoid damaging the developing adult tooth.
- Dental radiographs pre- and postextraction are critical.

Class I malocclusions

DEFINITION
This is defined as an occlusion with normal jaw lengths (scissors bite), where one or more teeth are out of alignment[2,4,7].

ETIOLOGY AND PATHOGENESIS
Class I malocclusions are typically considered nongenetic[2,4,13]. However, there is a high incidence of some syndromes in certain breeds (e.g. mesiocclusion of the maxillary canines in Shetland sheepdogs) which does indicate a genetic predisposition in some cases[2,13]. Class I malocclusions can result from many causes such as lip/cheek/tongue pressure (or lack thereof), as well as significant systemic or endocrine issues[4]. Finally, neoplastic or cystic formation may also result in tooth deviation[4]. Displacement in some situations was previously believed to result from retention of the deciduous teeth. However, research in the human field shows that deciduous tooth retention is *caused by* improper eruption of the permanent teeth[2].

CLINICAL FEATURES
With a class I malocclusion, the jaws are of the correct length with a scissors bite, but one or more teeth are out of alignment (tipped [**127**] or rotated [**128A, B**])[2]. Most cases of class I malocclusions are cosmetic only and do not cause any deleterious effects to the patient. However, there are instances of pathology occurring secondary to the maloccluded tooth.

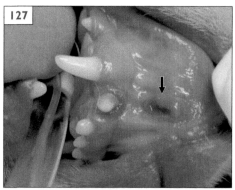

127 Mesiocclused maxillary right third incisor (103). Note trauma to the buccal mucosa (arrow).

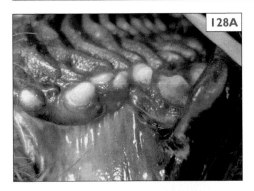

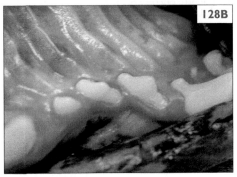

128A, B Rotated maxillary premolars in a dog.

As a result of the malpositioning, teeth may be slightly infraerupted or crowded. Infraeruption will result in a pseudopocket on the affected tooth. The combination of crowding and infraeruption often contributes to the early onset of significant periodontal disease in the area[2]. Oftentimes, periodontal disease may be the only untoward effect caused by the malocclusion. However, if occlusal trauma is present, it can result in severe palatine damage (potentially causing an ONF) or periodontal damage to the opposing tooth[5,14]. An additional problem that may occur secondary to the occlusal trauma is traumatic pulpitis of the opposing tooth[5], which may result in endodontic disease and abscessation[17].

There are two common class I malocclusions (base narrow mandibular canines and mesioccluded maxillary canines) that often have significant traumatic ramifications. These are discussed in detail in their own sections.

DIFFERENTIAL DIAGNOSES
- Any other cause of tooth movement (i.e. trauma, cyst, periodontal disease).

DIAGNOSTIC TESTS
Visual examination is diagnostic. However, dental radiographs should be exposed prior to definitive therapy.

MANAGEMENT
Depending on the presentation, class I malocclusions may be cosmetic only, or may cause periodontal or traumatic disease. In cases of traumatic or periodontal disease, therapy is mandated. In strictly cosmetic cases, treatment is not recommended. There are several options for treatment of maloccluded teeth, which include: orthodontic movement of the tooth, coronal amputation and vital pulp therapy, or extraction(s)[4].

Orthodontic therapy should not be performed in patients destined for a show career, or for cosmetic purposes only. This type of therapy should be reserved for cases of traumatic malocclusions where extraction or coronal amputation is either impractical or declined by the client. Orthodontic therapy involves the use of an appliance, which can be created in-house or by an orthodontic lab[2,4]. There are numerous types of appliances available depending on the case. Orthodontic correction should only be performed by an experienced clinician and with a very committed owner. Methods of correction which are more expedient and reliable include either extraction, or coronal amputation and vital pulp therapy of the offending tooth or teeth[2,4,5].

KEY POINTS
- Class I malocclusions are typically considered nongenetic; however, there are conditions that appear to have a genetic predisposition.
- Secondary crowding and infraeruption can hasten the onset of periodontal disease.
- Class I malocclusions may create orthodontic problems and secondary lip/tooth/gingiva trauma.
- Orthodontic therapy for this condition may be effective, but is complicated and extensive.

Mesioversed maxillary canines (lance effect)

DEFINITION
Mesioversion of the maxillary canines is a malocclusion that occurs in a patient with normal jaw lengths, where one or both of the maxillary canines are tipped in the mesial direction[2,4].

ETIOLOGY AND PATHOGENESIS
This is classified as a class I malocclusion[18], which is typically considered nongenetic[13,15]. However, the high incidence in certain breeds (Shetland sheepdogs and Persian cats) indicates a genetic predisposition in these breeds[2,13]. Mesioversed maxillary canines can result from many causes such as lip/cheek/tongue pressure (or lack thereof) as well as significant systemic or endocrine issues[4]. In rare cases, it may also result from excessive tugging on a toy early in life[13]. This occurs only in extreme cases, however, and should be seen in conjunction with incisor mesioversion[13]. Finally, neoplastic or cystic formation may result in tooth deviation[4].

This mesioversion was previously believed to result from retention of the deciduous maxillary canines. Since the permanent maxillary canines erupt mesial to the deciduous teeth, this made sense and in rare cases may be true. However, research in the human field shows that deciduous tooth retention is *caused by* improper eruption of the permanent teeth[2]. Consequently, the lance effect condition may be due to many causes, but heredity is the most likely[2,5,13].

CLINICAL FEATURES
Shetland sheepdogs and Persian cats are strongly overrepresented, followed by Scottish terriers and Italian greyhounds[2]. Lance effect is generally diagnosed at about 6 months of age (often during anesthesia for neutering). The patient's jaws are of the correct length with a scissors bite, but the maxillary canines are mesioversed (**129**). One or both maxillary canines may be out of alignment. Due to the malpositioning, these canines are often slightly infraerupted. This infraeruption will result in a pseudopocket on the maxillary canine, which may hasten the development of periodontal disease on that tooth. In extreme cases, the maxillary canine will come into contact with the maxillary lateral incisor. The combination of crowding and infraeruption often results in the early onset of significant periodontal disease in the area (**130, 131**)[2]. This mesioversion also often results in the mandibular canines being deflected labially (**132**). The labiocclusion may

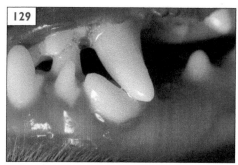

129 Mesiocclusion of the maxillary left canine in a dog. (Courtesy of Dr. Brett Beckman.)

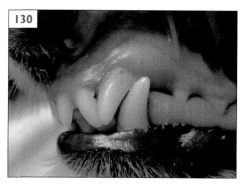

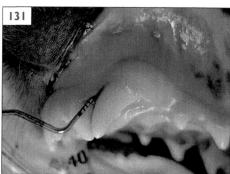

130, 131 Significant periodontal inflammation secondary to the crowding caused by the mesiocclused maxillary canine in a dog.

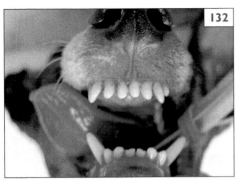

132 Labioversed mandibular canines in a dog with bilateral mesioocclused maxillary canines.

cause the upper lip to catch on these teeth, creating lip ulcers and oral pain[2].

DIFFERENTIAL DIAGNOSES
- Any other cause of tooth movement (i.e. trauma, cyst, periodontal disease).

DIAGNOSTIC TESTS
Visual examination is diagnostic; however, dental radiographs should be exposed prior to definitive therapy.

MANAGEMENT
There are several options for treatment of mesioversed maxillary canines. These include: orthodontic movement of the tooth, coronal amputation and vital pulp therapy, or extraction(s)[4].

Orthodontic therapy typically involves the use of orthodontic buttons and elastics[2,4]. The buttons are attached to the maxillary canine, and the distal attachment is generally a combination of the maxillary fourth premolar and first molar. Healthy root structure of these two teeth is required to provide sufficient anchorage[4] to allow movement of the large maxillary canine without displacing the anchor tooth/teeth. Other maxillary teeth as well as the mandibular molar can also be used in various combinations for anchorage. Orthodontic movement is a long-term therapy which can be very difficult, especially if the patient is orally inclined as this may result in lost buttons. Another possible complication is the interlock of the maloccluded mandibular canines, which blocks the distal path of the maxillary canine. In these cases, the patient must wear an uncomfortable bite block device until the tooth is cleared. This orthodontic correction should only be performed by an experienced clinician and with a very committed owner.

A much more expedient and reliable method of correction is either extraction or coronal amputation and vital pulp therapy of the offending tooth or teeth[2,5]. If the mandibular canine is not affected, extraction of the lateral incisor and homecare may prove curative for the crowding and secondary periodontal disease. If the mandibular canine is affected, extraction of the maxillary canine and orthodontic movement of the mandibular canines with elastic ligatures is often performed[4].

KEY POINTS
- This is considered a genetic trait in Shelties and Persians.
- The secondary crowding and infraeruption causes periodontal disease for the maxillary canine +/− lateral incisor.
- The lance effect condition may create orthodontic problems in the mandibular canines and secondary lip trauma.
- Orthodontic therapy for this condition is effective; however, it is complicated and extensive.

Base narrow canines

DEFINITION
This is a class I malocclusion. In class I malocclusions, the patient has a normal maxillary/mandibular relationship; however, a tooth (or teeth) is out of alignment[4,18]. In this case, the mandibular canines are linguoversed resulting in palatine trauma.

ETIOLOGY AND PATHOGENESIS
This is classified as a class I malocclusion, and thus is classically considered nongenetic[13,15,19]. However, due to the increased incidence in some breeds (especially doliocephalic breeds), the base narrow condition is often considered hereditary[2].

This condition was previously believed to occur secondary to retained deciduous mandibular canines deviating the permanent canines lingually[13]. However, research in the human field shows that the deciduous teeth are actually retained *due to* an improper eruption pathway of the permanent teeth[2]. Another possible etiology is trauma (early in life) causing the tooth bud to be misaligned. A less common cause may be a cystic structure which has developed early in the patient's development[4]. Finally, it has been reported that a malpositioned mandibular first premolar or lateral incisor can interfere with the normal eruption path[20].

CLINICAL FEATURES
Standard poodles and all doliocephalic breeds anecdotally appear to be overrepresented, although no published papers exist at this time. Patients with this condition generally do not show any clinical signs; however, oral pain and bleeding may be noted. The jaws are the correct length and in a scissors bite except for the canines being linguoversed (**133**). One or both mandibular canines will be out of alignment and causing palatine trauma. This problem is generally noted at about 6 months of age, but it was likely present in the deciduous dentition as well. Regardless of the lack of clinical signs with base narrow canines, these patients are uncomfortable[5]. Depending on the severity of misalignment, the malocclusion can result in severe palatine damage (on occasion causing an ONF [**134**]) or periodontal damage to the maxillary canine[5,13,14].

An additional problem that may occur secondary to the occlusal trauma is traumatic pulpitis of the mandibular canine[5], which may result in endodontic disease and abscessation[17].

DIFFERENTIAL DIAGNOSES
- Any other cause of tooth movement (i.e. trauma, cyst, periodontal disease).
- Class II malocclusion.

DIAGNOSTIC TESTS
Visual examination is diagnostic; however, dental radiographs should be exposed prior to therapy.

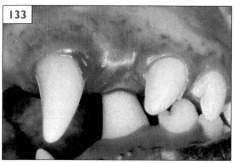

133 Base narrow occlusion of the mandibular right canine resulting in palatine trauma.

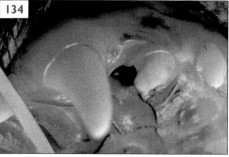

134 Oronasal fistula secondary to a base narrow occlusion.

MANAGEMENT

There are numerous options for treatment of base narrow canines. These can be separated into two distinct categories: orthodontic movement of the tooth or removal of the source of trauma.

If the malocclusion is minor and diagnosed early, a wedge of the maxillary gingiva can be removed to guide the tooth into the correct position[4]. In addition, composite crown extensions can be added to the canines to encourage buccal movement. Ball therapy has been used with success by some dentists, which is inexpensive and noninvasive[21]. Finally, surgical movement of the tooth has proven successful in some cases[22].

Orthodontic therapy has an excellent success rate for this condition. The most common means of achieving the desired movement is via an incline plane[2]. This can be formed in the patient's mouth with dental acrylics or by an orthodontic lab using stone models which are created by the veterinarian (**135**)[4]. If the owner desires a one step therapy, removal of the source of trauma can be achieved in several different ways. It is best achieved via coronal amputation and vital pulp therapy[4]. When performed skillfully, this procedure has an excellent success rate but the client must be made aware of the need for follow-up radiographs[4,23]. Alternatively, the tooth may be extracted, but due to the size of the tooth and the importance of the mandibular canines in tongue retention and esthetics, this is generally not the treatment of choice[2].

KEY POINTS

- Patients will often show no clinical signs, but they are in pain.
- Base narrow canines can cause severe periodontal disease or ONF.
- This is a very treatable problem.
- Many treatment options exist depending on age of patient, presentation, and owner's goals.

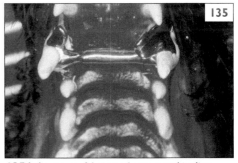

135 Laboratory fabricated cast metal incline plane for a base narrow condition in a dog.

Class II malocclusion (overshot, mandibular brachygnathism)

DEFINITION
A class II malocclusion in the EH Angle classification system is defined as the lower molar positioned distal to the upper molar[18]. This is a jaw length discrepancy where the mandible is shorter than the maxilla, with the mandibular premolars distal to the maxillary[7,19].

ETIOLOGY AND PATHOGENESIS
Class II malocclusions are considered a primarily genetic condition[15]. Class II malocclusions occur due to a discrepancy of the dentofacial proportions[4]. This discrepancy of proportions often results from line breeding for a specific size and shape of the head. Other factors which contribute to malocclusion incidence include: the great variety in the size and structure of canine maxilla and mandible as well as the variation of tooth size between breeds, in combination with cross breeding[2,12]. Further evaluation of these findings support that the malocclusions likely occur secondary to the degree in which achondroplasia is expressed within the patient[19].

Early trauma with bone scarring or physeal closure may also result in this condition; however, this should be historically supported[19]. Furthermore, trauma is generally unilateral and should result in a class IV (as opposed to class II) malocclusion. Trauma or other conditions which result in muscle or soft tissue contracture/scarring, laxity, or loss, can disrupt the orthodontic equilibrium and result in a malocclusion[19]. Other nongenetic causes, such as severe infection or nutritional diseases, should affect both jaws equally[4].

CLINICAL FEATURES
The typical presenting complaint is that the mandible is shorter than the maxilla and the mandibular canines are striking the palate (**136**). In general, this will occur medial to the maxillary canines, but in severe cases the mandibular canines can rest distal to the maxillary. The mandibular incisors will be slightly to significantly behind the maxillary, and there may be a loss of normal premolar interdigitation. Rhodesian ridgebacks and Labrador retrievers appear overrepresented. Class II malocclusions are generally present in the deciduous dentition and,

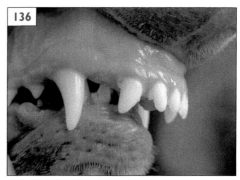

136 Class II malocclusion in a dog.

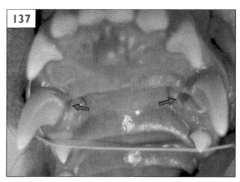

137 Palatine trauma (arrows) secondary to the class II malocclusion in 136.

if diagnosed early, the deciduous mandibular canines should be extracted at this time (see deciduous malocclusions, page 97).

The permanent teeth will begin to impact the palate at approximately 6 months of age. Depending on the severity of the misalignment, a class II malocclusion can result in severe palatine damage (on occasion causing an ONF) or periodontal damage to the maxillary canine (**137**)[5,14]. An additional problem that may occur secondary to the occlusal trauma is traumatic pulpitis of the mandibular canine[5], which may result in endodontic disease and abscessation[17].

DIFFERENTIAL DIAGNOSES
- TMJ dislocation.
- Bilateral mandibular fracture.

DIAGNOSTIC TESTS
Visual examination is diagnostic; however, dental radiographs should be exposed prior to therapy.

MANAGEMENT

There are three options for treatment of a class II malocclusion[4]. The most common form of therapy is coronal amputation and vital pulp therapy of one or both of the mandibular canines (**138**). This is due to the fact that it is less traumatic and disfiguring than extractions[5]. When performed skillfully, this procedure carries an excellent success rate[23]. The tooth is aseptically prepared and amputated with a dental bur. This procedure exposes the dental pulp and therefore protection is required, which is performed via vital pulp therapy. A restoration alone, or no therapy, is not sufficient. The client must be made aware of the need for radiographic follow-up[24].

A second option for therapy if the malocclusion is mild, is orthodontic therapy. The typical appliance created in these cases is an incline plane device[4,5]. The prognosis for success is typically reduced when compared to base narrow canines, and the appliance design and creation is often more technical.

The final method of correction involves extraction of the tooth or teeth causing occlusal trauma. If the involved teeth are incisors, this is the preferred therapy. However, due to the size of the mandibular canine teeth as well as their importance in tongue retention and esthetics, this is generally not the treatment of choice with these teeth[2,5]. Finally, the maxillary canine may be extracted and buccal cortical bone removed to allow the mandibular canines to move labially into the space previously occupied by the maxillary canines[5]. The biggest concern with this therapy is dehiscence of the extraction site due to trauma from the mandibular canines.

KEY POINTS

- Patients with class II malocclusions often show no clinical signs, but they are in pain.
- Class II malocclusions can hasten the onset of periodontal disease or create ONF.
- This is a very treatable problem.
- Coronal amputation and vital pulp therapy is generally the treatment of choice.

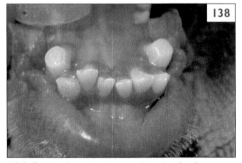

138 Coronal amputation and vital pulp therapy performed on the patient in **136**.

Class III malocclusion (undershot)

DEFINITION
A class III malocclusion is a jaw length discrepancy where the mandible is longer than the maxilla in a nonbracheocephalic breed[2,4].

ETIOLOGY AND PATHOGENESIS
Because this is a jaw length discrepancy, it is considered a genetic condition[2,4,13]. In fact, this malocclusion is particularly genetic in nature in human beings[25], and is due to a discrepancy of the dentofacial proportions[4]. This discrepancy in animals is often caused by line breeding for a specific size and shape of the head. The great variety in the size and structure of canine maxilla and mandible as well as tooth size between breeds, in combination with cross breeding have also resulted in malocclusions[2,12]. Further evaluation of these findings supports the theory that malocclusions likely occur secondary to the degree in which achondroplasia is expressed within the patient[19].

Early trauma with bone scarring or physeal closure may also result in this condition; however, this should be historically supported[19]. In addition, trauma is generally unilateral and should result in a class IV as opposed to class II malocclusion. Trauma or other conditions which result in muscle or other soft tissue contracture/scarring, laxity, or loss could disrupt the orthodontic equilibrium and result in a malocclusion[19]. Other nongenetic causes, such as severe infection or nutritional diseases, should affect both jaws equally.

CLINICAL FEATURES
In most instances, this malocclusion is present in the deciduous dentition and occasionally interceptive orthodontics may have been attempted (see deciduous malocclusions). The patient will present with the mandibular incisors and possibly canines rostral to the maxillary incisors (**139**). In addition, the maxillary and mandibular premolars may be incorrectly aligned. This may cause tooth-to-tooth trauma resulting in attrition (wear). The degree of displacement can range from very mild to severe. Very mild cases will result in the incisors meeting edge to edge which is termed a *level bite* (**140**). This is an accepted occlusion

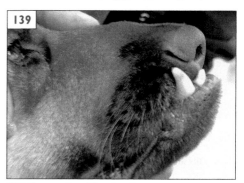

139 Severe class III malocclusion.

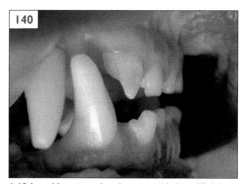

140 Level bite in a dog (a *very* mild class III). Note that the maxillary incisors occlude on the mandibular.

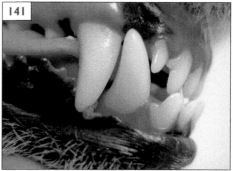

141 Reverse scissors bite in a dog (a mild class III).

standard; however, it is a destructive bite resulting in significant wear of the incisor teeth[13]. When the mandibular incisors are just in front of the maxillary it is termed a *reverse scissors bite* (**141**).

In most cases, there is no significant trauma associated with the class III (undershot) malocclusion, and the problem is strictly cosmetic. When traumatic problems are seen with this malocclusion, they present as soft tissue trauma to the mandibular gingiva from the maxillary incisors[5]. This often occurs distal to the teeth and causes transient pain. Over time, the body does appear to create a form of 'callus' in the area. On occasion, however, contact may occur in the gingival sulcus and create periodontal inflammation and disease. In these cases, therapy is mandated.

The most common reason for presentation results from the tooth-to-tooth contacts of the maxillary lateral incisors and mandibular canines[5]. Depending on the severity of the discrepancy, this can result in significant attrition to the mandibular canines, and may contribute to fracture of the tooth. An additional problem that may occur secondary to the occlusal trauma is traumatic pulpitis of the mandibular canine[5], which may result in endodontic disease and abscessation[17]. Finally, in some cases (especially felines) this malocclusion may result in upper lip ulcers[2].

DIFFERENTIAL DIAGNOSES
* Normal bite for the breed (brachycephalic breeds, i.e. pugs and bulldogs).
* TMJ dislocation.

DIAGNOSTIC TESTS
Visual examination is diagnostic; however, dental radiographs should be exposed prior to therapy.

MANAGEMENT
Many cases require no therapy as there is minimal to no trauma present and no discomfort for the patient. If lip, tooth, or gingival trauma is present, then vital pulp therapy, extraction, or rarely orthodontic movement of the offending tooth or teeth, should prove curative[2,4,5,13]. If the client wants to pursue cosmetic correction of the teeth, orthodontic correction may be possible depending on the severity of the discrepancy. A maxillary expander or arch bar can be created to move the maxillary incisors rostrally, or a mandibular arch bar or elastics can be used to move the mandibular incisors distally[4]. Remember to perform genetic counseling and obtain a signed consent form prior to any orthodontic correction.

KEY POINTS
* Apparent class III malocclusions may be normal for the breed.
* Class III malocclusions are generally a cosmetic issue only; however, lip catching, periodontal trauma, or tooth attrition may occasionally result as well.
* Coronal amputation and vital pulp therapy or extraction of the offending tooth should cure the occlusal trauma.
* Orthodontic intervention can correct mild cases.

Class IV malocclusion (wry bite)

DEFINITION
A class IV malocclusion is a jaw length discrepancy in which one of the mandibles is shorter than the other resulting in a shift of the mandibular midline. A true class IV malocclusion occurs when one mandible is longer than the maxilla and the other is shorter than the maxilla[4]. The remainder of wry bites are subsets of class II or III[4].

ETIOLOGY AND PATHOGENESIS
Class IV malocclusions are jaw length discrepancies and therefore should be considered primarily a genetic condition[15]. These are generally due to a discrepancy of the dentofacial proportions[2,4]. Early trauma with bone scarring or physeal closure is also reported to be a common cause of this form of malocclusion[2]. However, this should be historically supported[19]. Trauma or other conditions which result in muscle or other soft tissue contracture/scarring, laxity, or loss could disrupt the orthodontic equilibrium and result in a malocclusion[19]. Other nongenetic causes such as severe infection or nutritional diseases should affect both jaws (mandible and maxilla) equally.

CLINICAL FEATURES
Unless the client is a breeder/shower, the client will generally not discover the problem. It is most commonly diagnosed during a routine physical examination or under anesthesia for altering. The patient is usually outwardly normal and will eat and play normally. Occasionally anorexia or oral hemorrhage may be the presenting complaint. Oral examination will reveal that the mandible is out of alignment with the maxilla. The midline of the maxilla will not be even with the midline of the mandible (**142**). The uneven occlusion will result in one or both of the mandibular canines striking the soft tissue of the maxillary palate, gingiva, or lip (**143, 144**). This can lead to severe pain and infection, as well as periodontal disease, oronasal fistulas, and traumatic pulpitis depending on the location of the trauma[5,14]. The traumatic pulpitis may result in endodontic disease and abscessation[17]. Wry bite is often seen in combination with a class II malocclusion, with the mandibular canine on the shorter side situated distal to the maxillary canine.

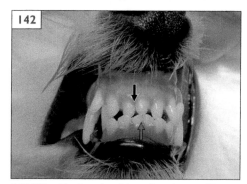

142 Wry bite in a dog. Note that the maxillary midline (black arrow) does not line up with the mandibular (red arrow).

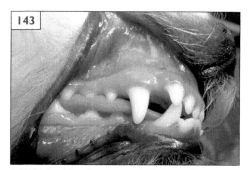

143 Right side of patient in **142**. Note the occlusal trauma.

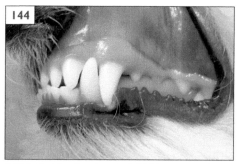

144 Left side of patient in **142**. Note normal canine interdigitation.

DIFFERENTIAL DIAGNOSES
- TMJ dislocation.
- Mandibular fracture.
- Class II or III malocclusion.

DIAGNOSTIC TESTS
Physical examination is diagnostic; however, dental radiographs should be exposed prior to therapy. If there is any doubt about the mandibular or TMJ integrity, radiographs or a CT scan/MRI should be considered.

MANAGEMENT
If there is no palatine, lip, or gingival trauma, this is strictly a cosmetic problem and therapy is not necessary[4]. Orthodontic correction can be considered following genetic counseling[4]. When occlusal trauma does exist (which is typical), there are three options for therapy[4]. The most common form of therapy is coronal amputation and vital pulp therapy of one or both of the mandibular canines[5]. When performed skillfully, this procedure carries an excellent success rate[23]. The tooth is aseptically prepared and amputated with a dental bur. This procedure exposes the dental pulp and therefore protection is required, which is performed via vital pulp therapy.

A restoration alone, or no therapy, is not sufficient. The client must be cognizant of the need for radiographic follow-up[24].

A second option for therapy if the malocclusion is mild is orthodontic therapy. The typical appliance created in these cases is an incline plane device[4,5]. In mild cases, it can be successful; however, in human dentistry, skeletal midline discrepancies are not considered treatable by orthodontics[19]. The prognosis for success is typically reduced when compared to base narrow canines, and the appliance design and creation is often more technical.

The final method of correction involves extraction of the tooth or teeth causing occlusal trauma. Due to the size of the tooth as well as the importance of the mandibular canines in tongue retention and esthetics, this is generally not the treatment of choice[2,5].

KEY POINTS
- Wry bite is typically a genetic problem.
- Rule out TMJ dislocation with history, physical examination, +/− radiographs.
- Coronal amputation and vital pulp therapy is the treatment of choice in most cases.

Cleft palate

DEFINITION
This is a midline defect of the maxillary bone (or secondary palate) which is congenital in nature. These clefts create a communication between the oral and nasal cavities.

ETIOLOGY AND PATHOGENESIS
Cleft palates are generally a congenital problem, although other palatine defects can occur secondary to trauma, neoplasia, or burns[4]. Congenital defects are seen in a wide variety of breeds in both dogs and cats and are typically sporadic[2]. Therefore, the majority of cleft palates are considered to be secondary to an intrauterine problem; however, breeding studies have shown a genetic link in some breeds[2]. In contrast, the majority of human cleft palates are considered to be hereditary. Some cases are easily traced genetically and some with more variability[10]. Cleft palates result from the failure of fusion of the palatal shelves[10]. This lack of fusion will create an epithelial lined communication between the oral and nasal cavity.

CLINICAL FEATURES
Congenital cases are typically diagnosed in very young puppies or kittens. These patients are generally unthrifty and underweight, as suckling is difficult due to the inability to create a vacuum[2,5]. Clefts are not externally evident, and patients are usually presented very early for sneezing and/or nasal discharge[2,5]. On occasion,

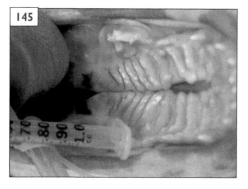

145 Midline cleft hard and soft palate in a dog. Note that the entire palate is affected.

a patient may be presented for respiratory problems such as aspiration pneumonia, which is a common sequela[2,5].

Oral examination will reveal a defect in the palate which communicates into the nasal cavity. Hard palate defects are almost invariably on midline and are generally associated with a midline soft palate defect (**145**)[2,5]. When the soft palate alone is affected, it may be on the midline or unilateral[5]. Unilateral hard palate defects have been rarely reported[5]. In most cases, there is no inflammation to the tissues and the defect appears regular. Congenital hard palate defects can also be associated with a cleft lip.

DIFFERENTIAL DIAGNOSES
- Trauma/burn.
- Neoplasia.

DIAGNOSTIC TESTS
Clinical appearance is generally classic. If there is any concern of an alternate cause of this condition, histopathology should be considered prior to surgical correction. Dental radiographs should be exposed to determine the extent of bony support.

MANAGEMENT
These cases can be exceedingly difficult and intensive to manage. The first challenge is to support the patient until it reaches sufficient size to undergo surgical correction[2,4]. This occurs at approximately 6–8 weeks of age, depending on the breed of the patient and the nursing skill of the owner[5]. Until this time, the patient must be carefully tube fed on a regular basis[4]. Tube feeding carries its own dangers, including regurgitation and aspiration pneumonia, or instant death if the tube is placed inadvertently into the airway. However, if the defect is not excessive and the owner is committed, surgical correction may provide an excellent long-term prognosis[5]. If the owner is willing, a multidisciplinary approach including an internist, a veterinary dentist, and potentially a nutritionist or anesthesiologist should be considered[10].

Although proper surgical correction has a high rate of success, the procedure is quite challenging due to many factors. These factors include the tension placed on the incision line during breathing and eating, tongue induced trauma to the sutures, and lack of pliability of the palate[4,5]. The major prognostic factor is not the length of the cleft, but rather the width. The wider the cleft, the more guarded the prognosis.

Many flap techniques have been devised for the correction of these clefts. The practitioner is encouraged to study and practice these techniques prior to attempting them on an actual patient. The major surgical goals include[2]:
- Cure the problem with the first surgery[5]! Each successive surgery becomes more difficult as scar tissue adds to the lack of pliability. Therefore, consider more aggressive surgical approaches in the initial surgery.
- Create closure without tension. This is critical, and can be aided by making large flaps (**146**).
- Ideally, the suture line is placed over bone rather than directly over the void, in order to avoid the trampoline effect.
- Use gentle tissue handling techniques to avoid damaging the fragile palatine vessels and tissues.
- All edges must be debrided, as intact epithelium will not heal to any other surface.
- Maintain the blood supply to the flap by preserving the palatine artery. (This runs parallel to the arcade approximately 0.5–1 cm medial to the teeth. (See **24, 25**)

Following creation of the flap(s), they are carefully raised and moved/rotated, to cover the defect and then sutured in place (ideally in two layers). If there is healthy maxillary/incisive bone, the donor site may be left uncovered to heal by secondary intention. A percutaneous endoscopic gastrostomy (PEG) or esophageal feeding tube (+/− a loose muzzle) should be considered in cases of large defects, to decrease the postoperative stress on the area.

KEY POINTS
- Cleft palates are a common cause of fading puppy/kitten syndrome, especially if presented with concurrent respiratory problems.
- These patients are very difficult to manage, requiring tremendous effort by the owner.
- Cleft palates are easier to correct in larger, more mature patients. Tube feeding should be instituted if possible, to delay surgery until 6–8 weeks of age.

- Surgical correction carries an excellent prognosis if the defect is not excessive (**147**).
- Make every effort to cure the problem with the first surgical procedure, as subsequent surgeries will be more difficult due to scar tissue formation.

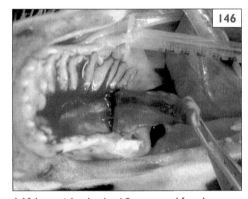

146 Large island palatal flap created for closure.

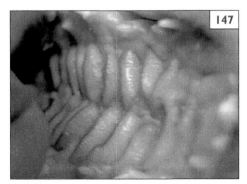

147 Three week re-check of patient in **145**. Note complete healing of palatal tissues.

Cleft lip (harelip)

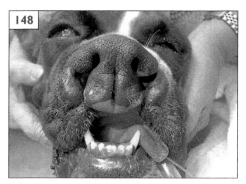

148 Bilateral cleft lip in a dog. (Courtesy of Dr. Mike Peak.)

DEFINITION
This congenital condition is caused by a failure of the primary palate to fuse, resulting in a fissure in the rostral lip[2,4,10].

ETIOLOGY AND PATHOGENESIS
While this lesion is congenital, it is not necessarily genetic. It has been reported in the veterinary literature to be secondary to intrauterine stress or trauma, rather than a genetic cause[2]. However, breeding studies, as well as reports from the human literature, suggest a familial tendency as offspring have been born to affected parents[2,10]. Cleft lip results from the two sides of the primary palate (incisive bone) failing to fuse normally[2]. This creates a defect which is off midline and can be unilateral or bilateral[5].

CLINICAL FEATURES
Cleft lip is a very rare problem and is easily identified in very young patients. It is externally obvious as a cleft or fissure in the rostral lip (**148**). Cleft lips can be bilateral, but they are most often unilateral, and if so it is virtually always left-sided[2]. There is generally no inflammation of the tissues and the defect appears regular.

Cleft lip lesions may exist alone or in combination with a cleft (secondary) palate and/or cleft soft palate[10]. When seen alone, this is a cosmetic problem only.

DIFFERENTIAL DIAGNOSES
• Trauma/burn.
• Neoplasia.

DIAGNOSTIC TESTS
No specific tests are required as clinical appearance is classic. If there is any concern of an alternate cause of this problem, histopathology should be considered.

MANAGEMENT
If the cleft lip is not associated with a cleft palate, it is a cosmetic problem only[5]. There are generally no deleterious effects. If the client wishes to have the problem corrected, properly performed surgery will result in a reasonable cosmetic appearance[2]. This surgery should be delayed to allow for patient growth and thus larger amounts of available tissue for surgical correction, as well as reduced anesthetic risk[5]. Surgical descriptions can be found in various dental texts.

KEY POINTS
• Cleft lip may present as a single lesion or in combination with cleft palate.
• Cleft lip as a single lesion is a cosmetic problem only.
• Surgical correction is curative, and can be done to improve cosmetic appearance.

Tight lip

DEFINITION
This is a condition where the rostral mandibular lip is very tight. This leads to a shrinking of the mandibular vestibule and often results in the lip being pulled over the mandibular incisors[2,4].

ETIOLOGY AND PATHOGENESIS
This is a genetic trait and is very common in the Shar-Pei breed[4,13].

CLINICAL FEATURES
The mandibular lip in the incisal area is pulled back towards the incisors. In many cases, the lip is pulled over the mandibular incisors and occasionally canines (149)[2,4]. In these cases, the lip is often significantly traumatized and will result in difficulty masticating[2]. Tight lip also commonly results in disto-occlusion of the mandibular incisors[2,13]. In severe cases, the lip may restrict mandibular growth and result in a brachygnathic (class II) bite[4].

DIFFERENTIAL DIAGNOSES
- Trauma or burns (may cause scarring of the buccal mucosa).
- Orthodontic disease (may mimic this disease in some cases).

DIAGNOSTIC TESTS
Visual examination is diagnostic.

MANAGEMENT
Surgical correction (*vestibuloplasty*) is the treatment of choice[2,4]. This will release the tension on the jaw and teeth as well as normalize the rostral mandibular vestibule. Surgery is initiated by incising the gingiva just apical to the attached gingiva of the mandibular incisors and canines. This incision should be made from frenulum to frenulum, exposing the entire rostral mandible including the canines. Following this, the soft tissue and muscular attachments of the rostral mandibular lip are dissected, leaving the lip hanging down into the natural position. The flap is then left to heal by secondary intention, thus re-establishing normal lip position. Depending on the surgeon, different options may be chosen as follows: the area may be left without sutures[13], it may be sutured down lower leaving the area bare[2], or a spacer may be placed in the defect[4].

KEY POINTS
- Tight lip can cause significant oral trauma and malocclusions.
- Early and aggressive surgical correction will allow for the best long-term outcome.
- This can be a very difficult problem to treat.

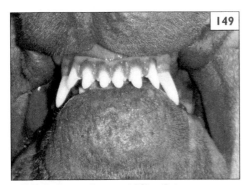

149 Tight lip in a 2-year-old Shar-Pei.

Hypodontia/oligodontia and anodontia (congenitally missing teeth)

DEFINITION[2,10,13]

Hypodontia is a condition where a few (one to five) permanent teeth are congenitally absent. Oligodontia is the lack of many (six or more) permanent teeth.

Anodontia is defined as the congenital complete lack of all permanent teeth.

ETIOLOGY AND PATHOGENESIS

This is typically a genetic condition which causes a defect in the development of teeth[10,13]. However, developing teeth are very susceptible to environmental forces (such as trauma, intrauterine disturbances, and medications). Thus developmental disturbances can result in a lack of a tooth or teeth in the permanent dentition[2].

The permanent tooth develops from a bud of the deciduous tooth (except for molars and first premolars which have no deciduous counterpart)[26]. Consequently, with a truly missing deciduous tooth, there will likewise be no permanent[2]. Keep in mind however, that the deciduous tooth may have been prematurely lost. Hypodontia of the deciduous teeth is exceedingly rare, but it is seen quite often in permanent dentition[10].

CLINICAL FEATURES

Patients lack one or more permanent teeth. Anodontia is extremely rare in veterinary medicine; however, hypodontia is very common in small breeds (especially bracheocephalic and Chinese crested/ Mexican hairless)[2,4,13]. The teeth most likely to be absent in these breeds are the premolars (especially first and second), incisors, and mandibular third molars[13]. Hypodontia may also be seen in the premolars of large breeds (especially Doberman Pinchers) in which case it is considered a serious fault[2,4]. It is very rare to see missing canine or carnassial teeth[2]. The most common presentation is an area of the arcade where one or more teeth are absent (**150**). It is not uncommon, however, to have a persistent deciduous tooth in the area due to the lack of the normal pressure from the erupting permanent tooth (**151**)[10].

DIFFERENTIAL DIAGNOSES
- Fractured tooth with retained roots.
- Previously exfoliated or extracted tooth.
- Embedded/impacted tooth.

DIAGNOSTIC TESTS

Dental radiographs are required to confirm that the teeth are truly absent (**152, 153**), either due to a congenital defect or previous exfoliation/extraction[4,5,13]. It is critical to rule out impacted teeth, as *dentigerous cysts* may develop around unerupted teeth (see page 118)[4,10]. In addition, fractured and retained roots should likewise be ruled out as these can result in endodontic disease (**154, 155**).

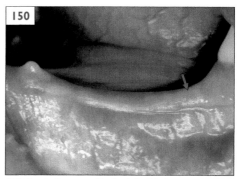

150 A missing mandibular left third premolar (307) (arrow) in a 10-month-old dog.

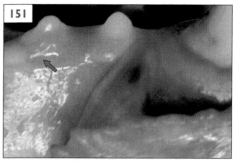

151 A persistent mandibular right second premolar (806) (arrow) in a 10-month-old dog.

MANAGEMENT

No specific therapy is necessary. Implants can be performed to improve masticatory function (carnassials), improve other oral functions (canines), or for esthetic reasons (incisors or canines)[10]. Implants should NOT be performed in patients destined for a show career.

KEY POINTS

- No specific therapy is necessary in most cases as this does not impair the patient.
- Dental radiographs must be exposed on all 'missing' teeth to rule out dentigerous cysts and retained roots.

- Implants can be used to improve function and/or esthetics.
- These conditions typically have a genetic cause and therefore implants should not be considered in patients that will be shown or bred.

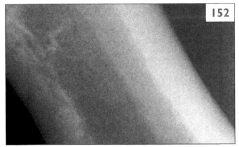

152 Intraoral dental radiograph of the patient in 150. Note the absence of a permanent tooth.

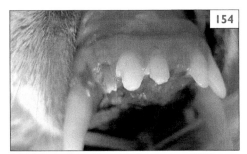

154 'Missing' maxillary left first incisor (201).

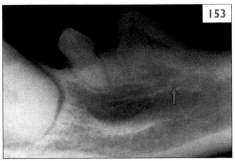

153 Intraoral dental radiograph of the patient in 151. Note the absence of a permanent tooth (arrow).

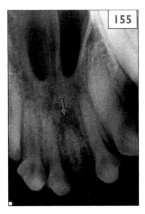

155 Dental radiograph of the patient in 154 reveals a retained and abscessed root (arrow).

Impacted or embedded (unerupted) teeth

DEFINITION[10]

Any tooth that has not erupted by the normal time is considered impacted. This is generally considered to be the time when the surrounding or contralateral teeth have already erupted. Teeth which have an identifiable physical barrier to eruption are considered impacted, and those without are considered embedded.

ETIOLOGY AND PATHOGENESIS

Delayed eruption or impaction can occur due to a variety of reasons. The most common cause is the presence of an overlying structure that interferes with normal eruption. This may be bone, soft tissue, or even tooth/teeth that interfere with the normal eruption path[13].

The most common soft tissue interference is an area of thick and firm gingiva called an *operculum*[4]. This condition is most often seen in toy and bracheocephalic breeds. Additional causes of soft tissue interference include neoplasms and cysts[10].

Deciduous teeth can impede eruption when they fail to exfoliate normally, and this is typically seen when they become ankylosed[27]. Permanent dentition can also block the eruptive path in cases of crowding or supernumerary dentition[10]. Crowded teeth may not only cause impaction, but also divergence of the developing tooth which may affect surrounding teeth (causing resorption) or other structures (i.e. the nasal cavity)[2]. Crowding is the most common cause of impaction in human beings[10]. Some cases of impaction are created by an errant direction of eruption[13]. Finally, if no identifiable cause of impaction is present, it may be considered due to failure of passive eruption (embedded)[10]. It should be noted that failure of passive eruption is a very rare condition; it is more likely that the impacting structure has not been diagnosed.

CLINICAL FEATURES

Impactions occur most commonly in the maxillary canine[2] and premolar teeth (especially PM1)[13]. It also occurs most often in toy and small breeds as well as brachycephalic dogs[2]. However, unerupted teeth can be found in any breed and can occur with any tooth[2]. Patients will generally have no overt clinical signs other than a missing tooth in a young animal (**156**).

Alternatively, there may be a persistent deciduous tooth past the time of normal eruption (see *Table 1*, p. 10). If missing teeth occur bilaterally, the cause is most likely true congenital absence; however, if this condition appears unilaterally, an impacted tooth should be strongly suspected. On occasion, an unerupted tooth may lead to the development of a dentigerous cyst (see page 118)[4]. Therefore, the presenting complaint may be a swelling in the area of a 'missing' tooth. However, dentigerous cysts are most often diagnosed however, during an oral examination under general anesthesia associated with a surgical or dental procedure.

DIFFERENTIAL DIAGNOSES

- Congenitally missing teeth.
- Previously exfoliated/extracted teeth.

DIAGNOSTIC TESTS

Dental radiographs should be exposed of any 'missing' tooth[5], as these will confirm the presence or lack of the permanent tooth (**157**)[4]. Furthermore, in cases where the permanent tooth is impacted, radiographs will determine if cyst formation has begun.

MANAGEMENT[10]

There are several options for therapy of impacted teeth:

- If an obstruction is present or suspected, an *operculectomy* may be performed[4]. This involves the removal of the barrier to eruption (soft tissue, bone, or tooth) via a surgical approach[28]. The procedure must be performed early, as once the root apex is complete (between 9 and 13 months depending on breed and tooth) passive eruption will not occur[13]. In humans, this procedure has been proven to be effective if performed promptly[29]. If this fails to resolve the problem, other therapy is required.
- Surgical extraction of the unerupted tooth is the preferred form of therapy, especially if the root apex is complete[4,30]. It is performed in order to avoid formation of a dentigerous cyst or other significant pathological condition. The incidence of these conditions is unknown in veterinary medicine; however, pathological changes were noted in 32.9% of cases in one human study[31].

- If the client is interested in having the tooth present in the mouth, orthodontic extrusion may be attempted[4,32]. This is a long and complicated process which is best handled by a specialist and only in extreme cases.
- In an older patient with no evidence of cyst formation, monitoring the tooth without therapy may be acceptable[4,13]. This is due to the fact that there are numerous complications that can occur during the extraction procedure, and these risks may outweigh the benefits[10]. If this is the selected method of treatment, regular radiographic monitoring is critical.

KEY POINTS
- Unerupted teeth are quite common in bracheocephalic breeds.
- Any missing tooth in a young animal should be radiographed to determine if there is an unerupted tooth.
- If caught early, operculectomy may be attempted to allow the tooth to erupt normally.
- Surgical extraction of the unerupted tooth is recommended to eliminate the possibility of creating a dentigerous cyst or other pathological condition.

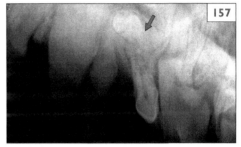

156 'Missing' maxillary right second premolar (106) (arrow) in a 3-year-old dog.

157 Dental radiograph of the patient in **156** reveals an impacted tooth (arrow).

Dentigerous cyst (follicular cyst)

DEFINITION
A dentigerous cyst is a fluid filled structure which develops from the separation of the follicle (or enamel forming organ) of an unerupted tooth[4,10].

ETIOLOGY AND PATHOGENESIS
Dentigerous cysts occur secondary to an unerupted (embedded or impacted) tooth[4]. They are almost always associated with permanent teeth, but they have been reported in association with deciduous teeth as well[10]. Enamel is formed and deposited on the developing tooth by the enamel forming organ, or follicle, which consists of cells called ameloblasts. The enamel is formed prior to tooth eruption. If the tooth erupts normally, the enamel forming organ is quickly worn away. When the tooth does not erupt, the ameloblasts persist and form a sac lined with epithelium[4]. This lining may not be productive, but commonly it will create fluid and thus result in cystic formation[10]. Not all unerupted teeth will develop dentigerous cysts. The incidence is unknown in veterinary medicine; however, pathological changes were noted in 32.9% of cases in one human study[31].

CLINICAL FEATURES
Small dentigerous cysts are generally asymptomatic, and often go undiagnosed without dental radiology. Radiographs should be exposed of any area with a missing tooth, as these cysts do grow and may result in significant bone loss and/or destruction due to the pressure applied. They are generally seen as swellings in the area of a missing tooth in a young patient (**158**). However, due to the typically slow growth of these cysts and the stoic character of veterinary patients, some cases are initially diagnosed in older patients[33]. These cystic growths can become quite large and disfiguring, requiring major surgical correction[4,10].

Additional potential problems associated with dentigerous cysts include infections and neoplasia. Dentigerous cysts may become infected, resulting in acute swelling and pain[10]. These cases are often misdiagnosed as abscesses. With regard to neoplasia, there are reports in the human literature that these cells can undergo a neoplastic transformation into an ameloblastoma[10,34]. Finally, squamous cell carcinomas have developed within dentigerous cysts[10].

DIFFERENTIAL DIAGNOSES
- Neoplasia.
- Abscess.
- Other cystic growths.
- Hematoma.
- Sialocele.

DIAGNOSTIC TESTS
Dental radiographs should be exposed of any 'missing teeth' to ensure that an early cyst is not developing[5]. Dental radiographs are generally diagnostic in these cases, revealing a unilocular radiolucent area that is associated with the crown of an unerupted tooth (**159, 160**)[10]. An aspirate obtained for fluid analysis and cytology will appear supportive of a cyst. Definitive diagnosis can be achieved with histopathological analysis of the cystic lining.

MANAGEMENT
Prognosis for these lesions is excellent if diagnosis and treatment are achieved relatively early in the disease course[10]. Surgical removal of the offending tooth and careful debridement of the cystic lining will prove curative[4,10,35]. This should be performed with the goal of removing the cyst *en bloc*. It is important to avoid leaving any of the cyst lining behind, as this could allow the cyst to reform. Early surgical intervention will result in the least invasive surgery possible. If the cyst has grown quite large, which is very common in veterinary patients, marsupialization can be performed as the initial step in therapy[10]. This will allow for a decompression of the cyst and result in a reduction of the bony defect. Complete removal of the cyst can then be performed via a less invasive surgery at a later date.

KEY POINTS
- All unerupted teeth should be radiographed to ensure that no cyst is forming.
- Infection and malignant transformation can occur.
- Early removal of tooth and cyst is curative and carries an excellent prognosis.

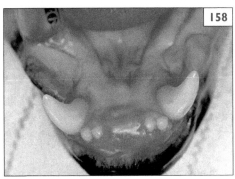

158 A smooth swelling in the area of missing mandibular incisors in a young cat is suggestive of a dentigerous cyst.

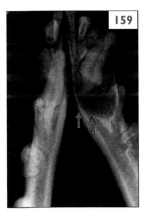

159 Dental radiograph of an unerupted mandibular canine reveals a large dentigerous cyst. Note the thin mandibular bone near the symphysis (arrows), risking a pathological fracture.

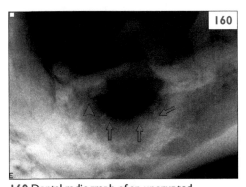

160 Dental radiograph of an unerupted supernumerary first premolar (305) (arrowhead) revealing a large dentigerous cyst (arrows). This underscores the importance of full mouth dental radiographs.

Odontoma

DEFINITION

An odontoma is an odontogenic tumor which contains both epithelial and mesenchymal cells[4,10,36].

ETIOLOGY AND PATHOGENESIS

Odontomas are classified as odontogenic tumors as they arise from the tooth forming cells and create fully differentiated dental tissues. The inductive process between the mesoderm and the odontogenic epithelial tissue leads to the development of specialized cells[36]. Ameloblasts create the enamel and odontoblasts the dentin[37]. The true etiology is unknown, but some mechanisms of creation or causes include: hyperactivity of the dental lamina[36], trauma, local infection, or hereditary/genetic changes[36]. Compound and complex odontomas may also have different pathogenic mechanisms[36].

Odontogenic tumors are rare in human and veterinary[37] patients, accounting for only 1.3% in humans[38] and 0.5 or 0.7% in companion animals[36]. Odontomas are the most common odontogenic tumor in humans[10], and this appears to be true in veterinary patients as well. No sex or breed predilection currently exist in the veterinary literature[39]. Odontomas are generally considered a benign tumor, and now are actually defined as a *harmatoma* (a developmental anomaly where relatively normal, although atypical, tissues exist in their normal location)[5,10,36]. The outward appearance is of a tumor. However, it must be noted that these lesions typically do not have *any* neoplastic characteristics[36]. While benign and slow growing, they can be expansile and create a mass effect in the oral tissues. Most experts believe these are benign, but a few label compound odontomas as neoplastic, based on several cases of recurrence following surgical excision[40,41]. Regardless of labeling, these lesions should be treated as expediently as possible.

CLINICAL FEATURES

Small odontomas are generally asymptomatic, and often go undiagnosed without dental radiology[36]. The most common clinical sign is an unerupted tooth, as the tumor will prevent its eruption[10,36]. Expansive lesions will present as swellings in the area of a missing tooth in a young dog (**161**). Due to the stoic character of veterinary patients, and the low incidence of intraoral dental radiography in veterinary practice, these growths can become very large, potentially very early in life[37,42]. On rare occasions, the odontoma can erupt into the mouth[36,43].

There are two subgroups of odontomas, *compound* and *complex*, which can usually be differentiated radiographically. However, some denticles are more organized than others and the distinction between compound and complex may be arbitrary[37].

DIFFERENTIAL DIAGNOSES
- Neoplasia.
- Abscess.
- Cyst.
- Hematoma.

DIAGNOSTIC TESTS
Dental radiographs should be exposed of any 'missing teeth' to ensure that an odontoma is not present[5]. Radiographs are generally diagnostic in these cases. A *compound* odontoma is comprised of numerous small tooth-like structures (denticles), often surrounding a somewhat normal looking tooth (**162**)[5,10]. A *complex* odontoma has all the requisite parts of a tooth present (enamel, dentin, pulp), but in a disorganized, amorphous mass[5,10]. Both types of lesion are generally surrounded by a well demarcated radiolucent area (which represents the oral soft tissue)[4,10,36]. Definitive diagnosis can be achieved with histopathological analysis.

MANAGEMENT
Prognosis for these lesions is excellent, especially if diagnosis and treatment are achieved relatively early in the disease course[5,10,39]. Surgical removal of all denticles and associated teeth as well as the fibrovascular stroma should prove curative[5,10]. This should be performed with the goal of removing the entire growth as well as the cystic lining. Surgical removal may be performed *en bloc*, but since these lesions are considered benign hamartomas, surgical enucleation is considered the treatment of choice due to its less invasive nature[5,36,37]. Regrowth is rare, but may occur in cases of incomplete excision. Early surgical intervention will result in the

least invasive surgery possible. Follow-up examinations and intraoral dental radiographs are recommended on a regular basis to ensure that there is no regrowth of tumor. This will allow for a more expedient therapy, if it becomes necessary.

KEY POINTS
- All unerupted teeth should be radiographed to ensure that an odontoma is not forming.
- This is a very benign lesion, but can grow quite large without therapy.
- Early removal is curative and carries an excellent prognosis.

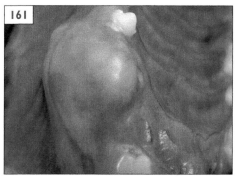

161 A large odontoma in the area where the maxillary left canine (204) sits in a 10-month-old dog.

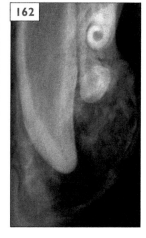

162 Intraoral dental radiograph revealing a compound odontoma surrounding the maxillary left canine (204).

Hairy tongue

DEFINITION
Hairy tongue is a condition in which long keratinous papillae are produced on the dorsal aspect of the tongue. These papillae become darkly stained and resemble hairs[4].

ETIOLOGY AND PATHOGENESIS
The true etiology is unknown. Hairy tongue is generally thought to be a genetic trait, although in humans most affected people are heavy smokers[10]. Other possible associated factors in humans include: antibiotic therapy, poor oral hygiene, radiation therapy to the head or neck, chronic systemic corticosteroid usage, and a general debilitation (especially with an overgrowth of fungal or bacterial organisms)[10,44]. In addition, a similar syndrome has been noted in people with the usage of certain antipsychotic drugs[45,46]. This condition likely results from either an increase in keratin formation or a decrease in keratin desquamation[10]. This condition has rarely been reported in small animals.

CLINICAL FEATURES
Long, thin, filiform papillae form on the dorsal surface of the tongue (**163**)[4]. These papillae closely resemble hair, especially if they become darkly stained, which often occurs early in life. The patient is usually asymptomatic, as this is a benign condition[10]. In severe cases however, it may result in halitosis or infection.

DIFFERENTIAL DIAGNOSES
- Severe fungal infection.
- Neoplasia.

DIAGNOSTIC TESTS
None are generally required as oral examination is diagnostic. If there is any question, biopsy and histopathology are recommended.

MANAGEMENT[10]
No specific therapy is usually required since this is a cosmetic condition only. Meticulous homecare is recommended to decrease oral infection. Any predisposing factors or medical conditions should be eliminated or addressed. In severe cases, tongue brushing or scraping may be attempted to promote desquamation.

KEY POINTS
- Hairy tongue does not involve true hair, but keratin fimbria which become darkly stained.
- No therapy is usually required.
- Homecare is recommended to decrease the level of infection.

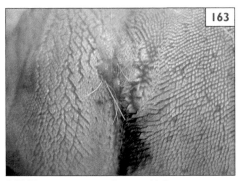

163 Hairy tongue in a 2-year-old dog.

Enamel hypocalcification (hypoplasia)

DEFINITION
Enamel hypocalcification is an enamel defect that occurs during tooth development[4,10].

ETIOLOGY AND PATHOGENESIS
Enamel is a very thin (<1 mm) material on the surface of teeth[47]. It is formed and deposited on the dentin of the developing tooth by the enamel forming organ which consists of cells called ameloblasts. Enamel is only formed prior to tooth eruption and cannot be naturally repaired after eruption into the mouth[10,13]. Hypoplasia/hypocalcification results from a malformation of the enamel during its development[4]. Ameloblasts are very sensitive to external stimuli and a host of factors can result in enamel malformation[10]. The malformed enamel will be easily lost, thus exposing the underlying dentin.

The most common acquired cause of enamel hypocalcification to one or several teeth in veterinary patients is trauma imposed on the unerupted tooth[2,10,13]. This can occur due to any external trauma, but is most often associated with the extraction of a deciduous tooth. In these cases, one or several adjacent teeth may be affected. The pattern of loss may include only the tip, one surface, or the entire tooth (**164**). Additional causes of this pattern of enamel hypoplasia are infection or inflammation from an overlying deciduous tooth[2,10]. In human dentistry this is known as Turner's hypoplasia. In veterinary patients this typically results from a fractured and abscessed primary tooth (see page 93).

A severe infectious or nutritional problem may also result in improper enamel production[4.] In these cases, most or all of the teeth are affected, but only in a small part of the crown, usually a horizontal circumferential strip[10]. Canine distemper was a common cause of this condition in the past[2]. Consequently, teeth with enamel hypoplasia were often termed '*distemper teeth*'. Widespread vaccination has greatly decreased the incidence of distemper, and therefore the resultant enamel hypoplasia has been rarely diagnosed in recent years. The recurrence of distemper and the recent outbreak of canine flu may once again increase the diagnosis of this condition.

Enamel hypoplasia may also result from a hereditary condition known as *amelogenesis imperfecta*[2,4,13]. This condition is associated with a decrease in the amount of enamel matrix applied to the teeth during development. In these cases, almost all surfaces on almost all teeth are involved (**165, 166**).

CLINICAL FEATURES
Patterns of affected teeth may present as anything from a single tooth to the entire dentition. Areas of enamel hypocalcification generally appear as stained a tan to dark brown

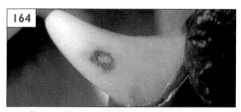

164 Enamel hypocalcification on the mandibular left canine (304) in an 8-month-old dog.

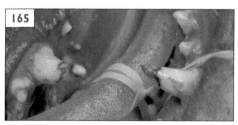

165 Widespread enamel hypocalcification (*amelogenesis imperfecta*) on the canines of a dog.

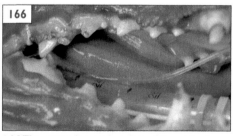

166 The premolars and molars of the patient in **165**.

(rarely black) color, and may appear pitted and rough[10]. The tooth surface is hard however, as opposed to the soft/sticky surface of a caries lesion. The areas of weakened enamel are easily exfoliated which then exposes the underlying dentin[10]. The dentin is a porous material and therefore becomes stained early on.

Dentin exposure results in significant discomfort for the patient[10]. Each mm² of crown surface contains up to 45,000 dentinal tubules, each of which communicate with the root canal system[48]. The following hydrodynamic mechanism of dentin hypersensitivity is the currently accepted explanation for pain associated with dentin exposure[4,49]. Dentin exposure changes the fluid dynamics within the dentinal tubules. The change in fluid velocity within the tubules is translated into electrical signals by the sensory fibers located within the tubules or subjacent odontoblast layer. These signals result in the sensation of pain (or sensitivity) within the tooth[48]. It is rare for veterinary patients to show this discomfort, but occasionally anorexia (typically partial) may be seen. In addition, these exposed dentinal tubules can act as a conduit for bacterial infection of the pulp (or root canal system), thus initiating endodontic disease[50].

Over time, the tooth responds to this exposure by laying down a layer of reparative dentin. There is no study that documents the time for an effective layer to be placed in veterinary patients. One human study found that reparative dentin is seldom found prior to 30 days following exposure of dentinal tubules, and completion of formation is generally around 130 days[51]. It is not known, however, if this layer of reparative dentin is effective in decreasing tooth sensitivity[48]. Therefore, treatment is recommended regardless of the patient's age. An additional means for protection of these teeth is the natural accumulation and mineralization of the surface layer which will occlude the tubules[4]. The time required for this is unknown, as is its overall effectiveness.

The roughness of the teeth will also result in increased plaque and calculus retention, which in turn leads to early onset of periodontal disease. For all of these reasons, prompt therapy of these teeth is critical to the health of the patient.

In cases involving widespread hypoplasia, it is common to find malformed roots (**167**)[4]. There is often very little root structure. While

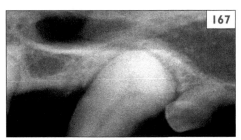

167 Severely underdeveloped root of maxillary left canine of the patient in **165**.

endodontic infection of these roots is rare, the lack of root structure will result in early exfoliation secondary to trauma or periodontal disease. The owner should be informed of this complication and be counseled on proper follow-up and homecare.

DIFFERENTIAL DIAGNOSES
- Caries.
- Crown fracture.
- Tooth malformation.

DIAGNOSTIC TESTS
Tactile probing of the dark areas with a sharp shepherd's hook explorer will reveal a roughened but hard surface. Dental radiographs should be performed to rule out endodontic disease and root malformation[4].

MANAGEMENT
Treatment is aimed at removing sensitivity, avoiding endodontic infection by occluding the dentinal tubules, and smoothing the tooth to decrease plaque accumulation. The most efficient and effective way to accomplish these goals is placement of a bonded composite restoration[2,10,13]. This composite restoration will also greatly improve esthetics[10].

The restoration process is initiated by removing the diseased dentin with a diamond or finishing dental bur or polishing disc. After the diseased dentin is removed, a commercial bonding agent is applied according to package directions. A two-step product is recommended in these cases, to allow for the application of additional layers of unfilled resin if indicated. Following the bonding agent, a microhybrid or flowable composite resin is placed, and roughly shaped to natural tooth contours and light cured.

After curing, the restoration is shaped and smoothed with a finishing/fine diamond bur or sanding discs. After the restoration is finished, a final coat of unfilled resin is applied for optimum smoothness and shine (**168, 169**). In small teeth and defects, an unfilled resin or fluoride varnish may be sufficient to decrease sensitivity and smooth the tooth. If the damage is severe and the client is interested in a permanent correction, crown therapy can be performed[7,13]. Alternatively, extraction may be performed; however, this is not the recommended course of therapy if the root structure is normal with no evidence of endodontic infection.

KEY POINTS
- If dentin exposure has occurred, these teeth are very sensitive for months and treatment should be performed as soon as possible.
- Composite restoration is the treatment of choice.
- Radiographs should be exposed to evaluate root structure.
- Traumatic extraction of deciduous teeth is a very common cause.
- New bonding agents are very strong. However, the restoration can be lost if inappropriate chewing is not controlled.

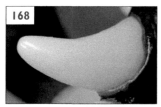

168 Composite restoration of the enamel defects seen in **164**.

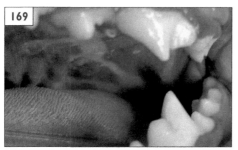

169 Composite restoration of the enamel defects seen in **166**.

Feline juvenile (puberty) gingivitis/periodontitis

DEFINITION
Juvenile periodontal disease is inflammation which occurs soon after permanent tooth eruption[4]. This can be further broken down into *feline hyperplastic gingivitis*, where the inflammation is confined to the gingiva, or *juvenile onset periodontitis*[4].

ETIOLOGY AND PATHOGENESIS
Etiology at this point is unknown. In humans there is a period of increased susceptibility to gingivitis in the pubertal period (puberty gingivitis)[10]. There does appear to be a genetic predisposition towards juvenile onset periodontitis in Somali, Siamese, and Maine coon cats[4].

CLINICAL FEATURES
Hyperplastic gingivitis results in significant inflammation which is confined to the gingiva and begins during the eruptive period. This inflammation consists of significant erythema and edema to the attached gingiva. Bleeding during mastication and on oral examination are common findings. While occasionally seen in dogs, this condition has a much higher incidence in cats, where the hyperplasia is a complicating factor (**170, 171**)[4]. It is generally a nonpainful condition for the patient, and halitosis is a common complaint. If untreated, this disease process can proceed quickly to periodontal disease, which may result in early infection and exfoliation of the teeth. The reader is encouraged to review the periodontal disease section of this book for more information on this aspect of the disease process.

As the patient matures, susceptibility appears to subside at approximately 2 years of age[4], which is the same pattern followed in the human disease[10]. Therefore, if treated aggressively the patient can enjoy normal periodontal health in the adult years.

Juvenile periodontitis, in contrast, will result in the rapid proliferation of plaque and calculus. This in turn results in significant early bone loss, periodontal pocket formation, and furcation exposure[4]. Treatment in these cases is often frustrating.

DIFFERENTIAL DIAGNOSES
- Lymphoplasmacytic stomatitis.
- Other infectious etiologies (fungal/viral).
- Neoplasia.

DIAGNOSTIC TESTS
Incisional biopsy should be considered to rule out other causes of gingival inflammation. Culture and sensitivity testing is generally nonrewarding, but may be of value in nonresponsive cases. Dental radiographs should be performed to evaluate bone quality. Finally, *Bartonella* testing may be beneficial in some cases, especially in nonresponsive patients.

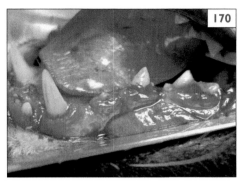

170 Hyperplastic gingivitis on the premolars of a 7-month-old cat.

MANAGEMENT
Early and frequent dental prophylaxis (even if minimal plaque is present) and diligent homecare are critical to decrease inflammation. Ideally, homecare consists of daily brushing. Other alternatives include chlorhexidine rinses and plaque control diets and treats. In cases where gingival hyperplasia is present, aggressive early gingivectomy is recommended to remove pseudopockets, decrease inflammation, facilitate the dental prophylaxis, and improve the effectiveness of homecare[4]. Finally, extraction of any significantly diseased teeth is warranted.

KEY POINTS
- Severe periodontal inflammation occurs during and immediately after eruption.
- Early dental prophylaxis, aggressive gingivectomy (if indicated), and homecare are mandated.
- With proper therapy, susceptibility will wane at about 2 years.
- If this condition does not at least partially respond to proper therapy, further diagnostics and subsequent therapy should be initiated.

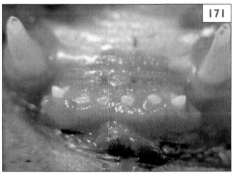

171 Hyperplastic gingivitis on the incisors of a 7-month-old cat.

Oral papillomatosis

DEFINITION
Oral papillomas are benign thickenings of the oral mucosa, which are supported by finger-like projections of the dermis resulting in numerous fronds[52].

ETIOLOGY AND PATHOGENESIS
Papillomas are most commonly induced by a virus (papovavirus)[4], but can be idiopathic as well[53]. They are transmitted most commonly by direct contact, but indirect contact may also be sufficient in some cases. There is generally a 2–6 month incubation time between exposure and clinical signs[54].

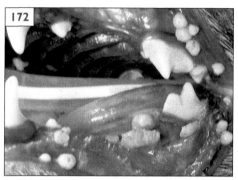

172 Viral papillomatosis in an 8-month-old dog.

CLINICAL FEATURES
Oral papillomas are most commonly seen in young dogs as white, gray, or flesh-colored masses on the oral mucosa[2,52]. They can be solitary or occur in bunches, and may be singular or spread throughout the mouth. They most commonly occur on the lips, palate, tongue, and/or oropharynx[4]. The classic appearance is pedunculated or cauliflower in shape (172). Sizes range from a few millimeters to a few centimeters, and may be associated with lesions on the skin or eyes[54]. Viral papillomas are generally self-limiting and will resolve over a period of time from weeks to months[4,52]. There are, however, reasons to initiate diagnostics and therapy in suspected cases of papillomatosis:
- Papillomas may grow large and interfere with mastication[4].
- They can become infected and result in significant local inflammation.
- Papillomas may mimic more aggressive tumors.
- Malignant transformation into squamous cell carcinoma has been reported[55].

DIFFERENTIAL DIAGNOSES
Oral neoplasia (especially papillary squamous cell carcinoma).

DIAGNOSTIC TESTS
Signalment and clinical signs are generally diagnostic. Biopsy (preferably excisional) is strongly recommended if the lesion is not absolutely classic in appearance[52].

MANAGEMENT
In most cases, no therapy is required as these lesions will spontaneously regress[2,4,52]. Following regression of papillomatosis, patients are generally immune to reinfection[52].

Surgical removal or debulking and histopathological analysis should be considered in cases where the masses are either severely infected, or are very large and interfere with mastication[4]. Histopathology (ideally excisional) should also be pursued if the growths are not regressing in the normal time span, or are not typical in appearance. This can be performed utilizing a standard surgical approach, cryosurgery, electrosurgery, or laser therapy[52].

Additional therapeutic measures which can be employed in persistent cases include vaccination, traumatic crushing, and chemotherapy[4]. However, vaccination has not been proven particularly successful and squamous cell carcinomas have been reported to arise at the injection sites[56].

KEY POINTS
- Papillomas are usually viral in origin.
- Lesions may be single or appear in bunches.
- Papillomas are generally self-limiting and require no therapy.
- These masses may mimic or transform into a malignancy, therefore, excision and biopsy should be considered in questionable cases.

Pathologies of the Dental Hard Tissues

Gregg DuPont

- **Uncomplicated crown fracture (closed crown fracture)**
- **Complicated crown fracture (open crown fracture)**
- **Caries (cavity, tooth decay)**
- **Type 1 feline tooth resorption (TR)**
- **Type 2 feline tooth resorption (TR)**
- **Enamel hypoplasia and hypocalcification**
- **Dental abrasion**
- **Dental attrition**
- **External resorption**
- **Internal resorption**
- **Intrinsic stains (endogenous stains)**
- **Extrinsic stains (exogenous stains)**
- **Primary endodontic lesion with secondary periodontal disease**
- **Primary periodontal lesion with secondary endodontic involvement**
- **Combined endodontic and periodontal lesion**
- **Idiopathic root resorption**

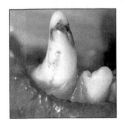
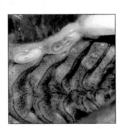
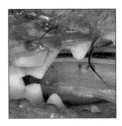
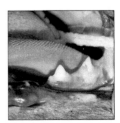

Uncomplicated crown fracture (closed crown fracture)

DEFINITION

A tooth fracture that does not result in direct pulp exposure. These fractures involve loss of enamel and some underlying dentin. (Tooth fractures that involve or expose the pulp chamber or root canal are termed 'complicated' fractures.)

ETIOLOGY AND PATHOGENESIS

Tooth fractures can result from excessive force applied to the crown of a tooth, or stresses that act on the tooth in a nonphysiological direction. A wide range of traumatic events can produce enough stress to fracture teeth. Uncomplicated crown fractures of canine and incisor teeth most commonly result from picking up rocks, or from contact with a hard surface while picking up other objects, but they can also result from impact against objects such as walls or other dogs' teeth, and from chewing on fences or crates. Uncomplicated crown fractures of premolar and molar teeth most commonly result from mild-to-moderate bite force on hard objects such as bones, rocks, and hard chew toys; however, they can also occur from a forceful bite on a rawhide toy.

Enamel is the hard, impervious, and smooth material covering the crown of the tooth. The hardness provides wear resistance to the tooth surface. The impervious nature of enamel protects the pulp from bacterial ingress and from dentin sensitivity that occurs when dentin is exposed to the oral cavity. The smooth surface of enamel provides some degree of resistance to bacterial adherence and plaque formation. In contrast to enamel, the underlying dentin is softer, is traversed by dentinal tubules leading directly to the dental pulp, and has a rougher surface. Exposed dentin wears faster, and exposed dentin tubules experience hydrostatic pressure changes on the cell processes that extend into them which create discomfort. Exposed dentin also accumulates plaque and calculus faster than intact enamel. When uncomplicated crown fractures occur to a tooth with healthy dentin and underlying pulp, the dentin can respond by producing additional tooth structure on the pulp (deep) surface. This is achieved by accelerating the production of tertiary, or reparative, dentin. This helps to protect the pulp by increasing the thickness of dentin between the fracture site and the pulp. However, if the pulp is compromised, severely traumatized, or the defenses are overwhelmed it can become infected or necrotic[1]. This will only be diagnosed via dental radiographs.

CLINICAL FEATURES

Fractured teeth are easily identified by the presence of an abnormal flattened area that is not caused by attrition or abrasion. Small fractures of incisal or occlusal cusps may appear as a slightly irregular incisal edge, or an abnormally shaped surface (**173**). Fracture facets that are angled toward the mouth may be difficult to identify on a routine oral examination, since the labial or buccal surface can appear nearly normal. Dental surfaces which are missing the enamel layer appear rough and dull due to exposure of the less mineralized subjacent dentin. Chronic fractures typically have a larger accumulation of plaque and calculus than intact teeth, and the exposed dentin is often stained. Gliding a dental explorer across the fractured surface demonstrates the rough quality, but should not drop into a depression in the area of regional pulp horns. Furthermore, there should be no visible holes into the pulp chamber. Exposed dentin tubules can cause dental sensitivity, but animals seldom exhibit outward signs of discomfort[2].

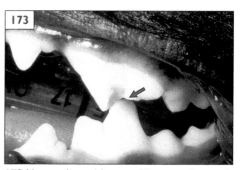

173 Uncomplicated fracture. The central cusp of the left maxillary fourth premolar tooth is abnormally shaped (arrow).

DIFFERENTIAL DIAGNOSIS
- Worn areas from abrasion due to aggressive play with abrasive toys.
- Worn areas from attrition, where the opposing dentition contacts and damages a tooth.
- Anomalous teeth that are malformed during their development.
- Complicated tooth fractures.

DIAGNOSTIC TESTS
Diagnosis is made on the clinical appearance of the fractured tooth. Abrasion lesions typically have a more regular appearance and a smoother surface. Careful evaluation of the occlusal relationships (with the mouth held closed and the teeth in full occlusion) rules out attrition from occlusal trauma against the opposing dentition. A sharp dental explorer passed over the area of the pulp horn moves unimpeded across the surface, verifying there is no pulp exposure. If the explorer drops into a hole in the center of the tooth, or if it stimulates any bleeding, then it is a complicated fracture.

MANAGEMENT
Very small chips in teeth of mature animals may not require intervention, other than a discussion with the owner about appropriate toys, treats, and activities to prevent further trauma. If the dentin is exposed, even small fractures should be radiographed. Larger areas of missing enamel, particularly in young animals, carry a greater risk of bacterial ingress through the exposed dentin tubules. These should be radiographed to evaluate the health of the pulp. If the pulp or root canal shows evidence of arrested development (necrotic pulp), internal resorption, external root resorption, or periapical bone loss, then the tooth requires root canal treatment or extraction, similar to a complicated fracture. If the radiographs show no abnormalities, then the dentin should be sealed with a dentin sealant. This is ideally an unfilled or lightly filled resin material, which is placed (following manufacturer's instructions), with the patient under anesthesia (**174**). If only a very thin layer of dentin remains covering the pulp, it may appear slightly pink in the area immediately over a pulp horn (center of the tooth) (**175**). However, as long as a dental explorer glides smoothly across, there is no direct pulp exposure and it is therefore still considered to be an uncomplicated fracture. In these cases, the dentin sealant should be covered by additional mechanical protection. The sealant acts as an 'indirect pulp cap' material; there is no need to

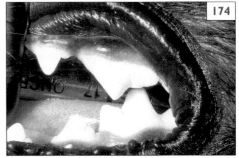

174 Appearance of the tooth in **173** after a sealant and a bonded composite restorative have been placed.

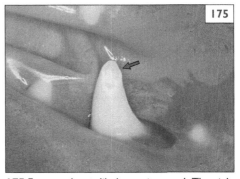

175 Fractured mandibular canine tooth. The pink spot in the center of the fractured face indicates very thin dentin covering the pulp (arrow). Note that a dental dam is placed around the tooth in this figure.

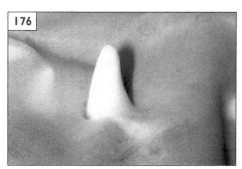

176 Post-treatment picture of the tooth in 175 after sealant and restoration (indirect pulp cap).

apply any other agent (such as calcium hydroxide or mineral trioxide aggregate [MTA]) to a near exposure. A bonded composite resin or other restorative should also be placed over the sealant material to provide additional mechanical protection (176). Follow-up radiographs should be taken in 1 year to evaluate the health of the pulp and periapical tissues, since bacteria may have invaded the pulp before the dentin was sealed.

KEY POINTS
- Tooth fractures that do not expose pulp can cause dentin sensitivity and may allow bacterial ingress to the pulp.
- Large uncomplicated crown fractures may benefit from placement of a dentin sealant.

Complicated crown fracture (open crown fracture)

DEFINITION
A tooth fracture that causes a direct exposure of the dental pulp. The pulp exposure most commonly occurs as an opening into the pulp chamber of the crown, but if the fracture extends into the root it can create an opening directly into the root canal.

ETIOLOGY AND PATHOGENESIS
Animal teeth are able to withstand very strong occlusal loads parallel to the tooth axis. However, large forces directed at an angle to the tooth axis can result in fracture of the crown. Exposure of the dental pulp occurs when a tooth fractures low enough on the crown to expose the dental pulp. This level moves apically with age as the pulp effectively 'recedes' over time as more dentin is produced throughout life. The most common causes of complicated fractures of incisor and canine teeth include automobile accidents, trauma against objects (walls, tables, cars) after 'missing a turn', fights with other animals in which their teeth make contact, receiving a kick from a horse or other large animal, attempting to catch rocks, getting a tooth caught while chewing and pulling on fences and crates, accidental contact with tennis rackets/golf clubs/baseball bats during play, and falling or jumping from heights onto hard surfaces (a very common injury to the canine teeth of cats and ferrets). Dogs frequently use their teeth for prehension of hard objects or for opening gates and doors in ways that apply outward forces on the teeth. Some dogs also attempt to retrieve balls at the same time that an owner is about to launch them with a racket or club, resulting in significant trauma. Maxillary canine teeth in cats are particularly prone to fracture due to their extension beyond the lips. When a cat's face or chin strikes the ground, the upper canine teeth are often the first hard tissue to hit. In dogs, the upper fourth premolar and lower first molar teeth most commonly suffer a complicated crown fracture as a result of placing heavy biting forces on a hard object that is relatively flat or long. Rib or steak bones, hooves, or very hard toys with similar shapes

are the worst objects for causing this injury. As the dog bites down on the object, it levers sideways placing a buccal (vestibular, lateral) force on the upper fourth premolar tooth and a lingual (oral, medial) force on the cusp of the lower first molar tooth. This often causes a 'buccal slab fracture' of the upper fourth premolar tooth as a portion of the outside surface is cleaved from the tooth. If the fracture extends to the subgingival cemental attachment, the loose fragment may remain in position, being held in place by the periodontal attachment. Teeth with this kind of fracture often have pulp exposure in the center of the main cusp where a pulp horn extends coronally from the pulp.

CLINICAL FEATURES

Teeth that have suffered a complicated fracture appear similar to those with an uncomplicated fracture except that there is a direct opening into the pulp chamber or root canal. Often the opening is grossly visible as a pink, dark brown, or black circular hole in the center of the tooth on the fractured face (**177–179**). The hole can range from less than 1 mm across, to as large as 2 mm in a young dog. If the pulp is still vital, the hole will appear pink or red and will bleed when it is probed (**177**). If the hole is black, then the pulp is necrotic and an explorer will drop into the opening without eliciting any discomfort (**178**). The mobile retained fragment that sometimes remains in place when an upper fourth premolar tooth has suffered a buccal slab

fracture can conceal the pulp exposure and must be reflected or removed to examine the fractured face (**179**). When the pulp is exposed, there is no dentin over that region and therefore the pulp cannot readily repair itself by the deposition of tertiary, or reparative, dentin. Invariably, the pulp eventually becomes irreversibly inflamed or nonvital. Inflammatory mediators escape from the root canal into the periodontal ligament area through the apical openings (foramen in an immature animal, delta in a mature animal) and lateral canals, where they cause localized osteolysis. These lesions of endodontic origin (LEO) appear on a radiograph as radiolucencies around the root tip apex

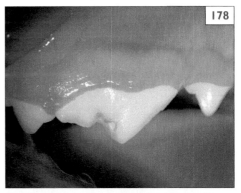

178 Complicated fracture of the right maxillary fourth premolar tooth with a nonvital pulp.

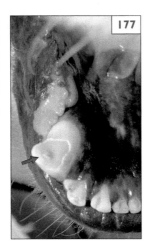

177 Complicated fracture of right mandibular canine tooth with an open pulp chamber and a vital pulp (arrow).

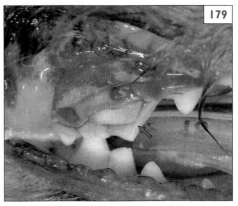

179 Buccal fracture fragment attached by the periodontal ligament (arrow).

or along the lateral aspect of a root (**180**). LEO lucencies can range from diffuse to very obvious, and from a slightly increased width of the periodontal ligament space to a very large defect. The lucency indicates the presence of a cyst, a granuloma, or an abscess[3]. Left untreated, the pathology often expands, extending along the path of least resistance to relieve the pressure. The result may be a red circle with a central draining fistula close to the mucogingival line (parulis) (**181**). Depending on which tooth is involved, endodontic disease can also manifest as a swollen mandible or a facial swelling just beneath the eye with or without a central draining tract. In cats, mandibular canine teeth often drain ventrally through the skin.

DIFFERENTIAL DIAGNOSIS
- Uncomplicated crown fracture with a near pulp exposure or irregular fracture face.
- Chronically worn teeth with central brown spots of tertiary dentin but no hole.

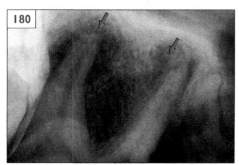

180 Large periapical radiolucencies (arrows) indicate endodontic disease.

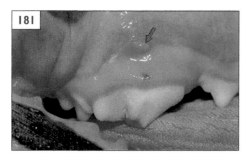

181 Necrotic pulp with drainage through a fistula at the junction between the gingiva and the mucosa (arrow).

- Dark material entrapped in a developmental groove.
- Anomalous teeth that are malformed during their development.
- Swelling from a foreign body or nondental infection.
- Oral tumor.

DIAGNOSTIC TESTS
A sharp dental explorer passed over the central spot drops into, catches on, or causes bleeding from a hole leading to the pulp. A radiograph may, or may not, confirm the presence of LEOs, depending on the duration of the fracture and other variables.

MANAGEMENT
When the pulp has been exposed in a mature dog or cat, it develops irreversible pulpitis or necrosis, requiring either root canal treatment or extraction. Strategic teeth or teeth that require a surgical approach for extraction (which is painful and invasive) should have root canal treatment if practical. These strategic teeth include the canine and carnassial (maxillary fourth premolars and mandibular first molars) teeth in dogs, and the canine teeth in cats. All teeth may be considered 'strategic' teeth to retain in show dogs. The permanent teeth of dogs less than 1 year of age have very large pulps and are weaker than mature teeth. For these patients, vital direct pulp capping is often done as a means of preserving pulp vitality to allow the tooth to mature. This involves removing 4 or 5 mm of coronal pulp, placing a medicament (generally MTA) on the pulp stump, and then placing a hermetically sealed restoration to prevent any microleakage. In animals over 1 year but less than 2 years of age, this procedure may be attempted depending on the length of pulp exposure and other factors, but becomes less important and carries a more guarded prognosis. Teeth treated in this manner should have follow-up radiographs annually, to determine whether definitive root canal therapy becomes necessary.

KEY POINTS
- Tooth fractures that expose the pulp in a mature animal must be treated with either root canal treatment or extraction.
- 'Wait and watch' is not an acceptable treatment plan.
- Immature teeth with recent pulp exposures may be treated with vital direct pulp caps.

Caries (cavity, tooth decay)

DEFINITION

A bacterial infection of the tooth that destroys enamel and dentin. Although caries is uncommon in dogs compared to humans and many other species of animals, it does occur. Reports on the prevalence vary widely[4]. This may be due to over-diagnosis of discolored but uninfected surfaces. An evaluation by a veterinary dentist of records from 435 dogs seen at a veterinary dental referral facility found a prevalence of 5.3%[5]. This clinical survey report provided a description of how caries lesions were diagnosed and differentiated from noncarious lesions. Dental caries has not been accurately documented in cats.

ETIOLOGY AND PATHOGENESIS

Commonly called 'tooth decay', caries most often affects the occlusal surfaces of the molar teeth, or the contact surfaces (the sides of the teeth that face towards the adjacent teeth). Root surfaces can also develop caries. Dental caries has been extensively studied in humans, but poorly studied in dogs. In humans, caries begins with the acidic destruction of teeth by acids that are produced when plaque bacteria ferment dietary carbohydrates[6]. There is also a clear genetic susceptibility factor. Therefore, caries is caused by a combination of genetic susceptibility, the presence of cariogenic bacteria (usually *Streptococcus mutans*, but also other *Streptococcus* spp. and *Lactobacillus* spp.), and an available source of fermentable carbohydrate. The initial lesion is a surface decalcification of the enamel caused by a drop in the pH. When the decalcification reaches subsurface enamel it appears as a white spot lesion. This is followed by extension of the bacteria into the dentin. Extension through the dentin can be rapid, leaving unsupported enamel (**182**). The undermined enamel collapses, forming an open cavity. Caries can only develop in areas which can develop plaque and accommodate stagnant food particles[7]. The occlusal surfaces of molar teeth have the highest caries risk in both humans and dogs[8]. There are a few factors that may contribute to the resistance of dogs to developing dental caries. Their occlusal surfaces have fewer pits and fissures than human premolar and molar teeth. Also, *S. mutans* is not a common inhabitant of canine oral microflora. Perhaps most importantly, the pH of dog saliva is more alkaline than human saliva. The acidity of the oral environment plays an important role in the initial acidic decalcification that starts the caries process[8].

CLINICAL FEATURES

Dark brown areas on the occlusal surfaces or contact (interproximal) surfaces of the molar teeth are suspect for dental caries. The affected surface often has a concave shape (**183**). Soft, darkened tooth structure that permits the penetration of a sharp dental explorer or

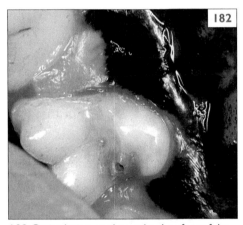

182 Caries lesion on the occlusal surface of the right maxillary first molar tooth. The enamel defect is small, but the underlying dentin defect is large creating a rim of unsupported enamel.

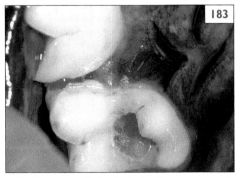

183 Concave cavity typical of caries.

excavator is confirmation that active caries is present. More advanced lesions destroy the tooth in an accentuated concave shape filled with debris and damaged dental tissue, eventually decaying through the entire crown of the tooth.

DIFFERENTIAL DIAGNOSIS

- Sclerotic or worn tooth surfaces caused by abrasion, attrition, or trauma.
- Intrinsic staining of occlusal surfaces.
- Fractured cusps.
- Tooth staining caused by ingested materials.

DIAGNOSTIC TESTS

Clinical observation of soft, dark tooth structure which can be penetrated by a dental explorer or sharp instrument is the pathognomonic sign. In humans, there is a trend towards visual diagnostic methods using caries detection (dyes, lasers, illumination systems), to avoid damaging the tooth surface by penetration with an explorer. However, in veterinary patients this is not a significant factor due to the large surface areas that are generally involved. Caries detection dyes that stain denatured collagen in dentin can be helpful, but they do not reliably distinguish between infected dentin that needs to be removed, and affected (but not infected) dentin that can be left behind. Practically, if the dentin can be easily removed with a caries curette, then it should be removed. If it is hard, it can be left. In dogs, radiographs are not helpful to diagnose the existence of dental caries, but radiographs are very important to determine whether the endodontic system has been infected.

MANAGEMENT

Teeth with caries lesions should be radiographed to determine the health of the endodontium. Carious lesions which do not involve the pulp are treated by removal of the infected dental tissue using an excavator, a dental drill, or air abrasion unit, followed by placement of a restoration. Bonded posterior composite resin fillings are probably the best material for this procedure due to their ability to preserve maximum tooth structure and to bond the crown and restorative together as a unit. However, amalgam is also a very functional restorative material (**184**). A circular lucency around any of the root tips is evidence of endodontic involvement. If the caries removal or cavity preparation instruments enter

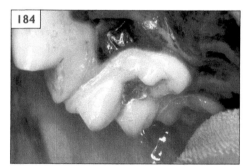

184 Amalgam restoration after removal of an occlusal caries lesion.

the pulp chamber during removal of the infected tooth material, that is also an indicator that the pulp is infected. An affected tooth with endodontic involvement should either be extracted or have root canal treatment prior to restoration (**185–187**).

KEY POINTS

- Dark brown lesions on the occlusal surfaces or contact surfaces of molar teeth in dogs may be caries lesions.
- If an explorer easily penetrates and sticks to this surface, then the tooth should be radiographed and treated with caries removal and restoration.

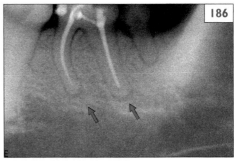

186 Radiograph of the tooth in **185** demonstrating caries-induced endodontic infection (periapical lucencies associated with both root apices, arrows) and endodontic treatment.

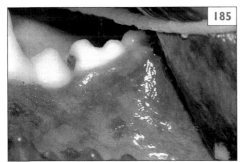

185 'Smooth surface' caries lesion on the interproximal surface of a left mandibular second molar tooth.

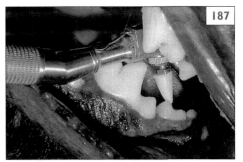

187 Finishing the posterior bonded composite resin restoration for the tooth in **185**.

Type 1 feline tooth resorption (TR)

(Feline odontoclastic resorptive lesions [FORLs], resorptive lesions [RLs], odontoclastic resorptive lesions, cervical lesions, neck lesions, and many other terms.)

DEFINITION

Noncarious odontoclastic destruction of cat teeth that does not result in replacement of the tooth roots by bone.

ETIOLOGY AND PATHOGENESIS

Feline dental TRs are described as either type 1 or type 2 depending on their radiographic appearance[9]. It is possible the two types could be different manifestations with a common etiology or may represent many different processes, but the separation into these categories is therapeutically useful. The periodontal ligament and roots remain distinct on radiographs of teeth with type 1 lesions, while the ligament and roots of teeth with type 2 lesions become radiographically indistinct as they are replaced by bone. Although there are many hypotheses, the cause of TRs in cats has not been proven. Inflammation associated with periodontal infection is a known cause of external root resorption in all species. This is a likely cause of many type 1 TRs. It is also probable that some type 1 TRs share the same etiology as type 2 lesions, but continued root resorption is prevented by inflammation or some other different physiological activity. Some apparent type 1 TRs may be in the process of becoming type 2 lesions but the radiographic changes to the roots are not yet visible. The incipient lesion is a defect in the cementum. Odontoclasts destroy dentin, and enamel is also lost to create a resorption lacuna. The crown ultimately fractures due to the weakened tooth, leaving the roots intact. The roots may act as a nidus of infection.

CLINICAL FEATURES

Type 1 resorptions commonly begin on the coronal third of the root, but can also begin further apically. However, they become first clinically visible on the crown as the internal resorption reaches the enamel. Cats with type 1 lesions often concurrently have periodontal disease and associated inflammation. Calculus may cover the lesion and may need to be removed before it becomes visible. The cervical defect that becomes apparent clinically often indicates a much larger subgingival defect. Hyperplastic inflamed gingiva often conceals the defect. Although many affected cats show no outward clinical signs, TRs have been reported to cause anorexia, ptyalism, lethargy, depression, dysphagia, halitosis, and discomfort.

DIFFERENTIAL DIAGNOSIS

- Type 2 TRs.
- Gingivitis or periodontitis without resorption.
- Furcation exposure in a multiroot tooth giving the appearance of a hole in the tooth.
- Gingival hyperplasia or mass lesion.
- Fractured or chipped tooth.

DIAGNOSTIC TESTS

Many TRs can become quite large before they show any clinical evidence. It is very important to perform a thorough oral examination on all cats since TRs are very prevalent. Clinical observation of a resorption defect on the teeth close to the gingival margin is pathognomonic for TRs. The lesion generally has a sharp enamel ledge around the periphery. Determination of whether a lesion is type 1 or type 2 requires a dental radiograph. The roots of teeth with type 1 TRs have an intact and identifiable periodontal ligament and a similar radiopacity to the roots of the adjacent teeth (**188**)[9]. Missing teeth should

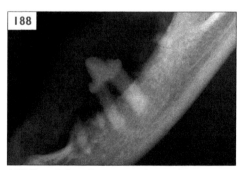

188 Type 1 dental resorptive lesions have destroyed the crowns of the third premolar tooth and the molar tooth. Both roots of the missing premolar and the distal (caudal) root of the molar tooth demonstrate normal radiodensity and a clearly identifiable periodontal ligament.

prompt radiographic investigation. Marked inflammation around teeth alerts the clinician to inspect the site with a dental explorer (**189**). Not all type 1 TRs are accompanied by gingivitis, so every TR must be radiographed (**190, 191**). Cats with an associated severe gingivitis should also be tested for diabetes, retrovirus, renal failure, and other conditions that can contribute to oral inflammation.

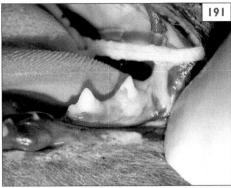

191 Clinical appearance of the mandible in **190**. The gingival tissue within the resorption defect appears noninflamed.

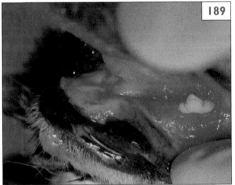

189 Clinical appearance of the mandible in **188**. Severe gingival inflammation is present.

MANAGEMENT

Extraction of the tooth is the only reliable treatment[9]. The roots are not being clearly replaced by bone as in type 2 lesions and often have associated pathology, so they must be completely removed.

KEY POINTS

- Radiographs are required to differentiate type 1 from type 2 TRs.
- Teeth with type 1 TRs must be completely extracted with no root remnants left in the alveolus. (See Appendix, p. 246 for explanation of the stages of tooth resorption.)

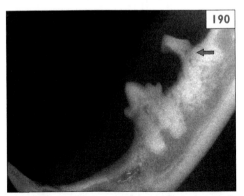

190 Radiograph of a mandible in which the third premolar (on the left) is missing due to previous extraction, the fourth premolar appears normal, and the molar (tooth on the right) has a large type 1 TR (arrow).

Type 2 feline tooth resorption (TR)

(Feline odontoclastic resorptive lesions, cervical lesions, neck lesions, invasive resorptions, and many others.)

DEFINITION
Noncarious odontogenic destruction of cat teeth that result in replacement of the roots by bone.

ETIOLOGY AND PATHOGENESIS
The etiology of type 2 TRs remains unproven. One popular theory involves the fact that cat teeth are not designed to masticate hard food. When sectorial teeth bite down on hard dietary materials, the food items can apply lateral forces to the crown tips. These forces are concentrated at the point where the unsupported crown meets the firmly supported root, causing an 'abfraction' injury[10]. This initial insult exposes dentin to the cells that begin odontolysis. Abfraction is also considered the cause for very similar lesions in humans. In addition to these lesions, humans also develop a different type of cervical lesion from aggressive tooth brushing with abrasive pastes. However, these lesions have a different and distinct appearance with a smooth sclerotic dentin. The abfraction lesions in human teeth appear clinically identical to feline TRs, and occur as both type 1 and type 2 lesions.

Another theory regarding the etiology of type 2 TRs involves the process of cementum repair. Normally the cementum develops microscopic areas of injury that repair without incident[11]. It has been proposed that high levels of dietary vitamin D may contribute to the marked resorption of roots in cats that develop TRs[12]. According to this theory the excess levels of vitamin D changes the normal physiological response of cementum repair to a pathological response of root resorption and replacement. Type 2 TRs show histologic evidence of simultaneous repair of the defect by osteoblasts at the same time that tooth structure is being resorbed by odontoclasts. Over time, the root is completely replaced by normal bone. The root canal and peripulpal dentin are often spared until late in the process. Surprisingly, in the absence of a concurrent complicated fracture, endodontic infection rarely occurs in type 2 lesions in spite of chronic exposure of pulp elements. A granuloma, which is often firmly attached to the dentin with thick collagen bundles, routinely fills the resorption lacuna.

CLINICAL FEATURES
The lower third premolar is commonly the first tooth to be affected. Type 2 TRs often begin at the CEJ close to the gingival margin, or 'neck' of the tooth[8]. Cats with one TR are at higher risk for developing additional lesions. Early lesions may appear only as localized, marginal gingivitis in a mouth that has very little inflammation in other areas. A sharp dental explorer will catch on the sharp enamel perimeter, differentiating a lesion from a normal furcation or periodontal pocket. Larger lesions will extend above the gingival margin (**192**). More advanced type 2 TRs often appear to have gingiva or granulation tissue growing up onto the tooth crown. This is particularly true of the canine teeth. The affected gingiva is commonly quiet and not inflamed, but can also be friable and inflamed (**193**). In end-stage lesions, the gingiva grows over the site. The alveolar ridge develops a convex shape in these areas, distinguishing them from tooth loss caused by periodontal disease or previous extraction. In humans, extraoral TRs (those that are completely subgingival in the sulcus or further apical on the root) often cause no discomfort[13]. Once they

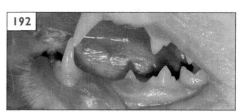

192 Left mandibular third premolar tooth with a type 2 TR. The inflammation at the site of the lesion is very localized. The gingiva around the unaffected teeth appears quiet and healthy.

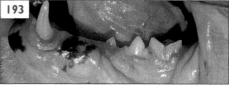

193 Marked gingivitis around the affected third premolar.

progress to extend into the oral cavity, they can become sensitive. It can be speculated that similar lesions in cats may cause comparable amounts of discomfort. Cats, however, frequently show no clinical signs[27]. The tissue filling the resorption lacuna would be expected to provide some protection from sensitivity.

DIFFERENTIAL DIAGNOSIS
- Type 1 TR.
- Gingivitis.
- Furcation exposure of a multirooted tooth.
- Fractured tooth.
- Gingival mass or hyperplasia.

DIAGNOSTIC TESTS
Clinical observation of a defect on the tooth surface, or gingival upgrowth onto the crown, is an indicator of a TR. Radiographically, the roots of teeth affected by type 2 TRs appear to be disappearing, i.e. they are less radiodense than the roots of adjacent teeth (**194–196**). The periodontal ligament disappears, and the root structure becomes hard to identify. In end-stage lesions, there is no longer any evidence of tooth structure visible on a radiograph, other than the signature convex alveolar ridge margin.

MANAGEMENT
Teeth with intraoral resorptions (lesions exposed to the oral cavity) should either be extracted or treated with crown amputation. Restoration of any TR carries a poor long-term prognosis due to the fact that the resorptive process continues, and that the visible intraoral lesion normally represents only a small part of the actual pathology.

Crown amputation of teeth with type 2 lesions results in less trauma to the patient, with faster and superior healing than full extraction[14]. Crown amputation can only be performed on teeth with confirmed type 2 TRs that show no periapical or periodontal bone loss and with roots that are becoming quietly radiolucent[15]. This surgical technique involves reflecting very small flaps on the buccal (vestibular) and lingual/palatal gingiva, and then using a new high speed bur to remove the entire crown to the level of the alveolar bone. Surgery is completed by placing one suture to close the gingiva, and applying gentle pressure for 20–30 seconds. Crown amputation should not be done for teeth with type 1 lesions, as pathology, inflammation, or infection should never be buried. Furthermore,

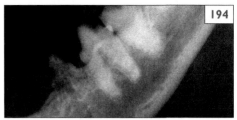

194 Radiograph of the cat in **193** showing type 2 TR. The roots of the third premolar tooth are less radiopaque compared to the normal roots of the fourth premolar tooth (center).

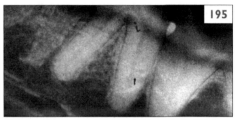

195 Mandibular third premolar tooth (left) has an advanced type 2 TR.

196 Mandibular canine tooth with a type 2 TR. The crown of the left mandibular (on the right of picture) has a lucency, and the root is less radiopaque than the contralateral canine tooth.

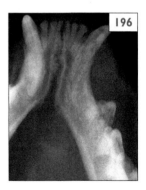

it should not be performed in patients with any evidence of inflammation in the caudal tissues between the upper and lower molar teeth (see diseases of the gingiva), or that are known to be positive for retrovirus.

KEY POINT
- Crown amputation is the treatment of choice when radiographs have proven a TR to be type 2 and other selection criteria are favorable (i.e. no periodontal or endodontic infection)[9].

Enamel hypoplasia and hypocalcification

DEFINITION

Defective or incomplete development of the enamel.

ETIOLOGY AND PATHOGENESIS

Enamel is formed in two stages by a layer of cells called ameloblasts. The first stage involves the production of all the enamel of the tooth as a partially mineralized organic matrix. The second step is the maturation and mineralization of the previously formed material. Interference with amelogenesis results in either the lack of enamel formation or abnormal enamel formation[16]. This occurs at the site of, and during the period of, the interference. Environmental, or chronologic, enamel hypoplasia is the type most commonly seen in dogs[4]. Environmental hypoplasia occurs when the patient experiences a systemic syndrome which damages the cells of the enamel organ or impedes their function. Any syndrome that affects the health of generalized epithelial tissues can potentially cause this. Local trauma or infection can also interfere with one or more teeth in a single location. Renal failure in young animals can result in hypocalcification due to secondary calcium deficiency during amelogenesis. In humans, the hereditary disorder amelogenesis imperfecta can cause enamel hypoplasia, hypomineralization, or hypomaturation[17,18]. The hypoplastic type results in generalized thin and irregular or pitted enamel. The hypocalcified type results in discolored enamel that is soft and crumbly. Finally, the hypomaturation type results in enamel that is normal in size and shape, is white and opaque, but easily chipped and can be pierced by an explorer[16,17]. Clinically, we see syndromes in dogs that resemble the hypoplastic and hypocalcified types, but these may be forms of early-insult environmental forms. These hereditary forms have not been documented in dogs.

CLINICAL FEATURES

Enamel is very hard and white with a smooth surface. Dentin is softer and tan with a rough surface. Chronologic hypoplasia is bilaterally symmetric. A very common pattern of affected enamel involves all the teeth except the four first premolar teeth. This indicates the insult occurred after the enamel was completed on the

unaffected teeth but before the enamel was formed on the affected teeth. This is associated with the timing of enamel formation at around 3 months of age when a puppy's maternal immunity wanes, increasing their risk for infections such as distemper and other viruses that can have this effect. Surfaces of teeth that lack enamel will appear rough and tan. Often, the area of missing enamel forms a band around the teeth with areas of grossly normal enamel above and/or below the band (**197**). Dogs can also have a complete absence of all enamel on all teeth similar to amelogenesis imperfecta (**198**). When the defect is caused by local trauma, only the small spot or region of trauma

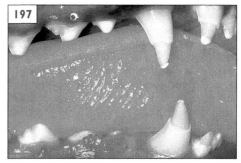

197 Environmental enamel hypoplasia. The linear band of affected enamel indicates the insult to amelogenesis occurred after the enamel was formed on the crown tips, and was resolved during formation of the marginal half of the crowns.

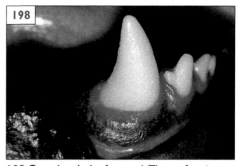

198 Complete lack of enamel. The surface is rough and softer than enamel. This is clinically similar to a hereditary form of enamel hypoplasia in humans.

will be affected (**199, 200**). The pattern of affected enamel indicates the timing of the insult. If the enamel that is present is poorly mineralized due to interruption during the later phases of formation, it can appear normal at first but be poorly attached and easily dislodged. Exposed dentin will accumulate plaque and calculus much faster than a normal tooth due to the plaque-retentive nature of a rough surface. Humans that have exposed dentin experience tooth sensitivity caused by hydrostatic intratubular pressure acting on the odontoblast cell processes[16,19].

DIFFERENTIAL DIAGNOSIS
- Odontodysplasia.
- Extrinsic staining.
- Intrinsic staining.
- Dental trauma from chewing abrasive material.

DIAGNOSTIC TESTS
The gross clinical appearance is diagnostic for abnormal enamel formation. Radiographs should be taken to evaluate endodontic health and to determine whether there has also been abnormal dentin formation, as would occur in odontodysplasia[8]. The roots of teeth affected with only enamel hypoplasia appear normal on radiographs, whereas hypoplastic or absent roots indicate a more severe problem.

MANAGEMENT
Affected teeth should be cleaned and all poorly attached enamel removed using an ultrasonic scaler. The exposed dentin is then acid etched to open the dentin tubules and a bonding agent or dentin sealant is applied to all affected areas to occlude the dentin tubules. This prevents tooth sensitivity and the ingress of bacteria to the pulp and, at least temporarily, provides a smooth surface[16]. For strategic teeth, placement of a layer of bonded composite resin provides a more enduring surface but may wear and chip over time and require replacement (**201**). Restorative treatment also provides an esthetic and mechanical improvement for large lesions. Hypoplastic teeth do not commonly have endodontic involvement due to the dentin defect, but if they do, endodontic treatment or extraction is indicated.

KEY POINTS
- Teeth with enamel hypoplasia rapidly accumulate plaque and calculus.
- Enamel hypoplasia also has the potential to cause sensitivity and pulpitis.
- Application of a dentin sealant, and possibly a surface restorative, can alleviate and prevent these problems.

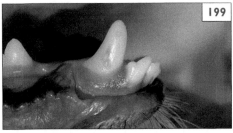

199 Focal enamel defects caused by local trauma during amelogenesis.

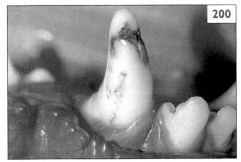

200 More severe trauma-induced enamel defects with secondary stains.

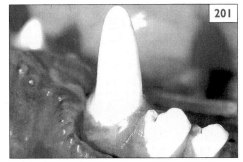

201 Postoperative appearance of the tooth in **200** after sealant and restoration.

Dental abrasion

DEFINITION

A dental abrasion is the loss of tooth structure through wear against materials other than the opposing dentition.

ETIOLOGY AND PATHOGENESIS

Rubbing the teeth against any hard or abrasive object wears them down. The more abrasive the surface and the more aggressive and/or constant the force, the faster the abrasion will occur. Dog teeth have much thinner enamel than human teeth. In addition, after the enamel has been worn through, the subjacent dentin is much less wear-resistant than the enamel. Abrasions in dogs typically result from biting or pulling against chain link fences or crate doors, chewing on flat items such as their skin or dirt, and excessive play with any abrasive toy such as tennis or rubber balls. When dirt or sand adheres to the toys, they become even more abrasive. Recently, more cases of excessive wear caused by owners scaling their pets' teeth are being seen.

CLINICAL FEATURES

The pattern of abrasional wear usually reveals the cause. Flattened tips of the canine teeth and premolar teeth indicate excessive wear on an object such as a tennis ball or rubber ball (**202, 203**). As the tooth wears, the pulp is stimulated to form tertiary (reparative) dentin, which is a darker color. As the worn surface extends into this dentin, a brown circular spot appears in the center of the worn face corresponding to the receding pulp cavity or pulp horn. If the abrasion proceeds slowly enough for the pulp to respond and effectively recede behind its 'bandage', the tooth may remain vital. The response can be dramatic; multirooted teeth can wear through the furcation, effectively 'cuspidizing' the tooth into two separate teeth while the pulp remains vital in each separate root. If the abrasion occurs more rapidly than the pulp can recede, the pulp is exposed and becomes infected and necrotic (**204**). Wear on the labial (lateral) tips of the canine teeth typifies abrasion from playing with a soccer ball or basket ball. Incisor teeth that are all (both maxillary and mandibular) worn at an angle facing labially (forwards) is a common feature of dogs with severe pruritis from a skin allergy. With allergic skin-biters, the pulps are often exposed yet typically remain vital. Although these pulps are alive, they are irreversibly inflamed, and the roots can become super-erupted as the apical tissues push them from their alveoli. A crescent-shaped wear lesion on the

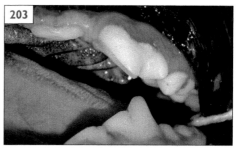

203 Close up of the curved abrasion on the mesial surface of the upper fourth premolar tooth.

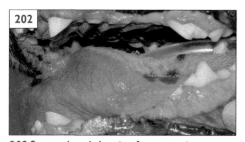

202 Severe dental abrasion from carrying a tennis ball. The distal (caudal) surface of the canine tooth and mesial (rostral) surface of the fourth premolar tooth have curved defects. The first three premolar teeth are worn flat.

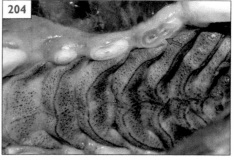

204 Abrasion has exposed the pulp on the third premolar tooth (arrow). The black holes are necrotic pulp tissue.

distal (back) surface of the canine tooth is a common finding in dogs that bite or pull on chain link fences or cage doors (**205**). This wear pattern weakens the tooth by thinning the crown, and creates a stress-riser at the junction of the apical third and middle third of the tooth, thus eventually fracturing off the coronal two-thirds of the crown. One of the most common abrasion lesions in humans is a cervical line lesion caused by aggressive tooth brushing with abrasive toothpaste[20]. Our veterinary patients do not routinely suffer from this problem, as unfortunately toothbrushing is not commonly performed. However, some owners can become quite aggressive with dental scalers during attempts to clean normal developmental grooves (**206**).

DIFFERENTIAL DIAGNOSIS
- Dental attrition.
- Fractured teeth.
- Developmental anomalies.
- Poorly erupted teeth.

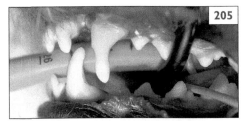

205 Fence-biting abrasion on the distal surface of the maxillary and mandibular canine teeth. There is also abrasion on the mesial surface of the maxillary canine tooth where the fence wears between the upper and lower teeth.

DIAGNOSTIC TESTS
Radiographs should be made of severely worn teeth to assess the endodontic health. Worn surfaces should be evaluated with a dental explorer to check for any pulp exposure.

MANAGEMENT
Dentin exposed through abrasion usually has a sclerotic surface that self-seals the dentin tubules, which prevents the sensitivity and risk of infection, in contrast to dentin exposed by fractures. Therefore, there is no need to seal the dentin. Behavioral modification, if possible, should be implemented to prevent continued damage. Abrasional wear can be decreased by varying the size, shape, and textures of toys which helps to spread the wear pattern to different teeth and surfaces. Timed, supervised play periods rather than unlimited carrying of favorite toys can also help to decrease the amount of wear. Pruritic patients should be treated for the cause of their pruritis. Fence-biters can be difficult to manage. Ideally they should not have access to chain link fencing or other materials that they can pull at with their teeth. Full coverage crowns, with a hard material like nickel chromium or titanium, will help slow the wear. However, obsessive ball-players can wear through these crowns over time. Full-coverage crowns will also slow the wear caused by biting fences and will protect the teeth from mid-crown fractures (**207**).

KEY POINTS
- Identification and elimination of the abrasive object and contributing behaviors are vital in stopping the process.
- Placement of a crown with a build-up of hard wear-resistant metal at the site of the abrasion will slow the damage.

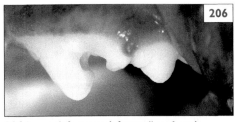

206 Large defect on a left maxillary fourth premolar tooth caused by abrasion by frequent and aggressive use of a dental scaler hand instrument by the owner.

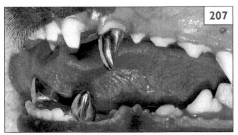

207 Crowns on all four canine teeth of a Jack Russell Terrier to slow the wear damage to the teeth.

Dental attrition

DEFINITION
The loss of tooth structure through wear against the opposing dentition during normal use or function.

ETIOLOGY AND PATHOGENESIS
The occlusal surfaces of teeth normally wear from contact against the opposing dentition and with abrasive food. In dogs and cats with normal occlusion, attrition is generally not clinically visible with the exception of the incisor teeth and the flat occlusal surfaces of the molar teeth. In older dogs, some attritional loss can occur on the labial aspect of the incisal ridge of the mandibular incisor teeth and the palatal aspect of the incisal ridge of the maxillary teeth. A level (or even) bite (mild mandibular mesiocclusion, class III malocclusion, or 'underbite') results in marked and progressive attrition of the incisor teeth. This is also true in humans[21]. Mild mandibular mesiocclusion also causes occlusal contact between the distal (back) surface of the maxillary third incisor teeth and the mesial (front) surface of the mandibular canine teeth, causing a flat or slightly concave worn area on the canine tooth and a curved loss of tooth from the back of the third incisor tooth. Various malocclusions will result in a pattern of attritional loss of tooth structure that is determined by the position and angle of the dental contact.

CLINICAL FEATURES
Incisor tooth attrition caused by a level (edge-to-edge) bite appears as flattened and angled occlusal surfaces of the incisor teeth, often with a 'wave' or 'step' pattern that corresponds to the shape of the opposing dentition (**208–210**). Incisor attrition from a normal scissors bite that slowly wears with advancing age appears as a wearing away of the palatal surface of the upper incisor teeth and the vestibular (labial) surface of the lower incisor teeth. A central brown spot corresponding to stained or tertiary dentin frequently appears in the center of the wear facet in the position where the coronal aspect of the pulp chamber once existed (**211**). The typical attrition of a mild mesiocclusion is seen as a very smoothly curved distal and palatal surface of the

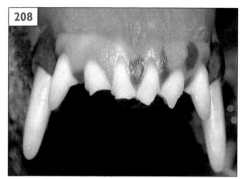

208 Attrition of maxillary incisor teeth. The incisal edge has an irregular pattern of damage that can be easily mistaken for fractures.

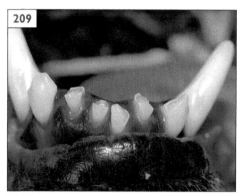

209 Severe wear of the crowns of the mandibular incisor teeth of the same dog as in **208**.

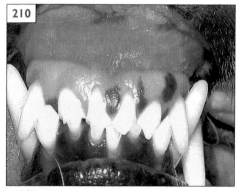

210 The jaws are held in maximal occlusion, showing the intercuspation of the maxillary and mandibular incisor teeth as they each wear against the opposing dentition.

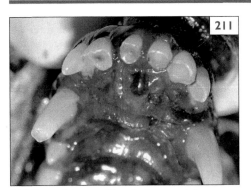

211 Four of the maxillary incisor teeth have marked attritional wear. The right first and second incisor teeth have necrotic pulps visible through the open pulp chambers. In contrast, the left first and second incisor teeth have apparently sufficient tertiary dentin.

contact tooth can be extracted to relieve the trauma and protect the more important contact tooth, but this is usually not necessary. Root canal treatment or extraction is indicated if there is pulp chamber exposure.

KEY POINTS
- Some amount of incisor and occlusal attrition is expected with age.
- The loss of tooth structure from attrition is accelerated or modified when malocclusions create areas of increased interdental contact.

third incisor teeth appearing thinner than expected with a sharp occlusal ridge. This is often accompanied by a wear facet on the lower third of the mesial (rostral) surface of the mandibular canine teeth.

DIFFERENTIAL DIAGNOSIS
- Dental abrasion.
- Fractured teeth.
- Anomalous teeth.

DIAGNOSTIC TESTS
Diagnosis is made through clinical observation. Holding the jaws closed in full occlusion will cause a perfect intercuspation of the worn occlusal surfaces with those of the opposing dentition. A dental explorer should be used to search for pulp chamber exposures.

MANAGEMENT
Intervention is generally not necessary unless the pulp chamber has been exposed. However, radiographs should be considered to rule out endodontic involvement. The dentin is sclerotic, similar to abrasion, and has an impervious surface. In cases where the traumatic occlusion is causing discomfort, the least important

External resorption

DEFINITION
Resorption that was initiated in the periodontal ligament or tissues surrounding the teeth.

ETIOLOGY AND PATHOGENESIS
External resorption is the process of breakdown of tooth substance by osteoclasts or odontoclasts in the periodontal ligament. Osteoclasts and odontoclasts may be the same cell. Odontoclasts are smaller with fewer nuclei, but this may be a result of the tissue being resorbed rather than an inherent difference in the cells. Regardless of the initiating cause, all root resorption is ultimately odontoclastic. Several mechanisms can initiate external resorption, including:

- Physiological resorption of deciduous tooth roots during normal exfoliation.
- Any source of chronic inflammation.
  - Lesions of endodontic origin, both root tip resorption and root resorption at the portals of exit of lateral canals along the root surface.
  - Periodontitis and purulent periodontal infections.
- Pressure resorption from adjacent structures such as impacted teeth or expanding cysts or tumors.
- Periodontal ligament trauma such as can occur with excessive orthodontic forces or reimplantation of avulsed teeth[22,23]. Root resorption is a common complication of orthodontic treatment in mature adult humans. At any age, excessive orthodontic force can induce inflammation in the periodontal ligament and cause damage to the ligament and cementum to stimulate resorption.
- Abfraction (see Type 2 feline tooth resorptive lesions, and Idiopathic root resorption) is also considered to be a type of external root resorption that progresses to an aggressive internal resorption.

CLINICAL FEATURES
External root resorption is not clinically visible unless the lesion extends up onto the crown of the tooth. However, external resorption can be initiated by some conditions that are visible intraorally such as periodontitis or endodontic disease from a fractured tooth. External resorption appears radiographically as variable areas of loss of exterior root structure. The normally smooth line of the root image will have a radiolucent defect extending into the root dentin. Inflammatory resorption from endodontic or periodontal infection is often accompanied by periradicular lucency of the bone in the immediate area (**212–215**). Pressure resorption is associated with a slowly expanding tumor or cyst, or a tooth exerting pressure against the root at the site. These are all easily identified clinically and/or radiographically. External root resorption is not inherently painful. However, periodontal abscess or endodontic infections and secondary inflammation from any process, can cause discomfort.

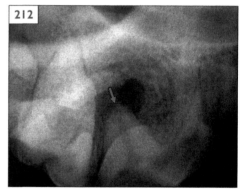

212 External root resorption (arrow) caused by inflammatory mediators exiting a diseased root canal. The adjacent lucency indicates bone destruction at the site of a lateral canal.

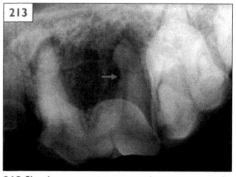

213 Slowly progressive external resorption with repair of the osseous defect (arrow).

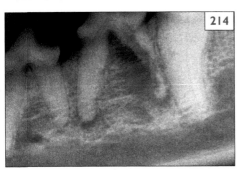

214 External root resorption from inflammation associated with periodontal infection.

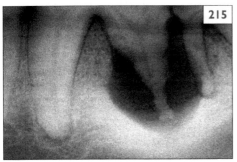

215 Severe external resorption on the distal root of the lower first molar tooth. This may be caused by inflammation from endodontic disease or from a periodontal infection.

DIFFERENTIAL DIAGNOSIS

- Radiographic pseudo-lesion caused by summation of overlying radiolucent structures such as foramina or fissures.
- Root surface calculus accumulation with bone resorption.

DIAGNOSTIC TESTS

Dental radiographs of fractured teeth, periodontally involved teeth, and oral swellings.

MANAGEMENT

Identify and remove or treat the cause of inflammation or pressure. Resorptions caused by lesions of endodontic origin are treated by root canal treatment or extraction (see Complicated tooth fractures). Intact teeth that are not fractured can also have endodontic disease, as significant external trauma can damage the pulp without fracturing the crown, causing irreversible pulpitis or pulp necrosis. Periodontal abscesses can be treated with open periodontal surgery or extraction. Dentigerous cysts are somewhat common in the mandible, particularly associated with embedded first premolar teeth. These can be very expansive and can cause dramatic root resorption as well as interference with the initial root formation. Complete removal of the cyst and its capsule will arrest the process of resorption. Tumors that cause external resorption will require removal of the affected teeth *en bloc* with the tumor and adequate margins. Impacted teeth that cause pressure resorption are less common in dogs and cats than in humans. This is a relatively common problem with human third molar teeth ('wisdom teeth'). It is sometimes seen in dogs with malpositioned canine teeth that can exert pressure on the third incisor teeth.

KEY POINTS

- External root resorption is caused by physiological or pathological processes occurring on the outside surface of the tooth root.
- Treating the inciting cause halts the resorption.

Internal resorption

DEFINITION
Tooth resorption which is initiated inside the pulp chamber or root canal.

ETIOLOGY AND PATHOGENESIS
Internal resorption is caused by inflammation of a vital pulp. Although mild pulpitis can stimulate an increased production of dentin, pulpitis can also cause localized spots of dentin resorption. The resorption occurs from the inside wall of the root canal or pulp chamber when the odontoblast layer has been disrupted and the pulp develops a granuloma[24]. Pulp is often necrotic coronal to the region of internal resorption. The resorption process can only occur while the area of pulp remains vital.

CLINICAL FEATURES
Internal resorption of the tooth crown can cause a 'pink spot' lesion where vital pulp tissue is visible through the remaining enamel. Severe internal crown resorption will weaken the crown and can eventually destroy the tooth. Internal resorption of the root canal is clinically unapparent and only found on radiographs. In humans, it is also asymptomatic and found on routine radiographs. A focal area of expansion in the root canal space or pulp chamber appears as an increased width or radiolucent defect over the pulp space (**216**). Some internal resorption lesions may not be readily visible until three-dimensional obturation with radiodense filling materials reveals the expanded area (**217**). This is one reason that chemical in addition to mechanical debridement is important during endodontic treatment, along with thermoplastic techniques during obturation. Conversely, in the same manner a lucency that appears to represent internal resorption can be shown to be unassociated with the root canal (**218, 219**).

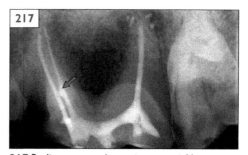

217 Radio-opaque obturating material has revealed an internal resorption lesion on the palatal root of the upper fourth premolar tooth (arrow). The resorption was not identified until the obturation phase of treatment.

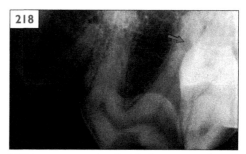

218 Lucency associated with the root canal of the distal root appears to be an internal resorption lesion (arrow).

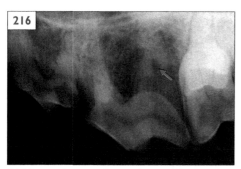

216 Internal resorption causing a mid-root lucency on the distal root of an upper fourth premolar tooth (arrow).

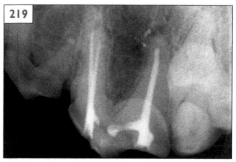

219 Postoperative radiograph shows no internal canal defect, and the slightly different tube angle moved the lucency away from the root canal space.

DIFFERENTIAL DIAGNOSIS

- External root resorption on the vestibular or lingual/palatal root surface.
- Summation effect of overlying radiolucent structures.

DIAGNOSTIC TESTS

All involved teeth should be radiographed. A second radiograph exposed from a different tube angle will differentiate the summation effect of an overlying external resorption or other structures from an internal resorption. An overlying lucency moves relative to the root canal, but an internal resorption preserves its association with the root canal.

MANAGEMENT

Root canal treatment will immediately halt internal resorption by removing the source of odontoclasts. Regional expanded spots of the root canal requires thermoplastic endodontic obturation to obtain a three-dimensional fill, or aggressive removal of coronal peripulpal dentin. Extraction is the other alternative.

KEY POINTS

- Internal root resorption occurs when a pulp is locally hyperplastic or vital but inflamed, destroying the dentin from the inside surface of the tooth.
- Endodontic treatment or extraction is curative.

Intrinsic stains (endogenous stains)

DEFINITION

Tooth discoloration from within the substance of the tooth.

ETIOLOGY AND PATHOGENESIS

The most common intrinsic stain seen in dogs is caused by a tooth receiving blunt trauma of sufficient force to cause pulp hemorrhage. Extravasated blood enters the dentin tubules where it degenerates. Intrinsic stains can also be caused by the deposition of substances not normally present in teeth from the circulation during tooth development. Tetracycline that is taken during tooth development causes a dark discoloration of the teeth that were developing at the time. This is caused by deposition of the tetracycline into the developing dentin and enamel[25]. Doxycycline produces less discoloration than tetracycline. In humans, excessive ingestion of fluoride during tooth development (flourosis) can cause discoloration and pitting.

CLINICAL FEATURES

A tooth stained by degenerating blood products following pulp hemorrhage appears pink immediately after the injury, and in time becomes darker brown or gray (**220**). Although dental pulp does have the ability to heal after injury if the damage was not too severe, most teeth with marked discoloration have suffered irreversible pulpitis that will progress to pulp necrosis.

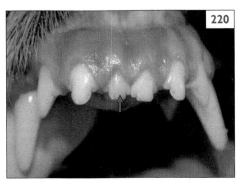

220 Previous pulp trauma. The crown of the right maxillary first incisor tooth (arrow) is darker than the adjacent teeth.

In cases of trauma, usually only one tooth is involved, but patients may present with more than one discolored tooth in the same area (**221**). Intrinsic stain caused by tetracycline or other incorporated substances affects all the teeth that were developing at the time of the exposure, and appears as varying degrees and shades of discoloration depending on the cause[25]. The enamel feels smooth and normal (**222**). In these cases, the stains are cosmetic without any effects on health, comfort, or function.

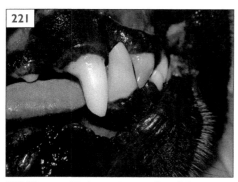

221 The mandibular canine tooth and the maxillary third incisor tooth are both discolored from previous pulp hemorrhage.

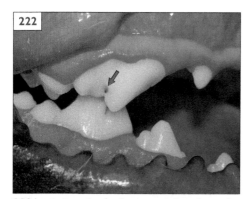

222 Intrinsic stain of unknown etiology (arrow). The stain is deep in the tooth and the enamel is smooth and normal.

DIFFERENTIAL DIAGNOSIS
- Extrinsic stains.
- Enamel hypoplasia.

DIAGNOSTIC TESTS
Clinical observation is diagnostic. The insult would have occurred previously and is likely only identifiable from the patient's history. Single teeth that have suffered pulp hemorrhage should be radiographed. Periapical or lateral radicular lucencies indicate endodontic pathology. A larger root canal diameter than the contralateral tooth indicates pulp necrosis. Radiographic evidence of a smaller diameter root canal space than the contralateral tooth indicates generalized pulpitis.

MANAGEMENT
Teeth with severe pulp hemorrhage are in general irreversibly inflamed or necrotic and should be treated with root canal treatment or extraction[26]. This is generally the case for individual teeth that are discolored due to traumatic pulp hemorrhage. For teeth that have become intrinsically stained by deposition of tetracycline or similar materials, intervention is not required. External bleaching and whitening techniques are ineffective. Internal (nonvital) bleaching can help esthetically, but this is not recommended for pets for several reasons. These reasons include: the need to devitalize healthy teeth, the necessity for multiple anesthetic episodes, and the fact that it weakens the teeth for cosmetic improvement with no health or functional benefit. Tetracycline staining can be prevented by avoiding its use in puppies or kittens less than 5 months of age or in pregnant animals.

KEY POINTS
- Intrinsic stains from pulp hemorrhage indicate a need for root canal or extraction.
- All intrinsically stained teeth should be radiographed.
- Generalized intrinsic staining is usually a cosmetic problem only.

Extrinsic stains (exogenous stains)

DEFINITION
Discoloration on the surface of teeth caused by factors or materials from outside the tooth.

ETIOLOGY AND PATHOGENESIS
Extrinsic stains can be caused by pigments in the diet or other ingested items, or by the by-products of bacteria in plaque. Regular and prolonged use of chlorhexidine products as an oral disinfectant can also cause extrinsic stains. Chewing on fencing or other metal objects can burnish a metallic stain onto the enamel surface.

CLINICAL FEATURES
Black, brown, green, silver or orange discoloration on the surface of the tooth is easily distinguished from the deeper intrinsic stain on close examination (**223**). Extrinsic stains are often darkest on the buccal/vestibular aspects of the premolar and molar teeth, with the exception of metal stains that can also be pronounced on the canine teeth and incisor teeth.

DIFFERENTIAL DIAGNOSIS
• Intrinsic stains.
• Enamel hypoplasia.
• Pulp hemorrhage.
• Abrasion.

DIAGNOSTIC TESTS
Clinical observation of topical stains on a normal enamel surface that can be scratched or polished off is diagnostic.

MANAGEMENT
Extrinsic stains can be removed using a rotary prophy angle with abrasive polish (**224**).

KEY POINTS
• Extrinsic stains are cosmetic in nature.
• They are easily removed by polishing.

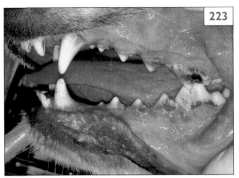

223 Extrinsic stains on the surface of the enamel.

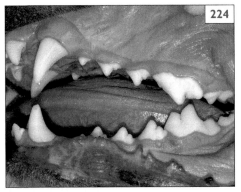

224 Extrinsic stains are easily removed with abrasive polish.

Primary endodontic lesion with secondary periodontal disease

(Endodontic-periodontal lesion, class I lesion.)

DEFINITION

Endodontic disease which has spread from the root apex along the periodontal ligament to establish a connection to the periodontal sulcus[8,27].

ETIOLOGY AND PATHOGENESIS

Chronic endodontic lesions establish drainage along the path of least resistance. This may be along the mucosa with an exit at the mucogingival line, or it may be into the nasal cavity or extraorally through the skin. On occasion, drainage may be along the periodontal ligament beside the tooth, eventually reaching the periodontal sulcus. Plaque and calculus then populate the defect, and the epithelial attachment migrates apically.

CLINICAL FEATURES

A cause of the primary endodontic disease is usually apparent, such as a crown fracture with pulp exposure or a discolored tooth from previous pulp trauma[27]. The periodontal attachment is healthy on all surfaces except the one area of drainage, so the tooth is nonmobile. Periodontal pocket measurement reveals an isolated abrupt and very deep periodontal pocket[27].

DIFFERENTIAL DIAGNOSIS

- Primary periodontal lesion with secondary endodontic involvement ('perio-endo' lesion).

DIAGNOSTIC TESTS

Dental radiographs show a radiolucent tract from the root apex along the root to the alveolar margin (**225**). There is no horizontal alveolar bone loss or radiographic evidence of periodontal disease other than the linear lucency along the root[27]. This is commonly known as a 'J lesion'[8]. Circumferential periodontal probing typically reveals a single very deep periodontal pocket with a narrow and abrupt sulcular orifice, while the remainder of the tooth has normal periodontal sulcus depth.

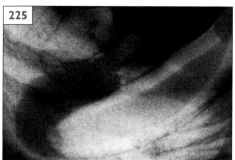

225 Endodontic-periodontal lesion. The large apical lucency extends coronally up the tooth towards the gingival margin. The radiograph shows convergence with the periodontium of the first premolar tooth. Clinically there was a deep periodontal pocket on the labial (lateral) side of the canine tooth that communicated with the endodontic defect. From DuPont G. and DeBowes L., (2009). *Atlas of Dental Radiography in Dogs and Cats*. p. 169, copyright Elsevier.

MANAGEMENT

Root canal treatment and appropriate periodontal treatment carries a good prognosis[8,27].

KEY POINT

- When the periodontal disease is secondary to a primary endodontic lesion, treatment has a good success rate.

Primary periodontal lesion with secondary endodontic involvement

(Periodontal-endodontic lesion, class II lesion.)

DEFINITION
Periodontal disease which has secondarily infected the endodontic system through the apical circulation, a lateral canal, or a furcation canal[8,27].

ETIOLOGY AND PATHOGENESIS
Root dentin is protected from infection by the cementum and surrounding tissues. When periodontitis destroys the cementum, infection can travel through any portal of endodontic access. Bacteria exposed to furcation canals, lateral canals, or the apical delta has access to the dental pulp[8,27]. The large surface area of unaffected roots on a multiroot tooth provide retention of the tooth even with severe chronic attachment loss on one or more other roots. This allows time for the bacterial infection to invade and kill the pulp while the tooth fails to exfoliate from the periodontal disease (**226, 227**).

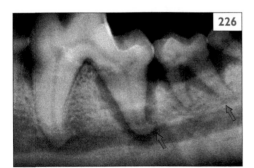

226 Perio-endo lesion. All three mandibular molar teeth have oblique, vertical, and horizontal bone loss, radiographic changes typical of periodontitis. The left mandibular first molar tooth (large tooth on the left) and the second molar tooth to the right have lucency extending to and around the root tip apex (arrows). There is periapical lucency around the root tips of the second root of each tooth, indicating spread of inflammation through the endodontic system.

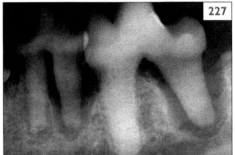

227 Perio-endo lesions. The left mandibular fourth premolar and first molar tooth each have one root completely devoid of attachment from periodontitis and bone loss, and a second root holding the tooth in position.

CLINICAL FEATURES

By the time periodontitis has progressed to this extent, teeth often (but not always) exhibit some mobility. Maxillary molars which have any mobility at all should be carefully evaluated periodontally and radiographically (**228, 229**). Periodontal probing reveals deep pockets and usually gingival recession typical of severe periodontitis. Periodontal disease that spreads to infect the dental pulp is a very common finding on both the maxillary and mandibular premolar and molar teeth of small breed dogs.

DIFFERENTIAL DIAGNOSIS

- Primary endodontic lesion with secondary periodontal disease (endodontic-periodontal lesion).
- Periodontal disease without endodontic involvement.

DIAGNOSTIC TESTS

Dental radiographs show alveolar bone loss typical of periodontitis, with oblique defects angled toward the roots. The infrabony pockets extend apically to meet an endodontic portal of vascular entry, and the root tips show periapical lucencies typical of endodontic involvement[27]. This endodontic pathology is seen with no other clinical evidence of a cause for endodontic disease (no fractured crown or pulp hemorrhage). Circumferential periodontal probing reveals multiple sites around the tooth of periodontal pocket formation, with a gradual deepening as the probe approaches the perio-endo defect.

MANAGEMENT

If the periodontal component is felt to be treatable, teeth can potentially be saved. In these cases, periodontal surgery combined with root canal treatment can be attempted but carries a poor prognosis[8]. Due to the severity of the periodontal component, extraction is generally the treatment of choice. Caution and gentle extraction technique are important when extracting mandibular canine and first molar teeth, since loss of mandibular bone can increase the risk of traumatic mandibular fracture during extraction. Multiroot teeth which have primary periodontal disease affecting only one or two roots can be salvaged by a combination of endodontic therapy and extraction. In these cases, endodontic treatment is performed on roots with healthy periodontal tissues; the tooth is sectioned and the periodontally affected crown-root segment or segments are extracted[8,27].

KEY POINTS

- Periodontitis that has become severe enough to infect the endodontic system is frequently associated with a periodontally hopeless tooth, necessitating extraction.
- In some cases, partial tooth extraction with root canal therapy on the periodontally healthy segment can salvage some tooth function.

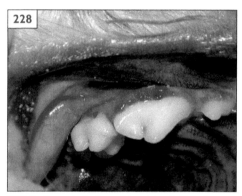

228 Perio-endo lesion with minimal clinical evidence. The right maxillary first molar tooth has some gingival recession and furcation involvement indicating periodontitis.

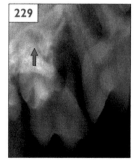

229 The radiograph of the tooth in **228** shows bone loss from periodontal disease extending around the apex of the mesio-buccal root, and a periapical circular lucency typical of endodontic disease around the palatal root tip (arrow).

Combined endodontic and periodontal lesion

(Class III periodontal-endodontic lesion.)

DEFINITION
These lesions have both an endodontic and periodontal component in which both lesions coevolved simultaneously and have merged[8,27].

ETIOLOGY AND PATHOGENESIS
The true combined lesion occurs when a patient develops periodontal disease and endodontic disease independently. As the pocket epithelial attachment migrates apically and the endodontic lesion dissects coronally, they meet along the periodontium.

CLINICAL FEATURES
This is a very unusual finding in animals. Endodontic disease in animals is generally traumatic in nature and uncommonly related to caries. When a periodontally compromised tooth sustains trauma, it often exfoliates rather than fractures. Conversely, dogs which are most prone to fracturing teeth are those that use them vigorously, helping control severe periodontitis through self-cleaning mechanisms.

DIFFERENTIAL DIAGNOSIS
- Primary endodontic lesion with secondary periodontal disease.
- Primary periodontal lesion with secondary endodontic involvement.

DIAGNOSTIC TESTS
Dental radiographs show changes typical of both periodontal disease and primary endodontic disease (**230**). There is generally an apparent cause for endodontic disease other than the periodontal disease (i.e. a fractured crown with exposed pulp, crown discoloration)[8,27]. Circumferential periodontal probing demonstrates areas of gently deepening periodontal pocket depths, and at least one site where the pocket is very deep.

MANAGEMENT
Root canal treatment and periodontal surgery can be attempted. However, it carries a guarded prognosis, depending on the severity of the periodontal disease and the ability of the owner to perform home oral hygiene[8,27]. Extraction is generally the appropriate treatment.

KEY POINTS
- True combined lesions are very rare.
- They can be treated with success, depending on the periodontal disease component.
- If the periodontal component is severe, extraction is the best alternative.

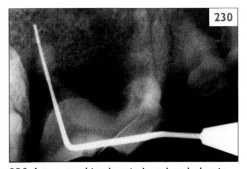

230 A true combined periodontal-endodontic lesion has two simultaneous problems that meet to form a single defect. True combined lesions are very unusual in animals. (Courtesy of Dr. Brook Niemiec.)

Idiopathic root resorption

DEFINITION

These are dental tooth resorptions (TRs) with no known etiology or identifiable cause. Although feline dental TRs are technically included in this category, the feline lesions are generally considered separately from those in dogs, humans, and other species.

ETIOLOGY AND PATHOGENESIS

Many TRs have unknown or unproven causes. Some examples in the human literature include cervical root resorption, invasive resorption, supraosseous extracanal resorption, and noncarious cervical lesions. These are separate from cervical lesions caused by tooth brush abrasion. A number of dental professionals now believe that some of these lesions in people are caused by abfraction. Abfraction occurs when lateral forces act on the teeth, for example those caused by malocclusion of parafunctional habits. Lateral forces cause microflexure of the crown. Stresses are concentrated at the cervical area where the unsupported crown joins the roots which are firmly supported by the alveolar bone, resulting in damage to the cementum and to the tooth. Whether abfraction is a factor for animals has not been proven, but seems likely. Idiopathic resorption in dogs appears identical to dental TRs in cats. The pulp is frequently spared, and some roots apparently disappear similar to type 2 TRs in cats, while others remain normal in the unaffected areas similar to type 1 TRs in cats. A granuloma firmly fills the resorption defect, and this granuloma can be friable and inflamed or firm and fibrotic. The lesion progresses to weaken the tooth which eventually fractures.

CLINICAL FEATURES

Lesions do not become clinically apparent until late in the course, eventually appearing at the gingival margin or as internal resorption under the enamel of the crown. Sharp enamel ledges border the enamel margins of the defect. Lesions are often found radiographically, with severe root involvement but minimal or no crown involvement (**231, 232**). If the spreading internal component of resorption undermines enamel, the lesion can initially appear as a pink spot on the crown. Patients frequently have more than one tooth affected with root resorption. This has also been reported in people[28]. Furthermore, in people, subgingival lesions are frequently found as incidental findings and are asymptomatic[29].

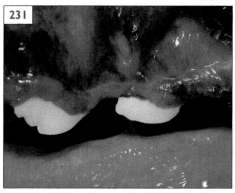

231 Idiopathic root resorption. Clinically the crowns of these maxillary second and third premolar teeth have coronal abrasional wear, but show few outward signs of resorption.

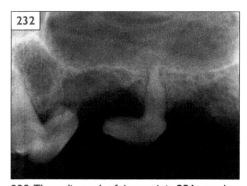

232 The radiograph of the teeth in **231** reveals extensive root resorption similar to type 2 resorption in cats; the distal (caudal) root of the second premolar tooth and the mesial (rostral) root of the third premolar tooth appears to have quietly disappeared.

DIFFERENTIAL DIAGNOSIS

- Cervical abrasion (**233**).
- Inflammatory resorption from periodontal inflammation.
- Caries.
- Crown fracture.
- Gingival mass.
- Gingival hyperplasia.
- Inflammatory resorption (either endodontic or periodontal origin).
- Pressure resorption from an expanding space-occupying lesion.

DIAGNOSTIC TESTS

Subgingival investigation with a dental explorer detects a deep defect on the root surface that bleeds easily. The explorer may also catch on the enamel margin. Clinical observation of gingiva growing up onto a tooth and nestled into a defect should prompt radiographic investigation. Dental radiographs show lucencies or irregularities in the root with or without concurrent endodontic disease. The roots can seem to disappear in chronic cases.

MANAGEMENT

Subgingival lesions that are identifiable only on radiographs (extraoral) are most likely asymptomatic[29]. No treatment is required, but the owner should be advised of the finding and understand that the process will likely continue and eventually require treatment. Teeth with lesions that are clinically observable should be extracted. Ankylosis can make these extractions challenging, similar to type 2 TRs in cats. Endodontic treatment and restoration can also be performed, but the resorption process can continue around a restoration if there is any source of odontoclasts. Even after root canal treatment, odontoclasts can be recruited from the periodontal tissues.

KEY POINTS

- The term idiopathic root resorption is a term used for TRs in dogs that appear in every way similar to feline TRs.
- Some of these lesions appear identical to human 'abfraction' lesions.
- Subgingival lesions are typically asymptomatic.
- Lesions with an oral component may cause discomfort and the affected teeth should be extracted.

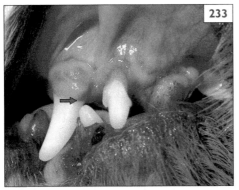

233 Cervical abrasion (arrow). This lesion is similar to toothbrush abrasion commonly seen in humans and is not resorption.

CHAPTER 6

Problems with the Gingiva

Linda DeBowes

- **Gingivitis**

- **Periodontitis**

- **Generalized gingival enlargement (gingival hyperplasia)**

- **Trauma**

- **Epulids**

- **Gingivostomatitis (caudal stomatitis) in cats**

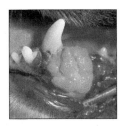 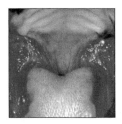 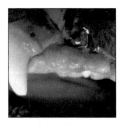 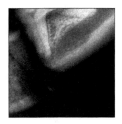

Gingivitis

DEFINITION

Gingivitis refers to any inflammation of the gingiva; however, the term is usually used to refer to plaque bacterial-induced gingivitis.

ETIOLOGY AND PATHOGENESIS

Plaque bacteria, a susceptible host, and the host's inflammatory response are all factors in the initiation and development of gingivitis. Bacterial plaque accumulates on the tooth surface and directly, as well as indirectly, stimulates a host inflammatory response. Supragingival plaque initially forms, and if not removed within a few days, it will initiate an inflammatory response within the marginal gingiva (marginal gingivitis). Bacterial plaque forms a biofilm that adheres tenaciously to the tooth surface providing protection against antimicrobial agents. Undisturbed supragingival plaque bacteria continues to mature and will extend subgingivally. Supragingival plaque is primarily a gram-positive aerobic bacterial population, whereas subgingival plaque bacteria are a more prominent population of gram-negative and anaerobic bacteria[1]. If subgingival plaque persists, it can lead to chronic gingivitis and the potential development of periodontitis.

Factors that enhance plaque accumulation will favor the development of gingivitis. Crowding of teeth, subgingival foreign bodies, trauma, roughened tooth surfaces, and restorations may all enhance plaque accumulation. Diseases or drugs that alter the host inflammatory response may also predispose to the development of gingivitis[2].

The level of the epithelial attachment of the gingiva to the tooth surface is not altered in gingivitis. This means that there is no attachment loss, no periodontal pocket formation, and gingivitis is completely reversible with removal of subgingival plaque[3].

CLINICAL FEATURES

Normal gingival tissues have thin and sharp margins, which are coral pink in color (unless normal pigmentation is different) (**234**). In gingivitis, plaque and calculus may be visible adjacent to the gingival tissues. The initial inflammation of the gingiva results in erythema and rounding of the gingival margins (**235–238**). As inflammation increases, the gingiva bleeds

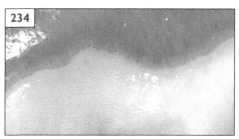

234 Normal gingiva, with thin, sharp margins.

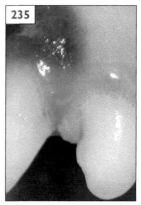

235 Normal gingiva over incisor, gingivitis (rounding of margins) in interdental papilla.

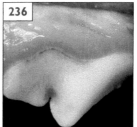

236 Mild plaque, calculus, mild gingivitis.

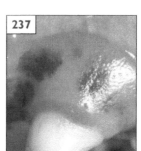

237 Marginal gingivitis, calculus.

more readily and the erythema may extend to the entire attached gingiva (**239–241**). The owners may report gingival bleeding by the animal during tooth brushing, when eating hard foods, chewing on hard objects, or playing with toys (**242, 243**). Halitosis is often a clinical feature of gingivitis. The depth of the gingival sulcus remains within normal limits, which is generally considered to be less than 3 mm in the dog and less than 0.5 mm in the cat[4]. The gingival sulcus may be increased in patients with periodontal disease limited to gingivitis, when chronic gingival inflammation results in gingival hyperplasia and pseudopocket formation.

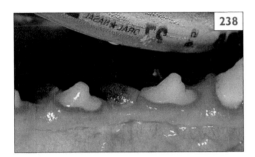

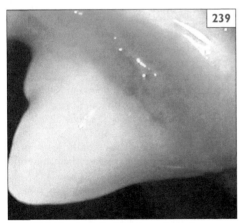

238, 239 Marginal gingivitis, rounded edges.

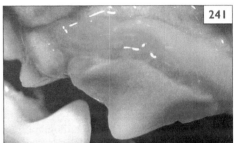

241 Gingivitis as evidenced by the severe plaque and calculus, gingivitis, erythema, and rounding of the gingival edges. Note that at the level of the first molar, the entire attached gingiva is inflamed.

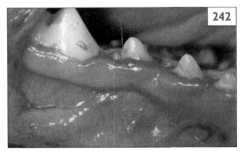

242 Gingival bleeding in advanced gingivitis.

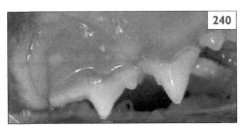

240 Gingivitis in a cat, with little attached gingiva. The entire attached gingiva may be inflamed.

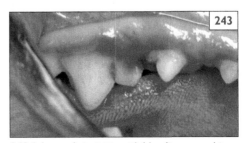

243 Advanced gingivitis, with bleeding on probing.

DIFFERENTIAL DIAGNOSIS

- Periodontitis.
- Subgingival foreign bodies.
- Subgingival root pathology (e.g. root fracture).
- Trauma.
- Tooth resorption.
- Neoplasia.

DIAGNOSTIC TESTS

Gingivitis is primarily a clinical diagnosis made after performing a complete oral examination. Gingivitis is diagnosed when the inflammation is limited to the gingiva, while the other parts of the periodontium (cementum, periodontal ligament, alveolar and surrounding bone) are not affected. A periodontal probe is used to evaluate the depth of the gingival sulcus and assess bleeding on probing. A dental explorer is used to probe the furcation area and to evaluate for subgingival calculus, tooth resorption, or other irregularities. Dental radiographs are indicated in the evaluation of tooth resorption, mobile teeth, or any firm swellings associated with the gingival inflammation. Infrequently, histopathological examination is indicated when it appears that the gingival inflammation may not be from periodontal disease.

MANAGEMENT

The approach to managing gingivitis includes treatment and prevention. Marginal gingivitis, with only supragingival plaque, can often be resolved with daily tooth brushing. If daily tooth brushing does not resolve the gingivitis, there is probably subgingival plaque or calculus that needs to be removed with professional cleaning. Plaque becomes mineralized within a few days, and is then referred to as calculus (or tartar). When plaque has migrated subgingivally, and/or calculus has formed, a professional cleaning is required. Physical removal of supragingival and subgingival plaque and calculus will result in resolution of the gingivitis.

Scaling of the teeth to remove plaque and calculus is done with mechanical and/or hand scalers. Mechanical scalers include piezoelectric and magnetostrictive scalers. The magnetostrictive scalers have either a stack-type insert or a ferrite rod. The tip of the magnetostrictive scalers with the ferrite rods move in a circular fashion and therefore have activity on all sides. This is in contrast to the magnetostrictive scalers with the stacks; these move in a figure-of-eight action and are active only on the sides of the tips. Piezoelectric scalers have ceramic crystals that are stimulated by an electric pulse causing the tip to vibrate. The tip of a piezoelectric scaler moves in a liner fashion back and forth and the sides of the tip are active[5]. The performance of the scaler may be adversely affected when the tip becomes worn, and replacing the tip will then be necessary[6]. The lavage fluid used to cool the instrument tip combined with the cavitational activity of the tip causes disruption of the weak and unattached subgingival plaque[7].

Important points to remember when using the mechanical scalers are[4]:

- Proper use of the mechanical scalers involves using the side of the tip to contact the tooth. The final 1–3 mm of the side of the tip provides the maximum vibration and therefore maximum efficiency for calculus removal.
- Do not place the pointed end of the tip of the instrument directly onto the tooth at a perpendicular angle. The tip of the instrument does not provide any beneficial action and if used against the tooth surface may cause damage.
- Heat is generated along the tip that may cause damage if the instrument is left on the tooth for too long (no more than 5–7 seconds per tooth is a general guideline).
- Water acts to cool the tip of the instrument as well as helping to remove the plaque and calculus.
- Be gentle so that the soft tissues are not damaged by the instrument.

Hand instruments which are commonly used include a scaler for supragingival use, and a curette for subgingival as well as supragingival use. Curettes have a rounded tip and edges, which are less damaging to the soft tissues than scalers. Hand instruments are used after the mechanical instruments have removed the majority of the plaque and calculus. Scaling with mechanical and hand instruments may roughen the enamel making it more plaque retentive. For this reason, the teeth should always be polished after scaling to smooth the enamel surface[4].

Polishing is done using a fine-grit polishing paste, applied with a polishing cup on a prophy-angle attached to a slow speed hand piece. Heat is generated when polishing the teeth, and therefore the polishing cup should be moved between teeth and not left on any one tooth for more than a few seconds. Polishing paste should be rinsed from the gingival sulcus. Rinsing the gingival sulcus also removes the unattached bacteria from the sulcus, so it cannot reattach following the procedure.

Air-polishing devices (APD) can cause gingival bleeding, sensitivity, and tissue damage that may take 6–12 days to heal. If an APD is used on the root surface it can cause substantial cementum and dentin loss. Complete plaque removal from the tooth surface can be performed in 5–20 seconds with this method. However, a study using dogs showed gingival damage occurring after 5 seconds of APD application, with more severe damage occurring at 20 seconds[8]. For these reasons, the use of APDs in dogs and cats is not recommended.

OraVet® (Merial), a plaque prevention barrier, may be applied as the last step of a professional dental cleaning. A study in dogs showed that when OraVet was applied as part of the professional cleaning and then followed up with weekly application of the homecare product, there was a decrease in both plaque and calculus accumulation as well as gingival bleeding over an 8 week period[9].

Home care is extremely important to prevent the rapid return of plaque and gingivitis. Plaque begins to accumulate within hours of a dental cleaning and if appropriate plaque control measures are not taken, the patient will again develop gingivitis. Daily tooth brushing is the gold standard for plaque prevention. It is usually only necessary to brush the buccal and labial tooth surfaces. This is much easier for owners to do than trying to open a dog or cat's mouth to brush the palatal and lingual aspects of the teeth. Other methods for plaque removal include manual removal using a gauze sponge or other device, feeding a dental diet or dental treats with proven dental benefits, and dental chew toys. Chlorhexidine is an excellent antimicrobial for decreasing plaque, and may be added to the home care regimen for certain patients. When advising owners on appropriate dental treats and toys, it is important to give precautions regarding potential adverse effects such as intestinal blockage if large pieces are swallowed, and fractured teeth if hard objects are given. Chewing on any hard object, that is either unbendable or that cannot be dented with a fingernail, may cause a tooth to fracture.

When evaluating the effectiveness of diets or treats that have dental claims, it is helpful to look for the Veterinary Oral Health Care Council (VOHC) seal on the package. The VOHC evaluates the research behind the various dental claims. The seal is awarded to those products which have passed the standards for a dental benefit as determined by the VOHC (http://www.vohc.org/). Even when oral hygiene is part of a regular home care program, oral examinations should be scheduled on an annual basis and professional cleaning carried out as necessary to maintain oral health.

KEY POINTS
- Gingivitis is preventable with plaque prevention.
- Gingivitis is reversible with treatment.
- Gingivitis should be treated to prevent progression.
- Gingivitis does not always progress to periodontitis.

Periodontitis

DEFINITION

Periodontitis is present when plaque bacterial-induced inflammation has affected the gingiva (gingivitis) as well as other tissues of the periodontium. The periodontium is made up of the tissues that surround and support the tooth including the gingiva, cementum of the tooth, periodontal ligament, and the alveolar and supporting bone.

ETIOLOGY AND PATHOGENESIS

Chronic periodontitis is an extremely common problem in dogs and cats[4]. Aggressive periodontitis (localized or generalized) is a severe form of periodontitis which is seen less frequently. Periodontitis is an infectious disease caused by plaque bacteria and the resulting inflammatory response in a susceptible individual. Gingivitis is present prior to the development of periodontitis. However, not all dogs and cats with gingivitis will develop periodontitis. Subgingival plaque bacteria develops into a population of primarily anaerobic gram-negative bacteria. Black pigmented anaerobic bacteria (BPAB) are commonly recognized as the primary putative periopathogens. A recently reported study identified *Porphyromonas gulae*, *P. salivosa*, and *P. denticanis* from periodontal pockets in dogs with periodontitis[10].

Subgingival plaque and bacterial products stimulate the local production and release of the proinflammatory cytokines interleukin-1 (IL-1) and tumor necrosis factor-α (TNF-α). Monocytes and lymphocytes are major sources of these cytokines. Lipopolysaccharide from the outer membranes of gram-negative bacteria induce the release of inflammatory mediators and cytokines such as prostaglandin E_2, IL-1α, IL-1β, TNF-α, and IL-8. Activated neutrophils release proteolytic enzymes and reactive oxygen species, both of which play an important role in the tissue destruction of periodontitis[11]. A study in humans demonstrated a hyper-reactivity of mononuclear cells and neutrophils in patients with adult periodontitis[11].

Together, all these factors result in destruction of the tissues surrounding the tooth. Initially, the epithelial attachment to the tooth loses integrity and migrates more apically as the disease progresses. As the epithelial attachment migrates apically, there will be an increase in the gingival sulcus depth. As disease progresses apically and the periodontal ligament (PDL) and alveolar bone are destroyed, the depth of the periodontal pocket increases unless there is gingival recession. Periodontitis is generally considered an irreversible process with an inability for regrowth of normal cementum, PDL, and alveolar bone. The progressive nature of this process will result in tooth loss if left untreated.

There are many different factors which may promote the development of periodontitis, including: crowded teeth (**244, 245**), persistent deciduous teeth (**246**), malocclusions, nonabrasive diet, periodontal trauma, foreign bodies, and genetic predisposition.

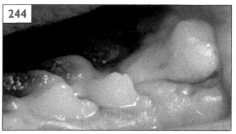

244 Rotated and crowded teeth may predispose to periodontal disease.

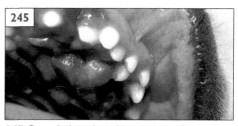

245 Crowded teeth and hair sulcular foreign body predispose to periodontal disease.

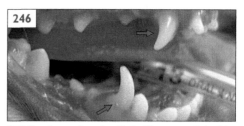

246 Persistent (retained) deciduous teeth in this toy breed dog has predisposed the patient to early onset periodontal disease.

CLINICAL FEATURES

In addition to gingivitis, gingival bleeding, and halitosis, the oral examination findings may include varying amounts of plaque and calculus accumulation, gingival recession (**247, 248**), furcation exposure (**249**), mobile teeth (**250–255**), missing teeth (**256**), and oral ulcerations (**257, 258**) (*254-258 over page*) .

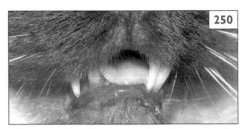

250 Cat with sudden onset of oral 'discomfort' and inability to close his mouth. Note the left maxillary canine is deviated towards the midline.

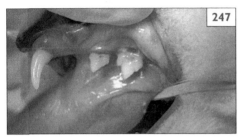

247 Localized periodontitis, severe gingival recession (attachment loss).

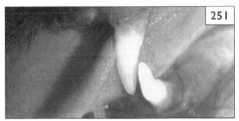

251 Left upper canine of patient in **250**, gingival inflammation, calculus accumulation, and bulge over the tooth root, mobile tooth (mesial to lower canine instead of in the normal distal position).

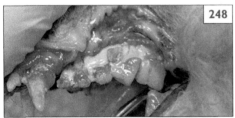

248 Generalized, chronic periodontitis, gingival recession, furcation exposure.

252 Dental radiograph of the patient in **250** revealing root and bone resorption and alveolar bone expansion secondary to chronic periodontitis.

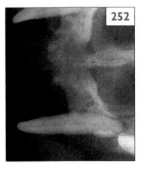

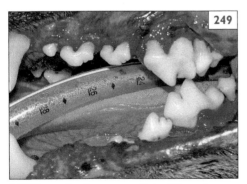

249 Generalized, severe periodontitis post scaling, severe attachment loss (gingival recession, furcation exposure).

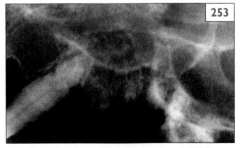

253 Dental radiograph of the patient in **250** revealing root resorption and alveolar bone expansion secondary to chronic periodontitis.

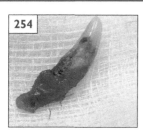

254 Extracted maxillary canine tooth. (Courtesy of Dr. Brook Niemiec.)

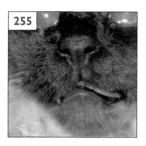

255 Following extraction of the left upper canine tooth the cat can comfortably close his mouth.

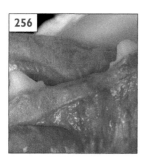

256 Missing tooth in a dog which was previously exfoliated secondary to periodontal disease. (Courtesy of Dr. Brook Niemiec.)

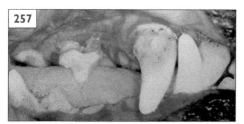

257 Buccal mucosal ulcerations in areas adjacent to the plaque and calculus in a patient with aggressive periodontitis.

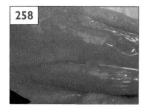

258 Sublingual erythema and edema in a dog with severe aggressive periodontitis.

Patients may have discomfort associated with periodontitis, and therefore may have changes in eating behavior such as decreased appetite, only eating soft foods, or not chewing on dry foods or treats (i.e. swallowing items whole). They may also become sensitive and not like to have their face touched or teeth brushed. In cases with extensive infection, the patient may be less active, a sign often misinterpreted by the owners as a sign of normal aging. The presence of sneezing (with or without nasal discharge) in a dog with periodontitis may indicate the presence of an oronasal fistula (**259, 260**).

In small and toy breed dogs, a fractured mandible may be the presenting complaint (**261**). In cases where periodontitis has resulted in severe bone loss around the mandibular teeth, especially the first molar, even minimal pressure (i.e. chewing on a hard treat, bumping into

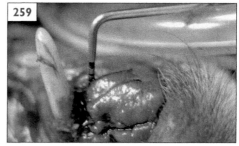

259 Mobile canine tooth, severe attachment loss on the palatal aspect forming an oronasal fistula. (Courtesy of Dr. Brook Niemiec.)

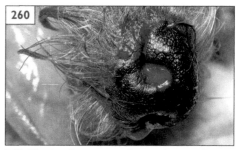

260 Bleeding from nares after probing a palatal pocket on the canine tooth, indicating an oronasal fistula.

something) can result in a mandibular fracture. For a further discussion on mandibular fractures see Chapter 8.

Another possible presenting complaint is a periodontal abscess. While oral abscesses are typically thought of as endodontic, periodontal abscesses are also possible (**262, 263**). For a further discussion on periodontal-endodontic relationships see Chapter 5.

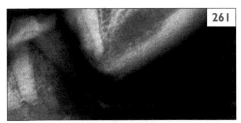

261 Dental radiograph of a pathological fracture secondary to severe periodontal disease in a small breed dog. (Courtesy of Dr. Brook Niemiec.)

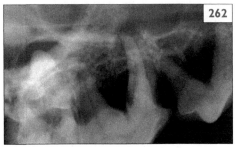

262 Intraoral dental radiograph of right upper fourth premolar in dog with periodontal abscess from chronic periodontitis.

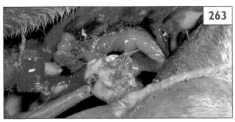

263 Dental picture of the case in **262**, removing exudates from the alveolus during periodontal abscess debridement.

DIFFERENTIAL DIAGNOSIS
- Immune-mediated disease.
- Neoplasia.
- Foreign body.
- Resorptive lesion.

DIAGNOSTIC TESTS
The periodontal probe is the most important tool used in the diagnosis of periodontal disease (**264**). Periodontal probes are available with different incremental markings and widths. A narrow probe with markings at the 1, 2, 3 mm level, up to 12 mm is recommended. There are automated and manual periodontal probes available. For clinical practice, a manual probe is a reliable probe[12]. Periodontal probes are used to measure pocket depth and attachment levels, as well as evaluate for the presence of plaque and calculus.

A diagnosis of periodontitis is made when there is attachment loss. The periodontal examination is done to evaluate the presence and degree of attachment loss (defined as probing depth greater than 3.0 mm in dogs and 0.5 mm in cats or gingival recession)[4]. A periodontal probe is used to evaluate the gingival sulcus around each tooth and measure any periodontal pockets (**265, 266**) (*overpage*). The depth of a periodontal pocket is measured from the cementoenamel junction (CEJ) to the epithelial attachment on the tooth. This must be done gently, so as not to penetrate the epithelial attachment. When the gingiva has receded, the attachment loss is determined by the sum of the gingival recession (measured from the free gingival margin to the CEJ) and the associated periodontal pocket (**267, 268**) (*overpage*). A dental explorer is used to determine the presence and amount of bone loss in the furcation area.

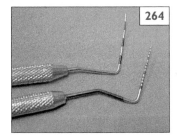

264 Periodontal probes, two of many varieties. (Courtesy of Dr. Brook Niemiec.)

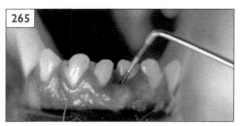

265 Periodontal probe in a deep pocket on the mandibular incisors of dog. Note the fairly normal appearing gingiva. This lesion would not have been identified without the probe. (Courtesy of Dr. Brook Niemiec.)

Dental radiographs are a critical diagnostic tool when evaluating the bone loss associated with periodontitis as well as complications such as endodontic disease (**269, 270**).

MANAGEMENT
Scaling and root planing (SRP) for mechanical debridement is the most important procedure in treating periodontitis[13]. SRP provides a favorable environment for periodontal tissue healing. Elimination or reduction of subgingival bacteria and toxic substances is also a primary

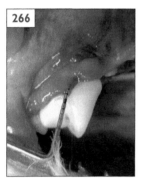

266 Significant periodontal pocket on the buccal aspect of the right maxillary fourth premolar in a dog. (Courtesy of Dr. Brook Niemiec.)

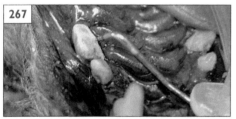

267 Significant periodontal pocket on the palatal aspect of the left maxillary second premolar in a dog. (Courtesy of Dr. Brook Niemiec.)

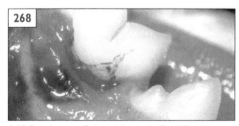

268 Focal area of gingivitis, periodontal pocket greater than 0.5 mm in a cat indicating periodontitis.

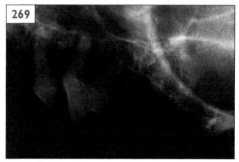

269 Dental radiograph of the case in **267** revealed severe bony loss surrounding the roots of the left maxillary first and second premolars (teeth were extracted). (Courtesy of Dr. Brook Niemiec.)

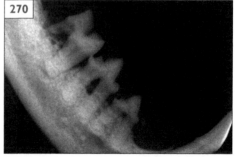

270 Dental radiograph of the case in **268** revealed severe bony loss surrounding the distal root of the right mandibular molar (tooth was extracted) as was the fourth premolar.

goal of treatment. The endotoxins on the tooth root are weakly adhered (previously thought to be deeply embedded in the root surface) and will be removed with ultrasonic instrumentation or hand instruments. These should be used with a light touch to avoid extensive dentin and cementum removal. Ultrasonic scaling, and the altered environment created by scaling, reduces the bacterial load in the subgingival area, thus returning the subgingival microflora to a population which is similar to that seen in healthy sites. However, the increased levels of subgingival bacterial population will return if supragingival plaque is not controlled. Therefore, follow-up home care is an essential part of the management plan.

Periodontal pockets which are 3–6 mm in depth may show enhanced periodontal attachment gains if a local antibiotic is applied following the SRP[14]. Doxirobe gel ™ (Pfizer) is a brand of doxycycline licensed for this application in dogs. When mixed and ready for use, it is a flowable solution of doxycycline cyclate equivalent to 8.5% doxycycline activity. A similar product for human use has shown significant reductions in anaerobic pathogens for up to 6 months after placement, as well as increased gains in clinical periodontal attachment with its use in humans[15]. A main advantage of local antibiotic treatment compared to systemic antibiotic administration is the ability to deliver a known concentration of drug at the site of infection while avoiding systemic and gastrointestinal side-effects.

Teeth which have pockets greater than 5–6 mm or furcation stages 2 or 3 require more advanced therapy for resolution of the infection[16,17]. This advanced therapy is typically periodontal surgery (including periodontal flaps) to visualize the root surface directly for effective cleaning, and/or guided tissue regeneration for bone height enhancement[18]. Teeth with severe attachment loss (> 50–70%) or mobility from periodontal disease should be extracted. Dental radiographs will confirm the extent of bone loss[19].

There are no 'evidence-based' guidelines for the use of antibiotics in treating periodontal disease in dogs or cats. The AVDC has a position statement on the use of antibiotics in dental disease that can be found on their web site (www.AVDC.org). The same is true for human dentistry[13]. Systemic antibiotic administration does provide benefits in the treatment of certain patients with periodontitis. In patients with deep periodontal pockets, the addition of systemic antibiotic treatment to the standard SRP treatment enhances attachment gain compared to those not treated with antibiotics[20]. Deciding which patients will have a sufficient enough benefit to warrant the administration of systemic antibiotics is not always a clear-cut decision. Patients with nonresponding or aggressive periodontitis are the most likely to benefit from systemic antibiotic administration. The choice of antibiotic is based on the spectrum of antimicrobial activity and the anaerobic nature of the periodontal pathogens. Therefore, amoxicillin-clavulanic acid, clindamycin, and metronidazole are frequently used because of their anaerobic spectrum of activity. In very severe cases, or cases refractory to empiric antibiotic therapy, a culture of the bacteria in the periodontal pockets may be indicated. The dosages and durations of antibiotic administration are generally based on clinical judgment rather than scientific evidence.

Nutritional support may be beneficial. Protein and other nutrients are important for maintaining healthy host epithelial defense and immune barriers. Therefore, a well balanced diet and vitamin supplementation is recommended for patients with poor nutritional status.

Prevention of supragingival and subgingival plaque accumulation is necessary to prevent additional attachment loss. The frequency of professional cleaning is recommended based on each individual patient's degree of periodontitis and success of the recommended oral home care program. A *Porphyromonas* vaccine (Pfizer, conditional license) may also be useful in preventing the development and progression of periodontal disease in dogs[21,22].

KEY POINTS

- Periodontal disease may be progressive if not treated.
- Periodontal disease is irreversible unless guided tissue regeneration techniques are utilized.
- Tooth loss is the end result of untreated periodontitis.
- Severe periodontal disease can result in pathological mandibular fracture.

Generalized gingival enlargement (gingival hyperplasia)

DEFINITION

Generalized gingival enlargement (gingival hyperplasia) is a proliferation of the normal cellular elements of the gingiva, primarily the connective tissue.

ETIOLOGY AND PATHOGENESIS

Generalized gingival enlargement (gingival hyperplasia) may be the result of nonspecific (chronic inflammation) or specific (drug-related and hereditary) causes. Chronic inflammation from local factors such as bacterial plaque and calculus can cause or exacerbate gingival enlargement. This hyperplastic tissue response in some patients may lead to generalized gingival hyperplasia.

Drugs that are known to be associated with generalized gingival hyperplasia include cyclosporine, calcium-channel blockers, and phenytoin[23,24]. Administration of these drugs results in the stimulation and growth of gingival fibroblasts. Discontinuation of the drugs may result in regression of the lesions. Hereditary (familial) gingival enlargement is commonly seen in certain breeds including Boxers and Collies.

CLINICAL FEATURES

The primary feature is a generalized increase in the bulk of the free and attached gingiva (**271–275**). The increase varies from mild to severe, and in severe cases the gingiva may completely cover the teeth. Gingival margins are rolled and blunted, and depending on the severity of inflammation, gingival bleeding and redness may also be present. The hyperplastic gingiva may form pseudopockets, which allow for subgingival plaque accumulation and gingivitis. Patients are usually asymptomatic unless the hyperplastic tissue is traumatized by mastication or other factors causing irritation.

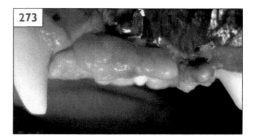

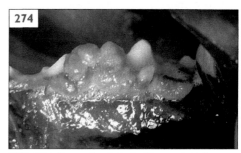

273, 274 Generalized gingival hyperplasia in a Boxer. (Courtesy of Dr. Brook Niemiec.)

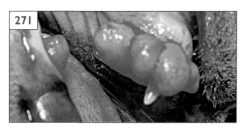

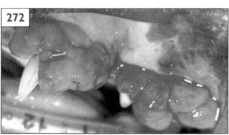

271, 272 Generalized gingival enlargement in a cat on chronic cyclosporine and calcium channel blocker therapy.

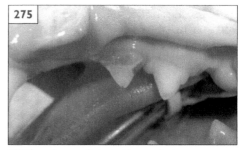

275 Local area of gingival hyperplasia over a resorptive lesion.

DIFFERENTIAL DIAGNOSIS
- Epulis.
- Fibroma.
- Peripheral odontogenic fibroma.
- Canine acanthomatous ameloblastoma.
- Neoplasia.
- Tooth resorption.
- Granuloma.

DIAGNOSTIC TESTS
Specific causes should be considered in breeds predisposed to gingival hyperplasia (genetic) and in patients receiving drugs associated with gingival enlargement. A definitive diagnosis is made with histologic examination of the tissue. The microscopic examination of the tissue shows increased fibrous tissue and superimposed inflammatory changes in tissue that otherwise appears normal. Dental radiographs should be normal except for the increase in soft tissue density of the enlarged gingiva.

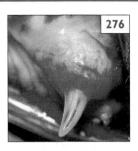

276 Patient in **271, 272** after gingivectomy surgery.

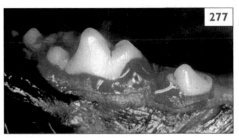

277 Patient in **273, 274** after gingivectomy surgery. (Courtesy of Dr. Brook Niemiec.)

MANAGEMENT
Management includes removal of plaque, calculus, and excess gingiva followed by continuous plaque removal strategies to decrease gingival inflammation. When removing excess gingiva, the goals are to return the contour of the gingiva to normal, to remove pseudopockets, and to return the gingival sulcus to a normal depth (**276, 277**). This author's preferred method for gross removal of excess gingiva is to use surgical blades. A fluted-bur is useful for fine contouring of the gingival margins after gross removal with a blade. Other options for generalized gingivectomy surgery include the use of gingivectomy knives, electrosurgery, or laser[25].

A minimum of 2 mm of attached gingiva should remain after the gingiva has healed from the gingivectomy. A periodontal probe is used to measure the gingival sulcus depth. The point of the probe can then be used to puncture into the gingiva at right angles marking the level on the gingiva where removal would leave about 3 mm in attached gingiva. Giving the extra 1 mm allows for a 2 mm gingival sulcus after healing and resolution of gingival inflammation. Once the proposed incision sites are marked, a number 15 scalpel blade is used to perform the gingivectomy. When making the incisions, bevel the gingival margins to create as normal a contour as possible. Several scalpel blades will be necessary because they are quickly dulled when incising the fibrous gingival tissue. Following the removal of the excess gingiva with the scalpel blades, the final contouring is done using a 12-fluted finishing bur on a high speed hand piece. When performing this step, it is very important not to damage the teeth or bone by direct contact with the contouring bur. Also, plenty of water is used as a coolant to prevent damage to the tooth, alveolar bone, and soft tissues from over-heating. Appropriate pain control measures should be taken in patients undergoing generalized removal of gingiva.

Gingival enlargements are expected to recur when the underlying etiology cannot be removed (i.e. hereditary, drug-related). Plaque control may slow the growth if the gingival inflammatory component is controlled.

KEY POINTS
- Histopathological diagnosis.
- Manage by removal of underlying etiologies when possible.
- Treat by removal of gingival enlargements.
- Plaque control is recommended postsurgery.
- Repeated treatment is often necessary.

Trauma

DEFINITION
Trauma to the gingiva and subsequent inflammation may result from chewing on foreign materials, interdental and subgingival foreign bodies, irritation from a malocclusion, or aggressive tooth brushing.

ETIOLOGY AND PATHOGENESIS
Foreign materials such as hair, string, plant material, wood, bones, and other items that become lodged between teeth or in the gingival sulcus, cause inflammation directly by their presence as well as by increasing plaque accumulation. Other causes of gingival trauma and inflammation include: brushing with a firm-bristled toothbrush, or using a hand-scaling instrument inappropriately on an unanesthetized patient.

CLINICAL FEATURES
The inflamed gingiva may be localized or generalized depending on the trauma. The foreign material causing the trauma may be evident on clinical examination (**278**), but in some cases general anesthesia is necessary to elucidate the cause (**279**).

DIFFERENTIAL DIAGNOSIS
- Periodontal disease.
- Immune-mediated disease.
- Neoplasia.

DIAGNOSTIC TESTS
History is important to determine whether the gingivitis may be secondary to trauma. The history should include all home care provided, chew toys offered or available, and habits/behaviors of the patient, including what they chew on.

MANAGEMENT
Removing the source of trauma is necessary to allow any existing periodontal disease to resolve (**280, 281**).

KEY POINTS
- If the source of trauma is not removed, severe periodontal disease may develop.

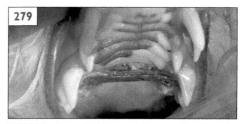

279 Wood caught between the maxillary fourth premolars in a dog. (Courtesy of Dr. Brook Niemiec.)

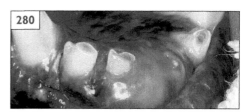

280 Gingival inflammation is apparent after removal of wood from the patient in **278**.

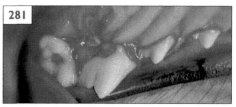

281 Gingival inflammation is apparent after removal of wood from the patient in **279**. (Courtesy of Dr. Brook Niemiec.)

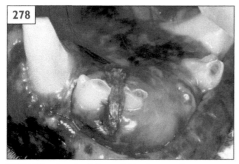

278 Wood material caught between the mandibular incisors in a dog.

Epulids

DEFINITION
Clinical term indicating a swelling of the gingiva in the area of the teeth. It is a clinical description, not a diagnosis. Fibromas, non-neoplastic odontogenic tumors, and neoplastic tumors may present as an 'epulis'.

ETIOLOGY AND PATHOGENESIS
The majority of epulids may be identified histologically as focal fibrous hyperplasia. Chronic gingival inflammation may play a role in their development. Canine acanthomatous ameloblastoma (previously described as acanthomatous epulis) is a soft-tissue tumor from neoplastic cells of ameloblast origin.

Peripheral odontogenic fibroma (previously described as fibromatous and ossifying epulids) is a benign neoplasm from odontogenic epithelium that may also exhibit evidence of mesenchymal induction (bone, osteoid, dentinoid, cementum-like materials).

CLINICAL FEATURES
An epulis is a tumor or mass of the gingiva in the area of the dental structures. Retrospective studies have shown that the majority of epulids can be classified as focal fibrous hyperplasia[26]. Acanthomatous ameloblastoma and peripheral odontogenic fibromas may present clinically as epulids. The rostral mandible, adjacent to the canine teeth, is a common site for these tumors (**282–284**) but they can occur anywhere in the mouth (**285**). The affected gingival tissue may appear firm or friable in appearance.

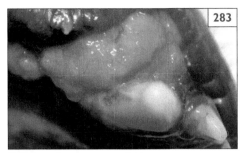

283 Acanthomatous ameloblastoma, same patient as **282**.

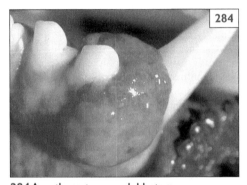

284 Acanthomatous ameloblastoma.

282 Acanthomatous ameloblastoma.

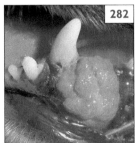

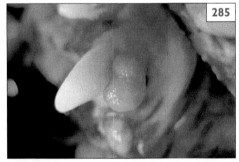

285 Acanthomatous ameloblastoma in maxilla. (Courtesy of Dr. Brook Niemiec.)

Peripheral odontogenic fibromas are slow growing and are commonly found around the maxillary premolars (**286**).

DIFFERENTIAL DIAGNOSIS
- Focal fibrous hyperplasia.
- Peripheral odontogenic fibroma.
- Peripheral or canine acanthomatous ameloblastoma.
- Pyogenic granuloma.

DIAGNOSTIC TESTS
Diagnostic tests should include dental radiographs and histopathology. A definitive diagnosis is obtained by histologic evaluation of a biopsy sample. An incisional or punch biopsy should be taken in the central area of the mass. Dental radiographs are necessary to evaluate the underlying tissues.

Canine acanthomatous ameloblastoma typically have radiographic evidence of local bone infiltration and tooth displacement (**287, 288**). Radiographic evaluation of peripheral odontogenic fibromas reveal no evidence of bony involvement (**289**), and may show areas of mineralization within the soft tissue mass.

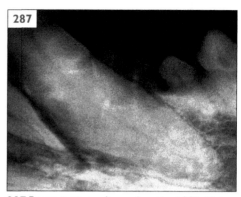

287 Preoperative radiograph, patient **282**. Note the significant bony reaction.

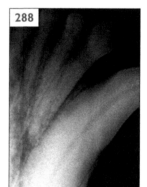

288 Dental radiograph from the patient in **284**. Note the mild bony reaction.

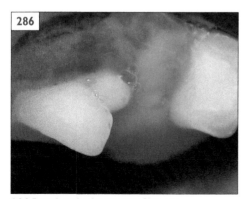

286 Peripheral odontogenic fibroma.

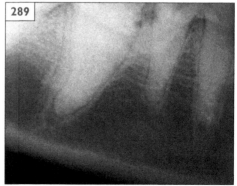

289 Dental radiograph from the patient in **286**. Note the lack of any bony reaction.

MANAGEMENT

Focal fibrous hyperplasia and peripheral odontogenic fibroma are managed by surgical excision. A marginal excision, with the plane of dissection located in the reactive zone around the tumor and its pseudocapsule, is generally curative. Treatment options for canine acanthomatous ameloblastoma include surgical excision and radiation treatment. Local recurrence following marginal excision is very common (**290, 291**) and, therefore, a wide surgical excision is recommended (**292**). The wide surgical excision should extend beyond the reactive zone of inflammation surrounding the pseudocapsule and include a 0.5 to 1 cm margin of 'normal' tissue to ensure complete excision[27].

Radiation treatment of canine acanthomatous ameloblastoma is another option; however, it does carry a low risk of radiation-induced carcinogenesis. A recent study reported a low incidence of 3.5% (2/57 dogs) and late onset of occurrence (5.2 and 8.7 years) of secondary tumors in the treatment field for dogs irradiated for oral acanthomatous epulis[28].

KEY POINTS

- Epulis is a clinical term, not a diagnostic term.
- Lesions that appear grossly similar can have markedly different biologic behavior.
- Histopathological diagnosis is necessary.
- Treat based on radiographic and histopathological diagnosis.

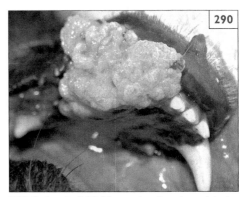

290 Patient in **282** 11 months after the original surgery, with regrowth of the acanthomatous ameloblastoma.

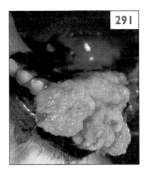

291 Regrowth of acanthomatous ameloblastoma 11 months after excision of the mass in **282**.

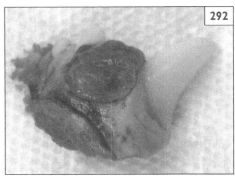

292 Excised tumor and surrounding tissue from the patient in **284**.

Gingivostomatitis (caudal stomatitis) in cats

DEFINITION

Gingivostomatitis is a clinical descriptive term indicating inflammation and proliferation of the gingiva and oral mucosa. Lymphoplasmacytic stomatitis is a histopathological description often identified from biopsy samples of oral tissue from cats with gingivostomatitis. The inflammation ranges from mild to severe, and typically increases with chronicity. In chronic cases, the tissues may also become ulcerated. Affected areas may include the gingiva, buccal mucosa, palatal mucosa, pharynx, mucosa in the back of the mouth in the area lateral to the palatoglossal arch, glossopalatine arch, and the tongue. The fauces is the archway between the pharyngeal and oral cavities formed by the tongue, anterior tonsillar pillars, and soft palate[29]. Inflammatory involvement of this area in the caudal portion of the oral cavity, with or without ulceration, is referred to as caudal stomatitis.

ETIOLOGY AND PATHOGENESIS

The etiology(s) of caudal stomatitis has not been identified. Multiple etiologies may exist that singularly, or combined, result in the clinical presentation of chronic caudal stomatitis. Viral infections, *Bartonella henselae* infection, altered immune status, and exaggerated inflammatory response to bacterial plaque have all been suggested as factors or cofactors[30].

Feline calicivirus can cause acute caudal stomatitis and has been isolated from these cats. Cats with chronic caudal stomatitis are more likely to be shedding feline calicivirus (FCV) and feline herpes virus 1 from the oral mucosa than cats without[31]. However, FCV has not been shown to cause feline chronic caudal stomatitis. FCV may be a contributing factor to the etiology or severity of chronic caudal stomatitis, but its role in this disease cannot be established until further studies are done. Most cats with chronic caudal stomatitis do not test positive for feline immunodeficiency virus (FIV) or feline leukemia virus (FeLV). However, FIV may play a role in the development of caudal stomatitis in some cases. Low salivary IgA levels in FIV-positive cats may predispose to oral diseases.

Bartonella henselae infection has been suggested as a possible factor in the development of feline chronic caudal stomatitis[32]. Cats positive for *B. henselae* and FIV have an increase in mandibular lymph node swelling and gingivitis compared to noninfected cats. The role of *B. henselae* in feline chronic caudal stomatitis remains an unknown and controversial issue at this time.

Cats with chronic caudal stomatitis have significantly higher serum IgG, IgM, and IgA concentrations and lower salivary IgA levels compared to healthy cats[33]. The decrease in salivary IgA concentrations may be a factor in the pathogenesis of this disease. In many cases of chronic oral inflammatory disease, a primary etiology other than periodontal disease is not identified. It has been speculated that these cats have an exaggerated inflammatory response to bacterial plaque.

CLINICAL FEATURES

Clinical signs in cats with caudal stomatitis include: halitosis, dysphagia, pawing at the mouth, reluctance to eat, anorexia, growling or crying when eating, weight loss, and decreased or lack of grooming (unkempt appearance). They may cry when yawning (or have stopped yawning), have excess drooling (**293**), blood tinged saliva, a change in temperament (aggressive or reclusive), and mandibular lymph node enlargement. Purulent material may be present in the oral cavity, as well as in the hair around the mouth, or on the paws if they have been trying to clean themselves.

Oral examination may be limited due to the painful nature of this condition. Usually, the

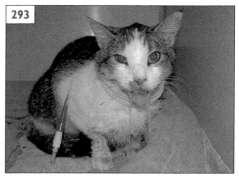

293 Hypersalivation in a cat with severe, painful caudal stomatitis. (Courtesy of Dr. Brook Niemiec.)

examiner can gently pull back the lips to get an idea of the inflammation present. If the mouth is then opened very slowly, oftentimes the entire oral cavity can be seen. The gingiva and oral mucosa will have varying amounts of inflammation, proliferation, and ulceration (**294–296**). Both gingivostomatitis and periodontal disease can present with severe gingival inflammation. *The main clinical sign that differentiates gingivostomatitis from periodontal disease is the presence of caudal stomatitis in cases of gingivostomatitis.* Very severe cases may have caudal tissue proliferation so extensive that the pharyngeal area is almost completely blocked (**297**). Oral tissues are friable and bleed easily. The distribution of proliferated and inflamed tissue is typically symmetric on both sides of the mouth (**298**).

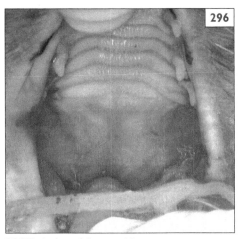

296 Typical caudal stomatitis.

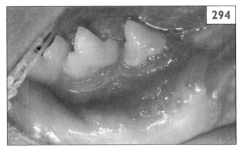

294 Severe buccal inflammation (stomatitis) with minimal plaque accumulation.

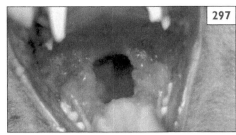

297 Severe bilateral caudal stomatitis. Note the significant blockage of the pharynx. (Courtesy of Dr. Brook Niemiec.)

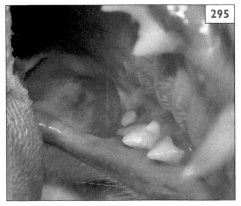

295 Caudal stomatitis.

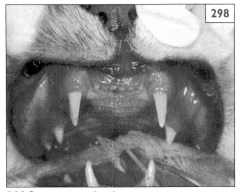

298 Severe generalized stomatitis in a young cat. Note the even, bilateral distribution.

DIFFERENTIAL DIAGNOSIS

- Squamous cell carcinoma/neoplasia.
- Eosinophilic granuloma complex.
- Periodontal disease.

DIAGNOSTIC TESTS

Caudal stomatitis is a clinical syndrome and does not indicate a specific etiology or diagnosis. Clinical diagnosis is made by visual inspection of the oral cavity[30]. Further diagnostic evaluation should focus on identifying any possible underlying factors or concurrent diseases. Diagnostic tests should include oral examination, dental radiographs when indicated (to evaluate for the presence of retained root tips, periodontal disease, or bony changes suggestive of neoplasia), and evaluation of FeLV and FIV status if unknown. Consider evaluation for FCV (reverse transcriptase polymerase chain reaction [RT-PCR] or virus isolation from oral swab) and *B. henselae* infection. If areas of asymmetric inflammation and ulceration are present, or if radiographic changes are suspicious for neoplasia, a biopsy should be taken and submitted for histopathology. If histopathology identifies lymphocytic-plasmacytic stomatitis, it is important to remember this is only a histologic diagnosis and does not indicate the specific etiology of the problem. A complete blood count and biochemical profile is indicated to evaluate for underlying and concurrent problems. Hyperglobulinemia, consistent with chronic antigenic stimulation, may be present.

MANAGEMENT

Resolution of the oral inflammation is the goal of treatment, but in some cases, maintaining a state of decreased inflammation is the best that can be achieved. Several treatments have been suggested, including: extraction of all premolars and molars, full mouth extraction, laser treatment to remove inflammatory tissue, chronic immune-suppressive treatment (i.e. cyclosporine, high-dose glucocorticoids, immuran), anti-inflammatory treatment (i.e. glucocorticoids, nonsteroidal anti-inflammatories), antibiotics, feline omega interferon (not available in the US), and nutraceuticals.

The most successful long-term treatment for cats with chronic caudal stomatitis is the extraction of all premolars and molars including the periodontal ligaments, and retained root tips (if present). Dental radiographs should be made to document extraction of all tooth roots. Extraction of the canines and incisors is indicated when the inflammation extends to include the gingiva surrounding them. If the buccal gingiva and mucosa over the canines remains or becomes inflamed following initial extractions, these teeth may also require extraction. Many cats do well without extraction of the canines; therefore, this author includes canines during the initial extraction procedure only when there is significant inflammation of the gingiva around these teeth. The reason for extraction of the premolars and molars is to remove the site of attachment for the bacterial plaque. This is based on the opinion that these cats appear to have an exaggerated inflammatory response to the plaque bacteria. The majority of cats will have an excellent response to this treatment requiring no chronic medical management (**299, 300**)[34].

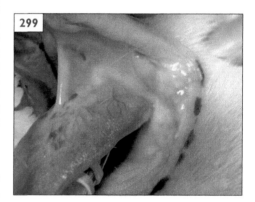

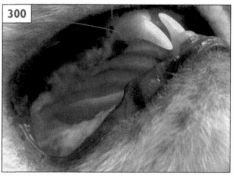

299, 300 Excellent response to a full mouth extractions in two cats. (Courtesy of Dr. Brook Niemiec.)

Owners will need to provide home care in order to decrease plaque accumulation on remaining incisors and canines. The oral inflammation usually resolves or improves within 3 to 6 weeks following the extractions. During this time, supportive medical management may be indicated. It is not necessary to treat minor residual inflammation in an asymptomatic cat.

Some cats gain only partial improvement and may require long-term medical management (**301**). These cats may respond well to low doses of immunosuppressive drugs and antibiotics. A small number of cats will not benefit significantly and require long-term medical management for bacterial infections and suppression of the inflammation. Fortunately, these are the minority of patients. These poor responders are typically patients with long-standing, chronic inflammation which has been treated with repeated high doses of glucocorticoids. Long-term repeated doses of glucocorticoids may have significant side-effects and are not recommended for treating these cats. The earlier the teeth are extracted, the better the outcome in most cases.

If a successful outcome is not achieved by extraction of all premolars and molars, it is typically because not all roots were extracted (**302–304**). It is also possible that continued plaque accumulation and inflammation is occurring on the remaining canines and incisors. Teeth that were not fully extracted or fractured teeth which have lost their crowns are the typical culprits, leaving root fragments behind. These fragments create continued inflammation and serve as an area for bacterial accumulation.

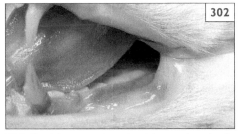

302 Caudal stomatitis with evidence of retained roots. (Courtesy of Dr. Brook Niemiec.)

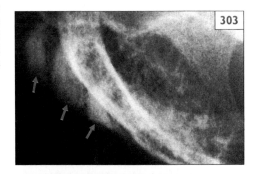

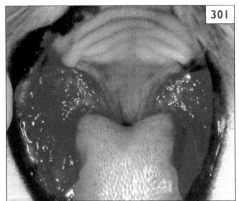

301 Persistent caudal stomatitis after a full mouth extraction.

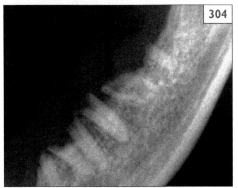

303, 304 Dental radiographs of the patient in **302** revealing the retained roots (arrows). (Courtesy of Dr. Brook Niemiec.)

Therefore, it is essential to remove all tooth roots. Curetting the alveolus to remove any remaining periodontal ligament has also been recommended. Antibiotic administration following extractions is recommended to help resolve the oral infection in severe cases. In some cases with slow improvement, it may be beneficial to treat with 2-week successive courses of clindamycin, amoxicillin-clavulanic acid, and metronidazole to resolve the residual infection/inflammation and return cats to normal eating behavior. Topical rinses, such as 0.12% chlorhexidine, may also be beneficial during healing. Analgesia is an important consideration in these patients. Appropriate pre-emptive analgesia should be given with the preanesthesia medications. Postoperative analgesia is managed very well with oral (buccal mucosal) administration of buprenorphine for 3–5 days.

Nutritional support is recommended in severe cases with prolonged inappetance, or severe inflammation that is slow to resolve following 'full-mouth' extractions. This may be easily provided with feedings through an esophageal tube. The improved nutrition supplied by enteral feedings may enhance healing.

In cases where owners are reluctant to have multiple extractions done initially, medical management can be attempted. The goals of medical management are to decrease bacterial plaque accumulation and to inhibit the associated inflammatory response. Concurrently with medical management, a complete oral examination and dental cleaning should be done. Any teeth with severe periodontitis and any retained root should be extracted.

Without extraction therapy (i.e. all premolars and molars), systemic antibiotics may result in various degrees of improvement in some cases. However, this is usually temporary, and some patients will relapse even while on antibiotic therapy. Appropriate antibiotic choices include: amoxicillin-clavulanic acid, clindamycin, metronidazole, and azithromycin. Topical rinses or gels (i.e. 0.12% chlorhexidine) may also be beneficial in some cats.

Glucocorticoids are the most commonly used drugs for suppression of inflammatory and immune response in these cats. Glucocorticoid administration results in clinical improvement in a greater number of cases than antibiotic therapy alone. Usually, glucocorticoids and antibiotics are used concurrently, at least in the initial treatment and during flare-ups. Long-term use of corticosteroids may have detrimental effects (see Chapter 7), and the lowest effective dose should be given. Either injectable (methylprednisolone acetate) or oral route (prednisone, prednisolone, triacimalone) may be used. Injectable treatment is usually recommended initially, because the patient's mouth is so painful that orally administered medications may be difficult for the owner to administer. This author typically treats with 15–20 mg methylprednisone SC per cat. This usually improves the cat's attitude and appetite within 24–48 hours, and the effects generally last for 3–6 weeks. This treatment regimen gives adequate time to stabilize the cat and schedule oral surgery. In very severe cases, it may be required every 3 weeks to maintain the cat's ability to eat and be comfortable. This should only be done as a last resort when an owner will not approve oral surgery (extractions) and there are no other options.

Alternatively, nonsteroidal anti-inflammatory drugs (NSAIDs) can be used to decrease the inflammation and improve the attitude and appetite in most cases. If a cat is not eating and is painful, NSAIDs can be used instead of glucocorticoids as a single treatment prior to a full-mouth extraction, if surgery is to be delayed for several days. Meloxicam is currently approved in cats and has been recommended as a onetime injection for acute control or can be administered orally on a long-term basis to control inflammation. When using NSAIDs, feline patients should be fully hydrated and have no pre-existing renal disease. Regular monitoring is recommended to detect any problems related to the NSAID administration, or emerging diseases that would contradict the use of these drugs. Even with these precautions, NSAIDs (including meloxicam) may have serious or lethal side-effects in cats and the owners should be advised of this prior to their use.

Cyclosporine A has been recommended as an immunosuppressive therapy for cats with chronic caudal stomatitis as an alternative to extractions and for those cats requiring additional medical management postextractions. It should be used with caution in cats with hepatic or renal disease. Reports indicate that cyclosporine A may help control a certain number of these cats. There is very little information currently in the veterinary literature documenting its therapeutic effect, but it may provide an alternative to long-term glucocorticoid therapy. The bioavailability of the two available forms differs. Atopica® (Novartis) is the veterinary product approved for use in dogs and Neoral® (Novartis) is the equivalent product for human use. Sandimmune® is an older cyclosporine product that is less bioavailable than the two newer forms. Therefore, the dose will depend on which form is used. Recommended doses for Sandimmune® are 4–15 mg/kg/day PO divided q 12 h and for Neoral® 1–5 mg/kg/day PO divided q 12 h. Serum cyclosporine levels should be monitored within 24–48 hours of beginning therapy, then weekly for a month, and then monthly to evaluate serum levels and maintain concentrations within a reported therapeutic range avoiding toxic levels. Additional blood tests to evaluate for side-effects should be done on a regular basis. The recommended therapeutic range reported for cats varies between 250–500 ng/ml and 500–1000 ng/ml[35]. Cats with high blood levels (1000 ng/ml) may develop anorexia. The expenses associated with the cyclosporine itself, as well as laboratory testing, can be cost prohibitive for some clients and should be discussed with the client prior to initiating treatment.

Lactoferrin, administered either orally or topically to the oral mucosa, may be beneficial in some patients, which are most likely to be those with mild inflammation[36]. Lactoferrin is normally found in mucosal surfaces and neutrophil granules, and it has antibacterial and anti-inflammatory properties. The topical application of lactoferrin (40 mg/kg of body weight) to the oral mucosa in seven ill cats with chronic caudal stomatitis resulted in clinical improvement, demonstrated by decreased pain and salivation, and increased appetite.

Anecdotally, coenzyme Q10 (30–100 mg daily) has successfully resolved or improved oral inflammation that persists following extraction of all premolars and molars. The response to treatment may take up to 4 months, and thus the initial trial period should be a minimum of 4 months.

Feline recombinant interferon omega (Virbagen; Virbac) may eventually be shown to be a good option for treatment; however, it is currently not available in the US. A case report has been published that presents a single case where Virbagen was used when treatment by extraction of all premolars and molars was determined to be unsuccessful. The authors report that after 6 weeks of treatment with Virbagen the stomatitis improved[37].

KEY POINTS
- The cause(s) of caudal stomatitis is/are unknown at this time.
- Complete extraction of all premolars and molars (+/– canines, incisors) provides significant benefit for most patients.
- Without extractions, most patients require intermittent or long-term medical management which may have significant side-effects.

Pathologies of the Oral Mucosa

Brook A. Niemiec

- **Oronasal fistula**

- **Eosinophilic granuloma complex**

- **Chronic ulcerative paradental stomatitis (CUPS) (kissing lesions)**

- **Immune-mediated diseases affecting the oral cavity**

- **Uremic stomatitis**

- **Candidiasis (thrush)**

- **Caustic burns of the oral cavity**

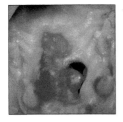
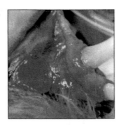
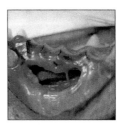
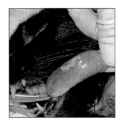

Oronasal fistula

DEFINITION
An oronasal or oroantral fistula is a defect in the gingival or palatine tissues and maxillary or incisive bone, which results in a communication between the oral and nasal cavities[1]. An oronasal fistula (ONF) is defined as a defect rostral to the mesial root of the maxillary third premolar, while a defect distal to that is considered an oroantral fistula[2].

ETIOLOGY AND PATHOGENESIS
There are numerous causes for this condition. These include periodontal disease, trauma, neoplasia, electrical/caustic burns, and iatrogenic secondary to oral surgery (especially extractions of maxillary canines)[1,3]. In addition, ONFs have been seen secondary to traumatic malocclusions[4,5], eosinophilic granulomas[6], and rhinolithiasis[7]. However, by far the most common cause, and the one that will be detailed below, is unchecked periodontal disease[8,9]. For a detailed description of periodontal disease and its therapy see Chapter 6.

The inflammation associated with periodontal disease will result in osteoclastic bone resorption. In the majority of cases, if left untreated (or under treated) the resorption will continue until the tooth exfoliates. However, some areas of the tooth (or roots of multirooted teeth) may become severely involved while other areas (or roots) retain the tooth in alveolar bone.

The fistula is created by periodontal disease progressing apically on the maxillary teeth. The most common tooth involved is the maxillary canine[8–10]. The roots of these teeth are adjacent and parallel to the nasal cavity, and are separated from it by only a thin sheet of bone[1]. Periodontal disease commonly destroys the thin plate of bone along with the normal attachment of the tooth. This results in a communication between the oral and nasal cavities. The bacteria in the mouth, along with food particles and other debris, will enter the nose through this fistula and create an infection in the nasal cavity (sinusitis). The infection will continue until the defect is surgically corrected.

CLINICAL FEATURES
Clinical signs of an ONF are chronic nasal discharge (blood or pus), sneezing, and occasionally anorexia and halitosis[9,10]. In some cases, the fistula can be seen easily on oral examination (**305**). The periodontal type, however, may not be clinically obvious on conscious examination. These fistulae can be definitively diagnosed by introducing a

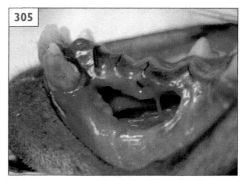

305 Large oronasal fistula in a Dachshund secondary to previous extraction of the maxillary canines.

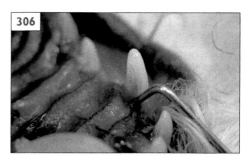

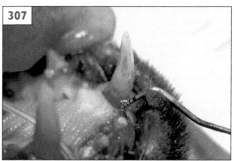

306, 307 Periodontal probe in an oronasal fistula from a maxillary canine in a dog (**306**) and a cat (**307**). Note the relatively normal appearing periodontal tissues.

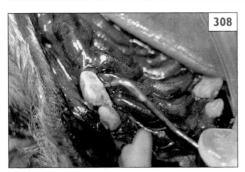

308 Camouflaged oronasal fistula from a second premolar.

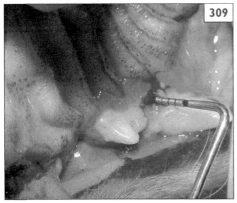

309 Oroantral fistula on a maxillary fourth premolar in a dog.

common in older, small breed dogs[10]. Chondrodystrophic breeds are strongly over represented[10]. However, any breed and age, as well as felines can be affected[1].

DIFFERENTIAL DIAGNOSES
- Trauma.
- Caustic or thermal burn.
- Neoplasia.

DIAGNOSTIC TESTS
Clinical appearance is classic and definitively diagnostic. If there is any concern of an alternate cause of this condition, histopathology should be considered prior to surgical correction. In addition, consider computed tomography (CT) if a more widespread problem is suspected. Dental radiographs should always be exposed to evaluate the surgical area; however, these should not be relied upon for diagnosis of the fistula.

MANAGEMENT
Periodontally induced
At this point, there is no viable recourse for this problem other than extraction of the tooth and closing the defect with a full thickness mucoperiosteal flap[9,11,12]. The single mucogingival flap techniques[9] (without a palatine flap) are sufficient in the vast majority of periodontally-induced cases, provided that the flap is large enough and vascularity has been maintained[11]. Very large or recurrent cases may require the performance of the double flap technique[1]. However, this author has used the single flap technique exclusively for the last 5 years with consistent success, even in cases where multiple (up to 9) previous surgeries on the same fistula have failed. The key is to create closure without tension. The reader is referred to an oral surgical/dental text for details of these procedures.

If deep periodontal pockets are discovered prior to development of the fistula (especially on the canines), periodontal surgery with guided tissue regeneration has proven very successful in salvaging the diseased dentition[1]. It is quite common for significant disease to be present on the contralateral tooth, thus it is very important to perform a full mouth evaluation.

periodontal probe into the periodontal space on the palatal surface of the maxillary teeth under general anesthesia (**306–309**). Often, no bottom will be found to the pocket. In addition, there may be blood visible in the nostril after probing. It is important to note that extensive periodontal pockets will occur prior to the formation of a fistula as these can be treated in alternative fashion to an ONF. Interestingly, this condition can occur even when the remainder of the patient's periodontal tissues are relatively healthy. This may include the other surfaces of the involved tooth. Periodontally-induced ONFs are most

Traumatic/neoplastic/caustic induced

These cases may be much more difficult to treat primarily due to their palatal location. The palatal tissues are inelastic and therefore require advanced flap techniques (rotational, split-U) to achieve a tension-free closure[6,13].

Exceedingly large fistulae, or chronic cases that have not responded to surgical closure, may be managed by alternate methods. These include silastic obturators[14] or creating a flap of the dorsal tongue tissue[15]. These techniques should not be used until other surgical means have been attempted or ruled out as insufficient.

KEY POINTS

- ONFs are most common in older small breed dogs, but can occur in any breed as well as cats.
- Suspect in any case of chronic nasal discharge (especially unilateral) or sneezing.
- Definitive diagnosis often requires probing under general anesthesia.
- Extraction of the affected tooth and closure with no tension is the current choice of therapy for periodontally-induced lesions.

Eosinophilic granuloma complex

DEFINITION

The eosinophilic granuloma complex (EGC) is a group of conditions which share a common etiology, as well as some histopathological features. While these lesions have been reported in dogs[16] (especially Siberian Huskies[17] and Malamutes[11]), they are much more common in cats. The discussion in this section will relate to cats, although the disease process is similar in either species[6].

ETIOLOGY AND PATHOGENESIS

The true etiology of these conditions is unknown. Local accumulation of eosinophils (and their release of inflammatory agents) is thought to initiate the inflammation and necrosis seen in most of these lesions[18]. The presence of eosinophils suggests that these lesions are secondary to an immune-mediated or hypersensitivity reaction[1]. This reaction may result from a local (food) or systemic (flea allergy or atopy) allergy[19], although these lesions have been seen in cases where allergic and infectious disease have been ruled out[20]. Additional causes may include a response to irritation, such as chronic grooming, or a traumatic malocclusion[1,21,22]. Finally, there appears to be a genetic predisposition to this syndrome[6,11,23].

CLINICAL FEATURES

There are several different clinical syndromes in this category, all of which may have oral manifestations. There may also be concurrent dermatologic manifestations.

Indolent ulcers

These are the most common oral manifestation of this disease process in cats[24]. They appear as red-brown lesions on the upper lip, at the philtrum, or around the maxillary canine teeth (**310**)[1]. These lesions can be unilateral or bilateral. Females are two to three times more likely to be affected than males. Some texts report that young cats appear to be predisposed[19], while others report that older to middle aged cats are predisposed[25].

Linear granulomas

This is the second most common oral form, and is the only true granuloma of the group. Lesions can be single or multiple throughout the mouth. The most common sites are the lips, gingiva, tongue, and palate. Linear granulomas are generally nonpainful, although they can occasionally become secondarily infected. The classic appearance is a raised, lobulated yellow-pink mass arising from the oral mucosa (**311**). However, they can also appear ulcerative (**312**) and in some cases, may cause severe damage to the oral mucosa and underlying bone. There have been cases reported of severe periodontal loss[26], ONFs (**313**)[6], and pathological fractures[27] occurring secondary to eosinophilic granulomas. Therefore, do not take these lesions lightly, and keep them in the differential list for aggressive appearing lesions.

Collagenolytic granulomas

These are most commonly seen in young female cats[19]. They appear as a firmly swollen, but not inflamed, lip in the rostral area of the mandible.

Eosinophilic plaques

When found in the mouth, they appear similar to the linear granuloma. These are very rare in the oral cavity, and are much more likely to be seen as a dermatologic lesion[24].

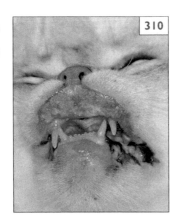

310 Indolent ulcer. (Courtesy of Dr. Mona Boord.)

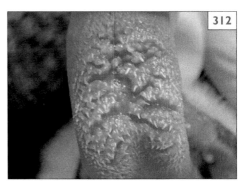

312 Ulcerative linear eosinophilic granuloma on the tongue of a cat.

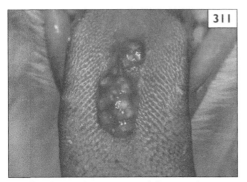

311 Productive linear eosinophilic granuloma on the tongue of a cat.

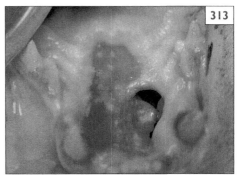

313 Large oronasal fistula secondary to an eosinophilic granuloma.

DIFFERENTIAL DIAGNOSES

If productive:
- Neoplasia.
- Gingival hyperplasia.

If ulcerative:
- Immune-mediated disease.
- Uremic toxicity.
- Caustic exposure.
- Trauma.
- Periodontal disease[26].
- Neoplasia[28].

DIAGNOSTIC TESTS

Histopathology should always be performed to confirm the diagnosis[1,26]. A complete blood panel should be performed to rule out any underlying disease. Following confirmation of the diagnosis, a thorough allergy evaluation should be conducted including food trial, flea treatment, +/− allergy testing (blood or intradermal).

MANAGEMENT

The acute disease process is best treated with corticosteroids. However, corticosteroids should not be used for long-term disease control, due to the significant systemic side-effects. The typical initial protocol is prednisone 2 mg/kg q 12 hours for 3–4 weeks[19,29,30]. Other corticosteroid options include intralesional triamcinalone (3 mg weekly) or methyl prednisone injections (20 mg q 2 weeks)[29].

Antibiotic therapy is required in some cases to induce remission or to treat secondary infection[19]. In addition, there are cases that appear to respond to antibiotic therapy alone[31,32]. Therefore, it is routine in our practice to treat mild cases initially with antibiotics alone and more severe cases with a combination of antibiotic and corticosteroid medications.

Thorough allergy testing (see Diagnostic tests) should be performed, especially in nonresponsive or recurrent cases. If an underlying allergic component is found, specific treatment can be instituted with a good rate of success[33]. Many cases remain idiopathic and require lifelong therapy[19]. Options for long-term medical therapy include antibiotics and cyclosporine.

Cyclosporine has recently been introduced as a veterinary labeled product for atopy and appears as effective as corticosteroids for atopic dermatitis in dogs and cats[34–37]. It has also been proven to be an effective medication for long-term therapy of oral eosinophilic diseases[38,39]. In addition, a lower incidence of severe side-effects may be expected in comparison to steroids[35]. This is especially valuable in cases requiring long-term therapy. Consequently, many dermatologists use this medication rather than corticosteroids for inflammatory skin diseases, including the EGC. When treating larger patients long term, the addition of ketoconazole may lower the necessary dosage of cyclosporine and subsequent cost to the client[40].

It is important to note that cyclosporine is currently not approved in cats and there are reports of opportunistic fungal and fatal protozoal infections associated with its chronic use[39]. Therefore, using the lowest effective dose (by tapering), and performing regular therapeutic levels as well as routine blood testing, are recommended.

Hormonal therapy is another medical option for treating these lesions[1], but the significant potential side-effects should make this the last option. Surgical removal of these lesions has been performed with some success, including laser and cryosurgery[1,41]. Finally, radiation treatment has been used effectively in some cases[41].

KEY POINTS

- This condition may be allergic in nature.
- Immunomodulatory drugs (corticosteroids or cyclosporine) and/or antibiotics are the mainstay of initial therapy.
- Allergy testing (flea control, hypoallergenic trial, intradermal skin testing) should be strongly considered, especially in resistant or recurrent cases.
- This condition may require life-long therapy if no specific cause is found.
- Cyclosporine (though off-label) appears to be the best long-term medical therapy.

Chronic ulcerative paradental stomatitis (CUPS) (kissing lesions)

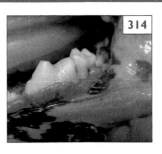

314 Gingival recession in a case of CUPS.

DEFINITION
CUPS is defined as an ulcerative, immune-mediated reaction of the oral tissues, typically of the buccal mucosa.

ETIOLOGY AND PATHOGENESIS
Because these lesions are characterized histologically by the predominance of lymphocytes and plasmacytes, CUPS is believed to represent an inflammatory rather than infectious etiology[42]. The antigen which stimulates the inflammatory reaction is presumed to be bacterial plaque[43]. It is believed that the switch from gram-positive to gram-negative bacteria (and their associated inflammatory antigens) seen in periodontal disease, may trigger the hypersensitivity reaction[42]. In layman's terms, this is an allergic reaction to bacterial plaque.

CLINICAL FEATURES
CUPS is most common in small dogs, especially white breeds; however, this condition can occur in any breed. Maltese and Cavalier King Charles Spaniels appear particularly susceptible[1]. Females appear more prone than males, and the age of onset is typically middle aged.

The presenting signs include: intense oral pain, fetid halitosis, and partial to complete anorexia[1]. Conscious oral examination is usually very difficult due to patient discomfort. Examination under general anesthesia will generally reveal significant dental plaque and calculus as well as gingival inflammation and recession (**314**). Oral examination will also reveal the classic sign of severe buccal ulceration where the mucosa contacts the dentition (kissing lesion) (**315–317**)[11]. The lesions are typically worst over the maxillary canine and carnassial teeth, and especially severe in areas of gingival recession. Depending on the chronicity and severity of the case, the entire buccal mucosa and occasionally the lateral edges of the tongue can become

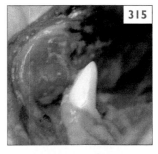

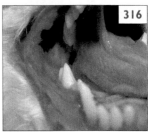

315,316 Kissing lesions on the caudal buccal mucosa. Patient in 316 had a dental prophylaxis 2 months previous and was receiving corticosteroids and antibiotics.

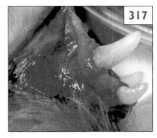

317 Kissing lesion associated with the maxillary canine.

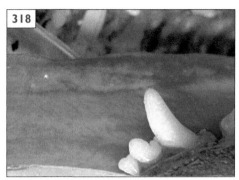

318 Kissing lesion on the lateral surface of the tongue.

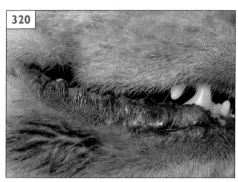

320 Intertrigo of the mandibular lip in a dog with CUPS.

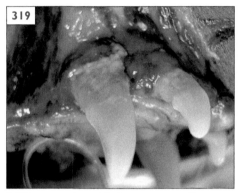

319 Creamy plaque/discharge on a maxillary canine with gingival recession.

involved (**318**). An additional common finding is white, loose, and creamy discharge on the teeth (**319**). Finally, it is not uncommon to see an intertrigo affecting the mandibular lip, due to a significant increase in drooling (**320**). In chronic cases, scarring of the buccal mucosa secondary to chronic inflammation may occur. This makes conscious and unconscious plaque control very challenging, thus early control of the problem is a priority.

Patients will often have a partial response to antibiotic or steroid therapy, in addition to a transient (weeks to months) recovery following a thorough dental prophylaxis. However, with either of these conservative modalities, relapse is usually imminent and generally complete[11,42].

DIFFERENTIAL DIAGNOSES[42]
- Neoplasia (most notably T-cell lymphoma).
- Immune-mediated disease (pemphigus, systemic lupus erythematosus [SLE]).
- Toxic burn.
- Fungal infection (*Candidiasis*).
- Uremic toxicity.
- Periodontal disease.
- Severe systemic infection, particularly *Leptospira canicola*[1].

DIAGNOSTIC TESTS
Prior to anesthesia, a complete physical work-up should be performed. This would minimally include a complete blood panel and urinalysis to rule out systemic disease. CUPS patients typically have an elevated total protein, (polyclonal) hyperglobulinemia, and possibly a mild neutrophilia[42]. Other preanesthetic tests should be added based on these test results, as well as the patient's signalment.

Clinical signs are classic; however, histopathology should be performed to support the clinical diagnosis. Bacterial and fungal cultures are generally mixed and unrewarding, but may influence antibiotic choices. Dental radiographs should be exposed to evaluate periodontal status. Finally, a response to therapy (complete dental prophylaxis) with early relapse is confirmatory.

MANAGEMENT

The key to managing this disease process is strict plaque control[42]. This management is best achieved by a combination of a strict homecare regimen, regular dental cleanings, and selective to full mouth extractions. Tooth brushing and chlorhexidine rinses (e.g. C.E.T. Oral Hygiene Rinse, Virbac Animal Health, Fort Worth) are the most effective means of plaque control. A dental diet (e.g. Hill Pet Nutrition, Topeka) can be used in addition to brushing or rinsing, or in cases of owner noncompliance. It should be noted that without strict home care this form of therapy will fail. Finally, a barrier sealant (e.g. Oravet™ Merial Ltd., Deluth) has shown some benefit in these cases when used consistently.

An important point to consider is that in the majority of cases, only a partial recovery will occur with even the strictest of home care. Resolution of most or all of the clinical signs may occur due to the stoic nature of the canine species, but there is generally some degree of continued inflammation (and pain). These cases can only achieve complete resolution with partial to full mouth extractions (**321**). During the first anesthetic event, a complete dental prophylaxis should be performed. In addition, all periodontally diseased teeth (especially those with gingival recession) should be extracted. Finally, histopathology +/− culture specimens should be obtained and submitted to a reference laboratory.

After the diagnosis is confirmed, remind the owner of the long-term and consistent commitment required for treating this disease process. In addition to home care, regular (several times a year) cleanings are necessary to control clinical signs in the majority of cases. If this is a concern, or home care is not possible, extractions of the maxillary canine and carnassial (as well as any other teeth involved) should be performed. Consequently, full mouth extractions are not unusual in these cases[1]. This form of therapy, while extreme, is curative in the vast majority of cases[11]. When full mouth extractions are performed, it is not uncommon for clients to report that their dog 'is acting like a puppy again'.

Medical therapy is generally unrewarding, but can be added to the strict plaque control measures (outlined above) in nonresponsive cases where owners are particularly resistant to extractions. These clients must be informed prior to initiation of therapy and at regular intervals

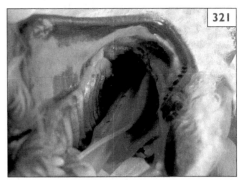

321 Patient in 316 1 month following left sided extractions. The right side was extracted during this anesthetic episode.

through the course of treatment of the side-effects and long-term complications that can result from these medications. Finally, regular blood and urine testing must be performed to ensure that untoward effects are not occurring. These factors, and the involved costs, need to be weighed against surgical therapy.

A combination of antibiotic and anti-inflammatory medications is typically used[42]. Antibiotic choices are amoxicillin-clavulonic acid, metronidazole, clindamycin, or tetracyclines. Glucocorticoids (prednisone) are the most effective of the anti-inflammatory medications; however, azathioprine or cyclosporine can be substituted in patients who cannot tolerate steroids.

KEY POINTS

- This is caused by an immune-mediated reaction to bacterial plaque.
- A thorough dental prophylaxis will induce a partial and temporary response.
- This condition is extremely painful.
- Medical management of CUPS is long-term and often unrewarding.
- Strict plaque control is the key to management.
- Extractions are the most definitive form of therapy.

Immune-mediated diseases affecting the oral cavity

DEFINITION

These diseases are caused by an inappropriate response of the immune system resulting in tissue destruction by its component cells[44]. Immune-mediated disease has been divided into two distinct types[44]. The first is primary immune-mediated, also called autoimmune, in which the antibodies are directed against normal body tissues. Examples of this are the pemphigus complex and bullous pemphigoid. In secondary immune-mediated disease, simply termed immune-mediated, the destruction is created by a reaction to something other than normal self antigens[44]. These syndromes include erythema multiforme, toxic epidermal necrolysis (TEN) and vasculitis. Discoid and systemic lupus erythematosus (SLE) may be primary or secondary depending on the case.

ETIOLOGY AND PATHOGENESIS

In primary (autoimmune) disease, antibodies develop against normal body tissues and induce lesions by passive transfer[44]. The development of autoimmune disease reflects a failure of the normal immune system control mechanisms. The exact mechanism of this loss of control is unknown, with many theories existing. Secondary (immune-mediated) disease is caused by antigens that are foreign to the patient. In general, these are drugs, bacteria, or viruses that create an immunologic response[44]. Antibiotics (especially sulfonamides[45], penicillins, tetracyclines, and aminoglycosides) are frequently implicated in secondary immune-mediated disease, as are numerous other medications[44]. Parasiticides have also been implicated in immune-mediated disease[46], and flea dips have been named as the cause of TEN in a dog and cat[47–49]. In addition, secondary cases have been reported in human and canine patients associated with malignancies, referred to as paraneoplastic pemphigus[50,51]. The most common malignancies associated with this syndrome are lymphoreticular neoplasms (lymphoma and leukemia)[52].

In either case, the auto-antibodies are directed towards the various parts of the molecular apparatus that bind epithelial cells together or connect the surface epithelium to the underlying connective tissue[52]. This loss of connection will result in the blistering or ulcerative type of lesion that characterizes this group of diseases. These lesions can become secondarily infected and, if left untreated, can result in the death of the patient[52].

CLINICAL FEATURES

Although typically considered dermatologic diseases, 90% of pemphigus vulgaris and up to 50% of bullous pemphigoid cases will have oral lesions[1]. These diseases are usually seen in older patients. History will generally include halitosis, dysphagia, decreased grooming, ptyalism, partial to complete anorexia, and lethargy[11]. Blood-tinged saliva may also be noted on occasion.

The classic vesicle is rarely seen in the oral mucosa, as early rupture often occurs secondary to oral trauma[52]. More likely, an ulcerative lesion will be noted within the oral cavity, especially along the mucocutaneous junction (**322, 323**)[11]. These can be single but are typically multiple and can be small, or large and coalescing. Skin lesions are often associated with the oral signs, especially other mucocutaneous areas (anus, genitals). In humans, it is typical for the oral lesions to be the first sign of the disease process (sometimes occurring over 1 year prior to cutaneous lesions), as well as the most difficult to treat[52]. Finally, signs of systemic illness may be seen in severe cases, especially secondary immune-mediated disease and SLE.

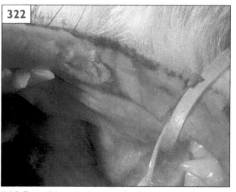

322 Pemphigus lesion on the lip margin of a cat.

DIFFERENTIAL DIAGNOSES
- Trauma/burn.
- Neoplasia.
- Uremic ulcer.
- CUPS.
- Intertrigo.
- Periodontal disease.

DIAGNOSTIC TESTS
A thorough history and physical examination (including the integumentary system and other mucocutaneous junctions) should be performed. Due to the possibility of systemic disease (especially with TEN and SLE), a complete blood panel should be performed prior to any further diagnostics or therapy. Diagnosis is confirmed by histopathology +/− immunofluorescence or immunohistochemical testing[11,44,52]. Ideally, this is performed on intact vesicles, but these can be difficult to obtain due to their fragility. If SLE is suspected, an ANA test should be performed. This is a highly sensitive test for SLE, although false positives do occur[44,53].

MANAGEMENT
The classic therapy for the primary form, or autoimmune disease (pemphigus complex, bullous pemphigoid, and SLE), is immunomodulation. This is typically achieved with corticosteroids. Many patients with predominantly oral lesions (especially the pemphigus complex) respond favorably to immunosuppressive corticosteroid doses (2–3 mg/kg BID for 10 days) tapering with response[11,52]. It must be noted that at these doses, severe side-effects (including death) are quite common[54]. For this reason, it is recommended to add steroid sparing agents such as azathioprine, to decrease the incidence of steroid-induced side-effects, especially in chronic cases[52,55]. Bullous pemphigoid is the most difficult autoimmune type to treat, and usually requires a combination of drugs to achieve remission, as well as long-term or life long therapy[44]. Levamisole has shown promise as an adjunct therapy for SLE[44].

Numerous new medications are being used with some to good success for these disease processes, particularly the pemphigoid complex. These include: tetracycline and niacinamide, cyclosporine[56], tacrolimus, mycophenolate mofetil, cyclophosphamide, chrysotherapy, dapsone[57], sulfasalazine, and intravenous immunoglobulin (IVIG)[44,58–60].

The key to treating the secondary forms (erythema multiforme, TEN, and vasculitis) is to identify and remove the inciting antigen. If this is performed, regression of the lesions generally occurs within a few weeks. During this time, supportive care (nutritional support, pain medications, and antibiotics) is critical. Corticosteroid usage is controversial at this time[61,62]. The major reason cited against their use is the high incidence of sepsis in these cases[44]. There may be an indication however, for corticosteroid use in drug-induced cases[44]. Cyclosporine and IVIG have also both shown promise in these cases[63–65].

KEY POINTS
- This is a rare set of diseases that commonly have oral manifestations.
- Immune-mediated disease should be considered with oral ulcerations in patients receiving recent drug therapy.
- A biopsy is required for definitive diagnosis.
- Drug reactions should be investigated early in the disease process.
- Treatment for most of these lesions involves immunomodulation/suppression.
- IVIG has shown promise as a form of treatment.
- Due to the difficulty in treatment and the significant side-effects of therapy, this is best treated by a specialist (Internal medicine or Dermatology).

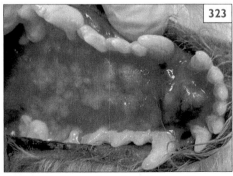

323 TEN lesion on the palate of a dog. (Courtesy of Dr. Craig Griffin.)

Uremic stomatitis

DEFINITION
This is a condition in which oral ulcers develop secondary to renal disease, as a result of the increase in nitrogenous wastes in the bloodstream[11,66].

ETIOLOGY AND PATHOGENESIS
The true etiology of the oral lesions is unknown[67]. It is known that the oral manifestations occur secondary to the increase in nonprotein nitrogenous waste levels in the blood due to renal disease. However, this does not happen in all patients[52,68]. Some believe that urease, an enzyme produced by oral microflora, degrades urea into ammonia within the saliva[52]. As the ammonia levels in the saliva increase, mucosal irritation, dehydration, and clotting abnormalities may develop as the normal mucosal protection is compromised[1,11].

Uremic ulcers are rare in human dentistry, and the majority of cases are associated with acute renal failure[52,67]. In humans, blood urea levels rarely get high enough to induce these changes with chronic disease. Uremic oral ulcers in people are typically seen when the BUN is over 300 mg/dl, (3 g/l) but can occasionally be seen at 200 mg/dl (2 g/l)[67]. There are no published studies in the veterinary literature, but one veterinary renal specialist notes that ulcerations are common in patients (particularly feline) with a BUN ≥ 200 mg/dl (≥ 2 g/l), and documented in patients with a BUN as low as 150 mg/dl (1.5 g/l)[69]. This is probably due to the increased level of oral infection in veterinary patients as compared to their human counterparts.

CLINICAL FEATURES
Animal patients with uremic stomatitis often present with an acute onset of anorexia, lethargy, and other signs of systemic disease. There may also be a history of chronic renal insufficiency, polyurea/polydypsia, or exposure to a toxin such as ethylene glycol[66]. Typical clinical findings include whitish plaque-like or ulcerative lesions in the mouth[52]. These lesions can occur anywhere, but in animal patients are most common on the ventrolateral aspect of the tongue (**324**), as well as the buccal mucosa[69]. In some cases, there may also be dark discoloration,

sloughing, and necrosis on the dorsorostal aspect of the tongue[11]. The mouth smells of uremic breath and a necrotic odor is also common[11,52].

DIFFERENTIAL DIAGNOSES
- Trauma.
- Neoplasia.
- Caustic burn.
- CUPS.
- Immune-mediated disease.
- Electric cord burn.

DIAGNOSTIC TESTS
A complete biochemical profile evaluated in light of a concurrent urinalysis should be diagnostic for severe renal disease. Other diagnostic tests are aimed at better defining the underlying renal component and identifying the etiology (if possible). If an oral biopsy is performed, histopathology reveals minimal underlying inflammatory infiltrate, a hyperplastic epithelium, and unusual hyperparakeratinization[70].

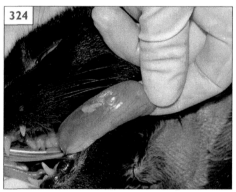

324 Uremic ulcer on the ventrolateral tongue of a cat.

MANAGEMENT

The key to managing these lesions is lowering the level of uremic toxins in the blood[71]. This is accomplished by rehydrating the patient, treating underlying etiologies, and providing supportive care, possibly including hemodialyis. If BUN levels are decreased significantly, the lesions will resolve quickly (typically less than 10 days)[52,69].

Treating any concurrent oral disease (e.g. periodontal) helps to decrease the infection and inflammation; however, these patients are not good candidates for elective anesthesia. Lavaging the mouth with dilute chlorhexidine or hydrogen peroxide solutions is reported to speed recovery of the lesions[52,67,69,71].

KEY POINTS

- Keep this on the differential list for oral ulcers.
- Acute onset is a common historical finding.
- Uremic ulcers respond rapidly to a decrease in BUN.
- The key to therapy is treating the renal disease.
- Lavaging with chlorhexidine helps to speed recovery.

Candidiasis (thrush)

DEFINITION

Candidiasis is a mycotic infection of the oral mucosa caused by *Candida albicans*.

ETIOLOGY AND PATHOGENESIS

The infectious agent in this disease process is part of the normal oral flora for many patients[72]. In fact, 30–50% percent of humans are asymptomatic carriers[52]. There are different strains however, and some seem more aggressive than others. In general, the disease is associated with immune compromise of the host (natural, infections, or drug-induced), or chronic antibiotic (or antifungal) therapy which alters the normal oral flora[11,52,72,73].

Diabetes mellitus and hyperadrenocorticism have been implicated in animals as well as human patients[72,74–76]. Humans infected with human immunodeficiency virus (HIV)[77] and human patients treated with radiation or chemotherapy for malignancies are at a higher risk due to compromise of the immune system[72,78,79]. Chronic corticosteroid usage is known to depress the immune system in animals[80]. This has been shown to be a risk factor for the development of opportunistic fungal infections, including candidiasis in humans and animals[72,81,82]. Consequently, dermatologic patients should be closely monitored for this disease due to the typical long-term steroid and antibiotic therapy. These medications should be used at a minimum, or more ideally, alternate drug therapies and specific antigen testing. Finally, patients using asthma inhalers which contain glucocorticoids are specifically susceptible due to the local suppression of the immune system[83,84].

CLINICAL FEATURES[52]

There are several different syndromes of oral candidiasis seen in human dentistry. The most common clinical form in humans is psuedomembranous 'thrush', which in fact is the only form reported in companion animals[11]. Thrush is characterized by the presence of adherent white plaques (that resemble cottage cheese) on the oral mucosa (**325** *overpage*). The plaques can be easily removed with a dry gauze sponge. Unless some other condition is affecting the oral cavity (e.g. radiation therapy), there is no bleeding, although the underlying mucosa may

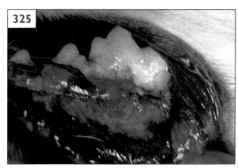

325 Candidiasis lesion in a dog.

be slightly erythematous. This is a nonpainful condition which creates no malodor, and thus outward clinical signs are generally not noted.

Systemic candidiasis has been reported in both the human and veterinary literature, and results in significant morbidity, as well as mortality in severely immune compromised patients[52,72,85].

DIAGNOSTIC TESTS
Diagnosis can be confirmed either by culture or cytology. Cytologic samples can be obtained with a swab and can be prepared either with a PAS stain[52] or India ink[11]. Cytology should reveal the hyphal stage of the organism, as this is the infectious stage[52].

DIFFERENTIAL DIAGNOSES
- Immune-mediated disease (pemphigus, SLE).
- CUPS.
- Periodontal disease.
- Other fungal infection.
- Uremic ulcers.

MANAGEMENT
The first step in management is to identify and treat any possible underlying cause effectively, such as diabetes mellitus or hyperadrenocorticism. In addition, if chronic steroid or antibiotic therapy is involved, this should be addressed by using other treatments/medications if possible. In cases with an underlying immune compromise, levamisole can be added to stimulate the immune system[86,87]. Specific therapy for the infection includes local and/or systemic antifungal therapy. Local therapy generally consists of rinsing with nystatin or clortrimazole[11,52].

Recent human studies have shown that a commercially available chlorhexidine gluconate rinse is effective in the prevention and treatment of candidiasis either alone or in combination with other topical rinses[88,89]. Topical rinsing allows for direct contact with the infectious agent with a minimum of side-effects. While topical therapy is very effective in human patients, it is difficult to apply in animal patients. Holding the medication in the animal's mouth for 1–2 minutes is often not achievable, and therefore systemic therapy is likely to be superior in all but the most tractable patients.

There are many systemic antifungal agents available for oral candidiasis including ketoconazole, fluconazole, and itraconazole. All are effective at once daily dosing. Itraconazole appears to be the current treatment of choice, due to increased hepatotoxicity of ketoconazole and increasing resistance to fluconazole[52].

Resistance of *Candida* spp. to traditional antifungals is becoming increasingly common. This is especially true in immune suppressed patients. In addition, systemic antifungal therapy can have serious side-effects. These concerns have led to increased interest in alternate therapies. Several new techniques which have shown promise in human studies may translate well into the veterinary field. These include a photodynamic compound (toluidine blue O)[90], lactoferrin[91], and lysozyme[92]. The latter two are naturally occurring, and much safer than most antifungals. In addition, these two therapies are delivered by a mucoadhesive patch which could potentially allow for effective topical therapy in veterinary patients[91,92].

KEY POINTS
- *Candida* is a fungal infection.
- This opportunistic infection is usually secondary to immune compromise or antibiotic therapy.
- Local infections are mostly an annoyance and easily cured with antifungal therapy[52].
- Antifungal resistance is emerging.
- Treat any underlying causes to avoid relapse.
- Check for drug interactions before prescribing systemic antifungals.
- Monitor liver enzymes, especially with ketoconazole.

Caustic burns of the oral cavity

DEFINITION
This is defined as oral damage caused by an exogenous toxin, usually an acid or base.

ETIOLOGY AND PATHOGENESIS
Oral caustic burns typically occur following an accidental ingestion of a caustic agent, but can also occur due to chewing on an object (i.e. battery). In addition, animals (especially cats) can be exposed during self-grooming[1]. There are reports which name flea dips as the cause of severe toxic sequela in a dog and cat[47–49]. Caustic agents which contact the sensitive oral mucosa cause almost instant ulceration in most cases. In some cases however, the actual clinical lesions will be delayed. Alkalis cause more extensive damage than acids, due to the liquefaction necrosis which occurs, which continues until the agent is removed or neutralized[93].

CLINICAL FEATURES
Caustic burns are most common in young dogs and puppies (especially large breeds)[1], but can be seen at any age, and in cats. History should include possible exposure to a caustic agent, but in many cases the clients have no knowledge of the incident. The history generally includes an acute onset of significant ptyalism and oral pain with partial to complete anorexia[11,93]. In addition, blood tinged saliva may be seen.

The most common oral finding is ulcerative lesions covered by a necrotic lining (**326**)[11,93,94]. On occasion, the presenting sign may be severe erythema throughout the mouth (**327**). Additional problems include respiratory compromise and vomiting. Some patients may demonstrate slight to severe systemic signs of poisoning, including shock. In humans, common sequelae to caustic ingestion are microstomia and esophageal strictures due to scarring of the severely damaged tissues[95–98]. In some cases, this may cause significant morbidity and possibly dysphagia.

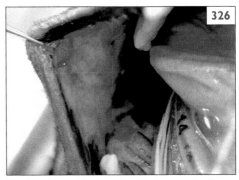

326 Widespread ulceration in the mouth of a dog following exposure to a base liquid.

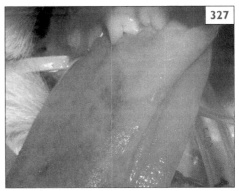

327 Significant erythema of the ventral tongue of a cat following acid exposure.

DIFFERENTIAL DIAGNOSES

- Trauma.
- Neoplasia.
- Uremic ulcer.
- CUPS.
- Immune-mediated disease.
- Electric cord burn.

DIAGNOSTIC TESTS

There are no specific diagnostic tests. A complete blood panel should be performed to asses the status of vital organs as well as to rule out uremia. Esophagoscopy is recommended in all cases as soon as possible (within 24–48 hours) to observe directly the extent of damage to the upper gastrointestinal tract[93,99,100]. If there is any doubt as to the etiology (especially in nonresponsive cases), a biopsy is recommended.

MANAGEMENT

Do not induce emesis in any case of caustic (acid/base) ingestion. In addition, do not give neutralizing acids or bases, as this can worsen the damage due to the exothermic reaction[93]! There are three main areas of concern for these cases: the mouth, the remainder of the gastrointestinal tract, and the patient as a whole.

The first step in therapy is to administer effective pain management, which should include opiates. Corticosteroid therapy should also be instituted to help decrease the inflammation and scarring[99–101]. Broad-spectrum antibiotics are warranted to combat any secondary infection[93]. All medications should be administered parenterally as oral medication should not be attempted. Fluid therapy, nutritional support, and other supportive care should be administered as needed[93].

The patient's mouth should be treated with dilutional therapy as soon as possible[100]. Water or milk are considered the liquids of choice[93,99]. This typically requires general anesthesia in animal patients, in order to avoid aspiration. Superficial areas of necrosis usually heal within 2 weeks. If lesions are severe, conservative surgical debridement should be performed to promote healing and prevent spread of the necrosis[52]. Dilutional therapy of the remainder of the alimentary tract should be performed if there is any evidence or possibility of ingestion. Again, water and milk are the preferred diluents[99]. Do not be overzealous in dilution

therapy as it could lead to vomiting. This will cause secondary exposure and may result in aspiration[100]. Activated charcoal is not recommended[93,99]. In cases of acid ingestion with minimal esophageal injury, gastric lavage and oral administration of aluminum hydroxide preparations are recommended[93]. Gastric lavage is contraindicated in cases of alkali ingestion[93].

KEY POINTS

- An acute onset is a key historical finding.
- Caustic oral burns are more common in dogs than cats.
- The key to therapy is lavage of the area to reduce concentration.
- Do NOT induce vomiting.
- Supportive care is necessary.
- Esophagoscopy is strongly recommended within 48 hours.

Problems with Muscles, Bones, and Joints

Kendall G. Taney and Mark M. Smith

- **Masticatory myositis**
- **Craniomandibular osteopathy**
- **Idiopathic trigeminal neuritis**
- **Temporomandibular joint luxation**
- **Temporomandibular joint dysplasia**
- **Fractures**
- **Traumatic tooth avulsion and luxation**
- **Root fractures**
- **Osteomyelitis**
- **Tumors and cysts**
- **Hyperparathyroidism**
- **Tetanus**
- **Botulism**

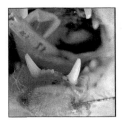
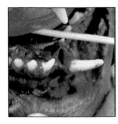
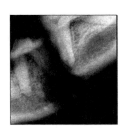
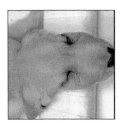

Masticatory myositis

DEFINITION
Masticatory muscle myositis (MM) is an autoimmune, focal inflammatory myopathy of the muscles of mastication that causes necrosis, phagocytosis, and fibrosis of the myofibers[1-3].

ETIOLOGY AND PATHOGENESIS
Masticatory muscle fibers have a distinct embryologic origin and contain type 2M fibers. These fibers differ histochemically and biochemically from muscle fiber types of the limbs[3-5]. This unique type 2M myofiber isoform is likely to be related to the different motor nerve branches that develop during embryologic development[6]. Autoantibodies against the specific type of myosin in these type 2M fibers are responsible for the immune-mediated reaction. The reason for the autoimmune response is still unknown. Some theories suggest that cross-reaction with self-antigens may be a causative factor[1]. Antibodies directed against bacterial antigens could potentially cross-react with these myofibers[7]. Inflammatory mononucleate cells infiltrate and phagocytose the muscle fibers causing necrosis and subsequent fibrosis[1,3]. Cellular infiltrates in MM selectively affect the muscles innervated by the mandibular branch of the trigeminal nerve, including the masseter, temporalis, pterygoid, tensor tympani, tensor veli palatine, and digastricus [1,5,8].

CLINICAL FEATURES
The disease has acute and chronic phases. During the acute phase, hypertrophy of the muscles of mastication with myalgia occurs. Pyrexia and enlargement of the mandibular and prescapular lymph nodes may be present. There is often an inability to open the mouth or conversely the jaws may remain open because of swelling, preventing complete closure. There may be exophthalmos from swelling of the pterygoid muscles behind the eyes[1]. Ocular signs are noted in as many as 44% of cases[9]. Vision disorder can be caused by stretching of the optic nerve from exophthalmos[1,2,3]. The disease can occur in any breed, but young, large breed dogs such as German Shepherds, Doberman Pinschers, Cavalier King Charles spaniels, and retrievers are overrepresented[1,3]. It does not appear to occur in cats. The disorder is generally bilateral but may appear unilateral if one side is more severely affected. The chronic phase is characterized by replacement of myofibers with fibrous tissue. This stage of the disease is irreversible and can result in continued and permanent trismus. The muscles of mastication become severely atrophied and enophthalmos may be present from atrophy of the pterygoid muscles[1] (**328**).

DIFFERENTIAL DIAGNOSES
Myopathies
- Leptospirosis.
- Toxoplasmosis.
- Neosporosis.
- Leishmaniasis.
- Hepatozoonosis.
- *Rickettsia* spp. infection.
- *Dirofilaria immitis* infection.
- *Clostridia* spp. infection.
- Systemic lupus erythematosus (SLE).
- Drugs toxins (cimetidine, trimethoprim-sulfadiazine, penicillamines).
- Thymoma.
- Lymphoma.
- Idiopathic disease.
- Trismus.
- Extraocular myositis.
- Generalized myopathy.
- Temporomandibular joint (TMJ) luxation, subluxation, or fusion from degenerative joint disease.
- Tetanus.
- Craniomandibular osteopathy.
- Retrobulbar abscess.
- Muscular dystrophy.
- Foreign body.

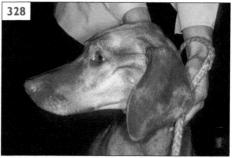

328 Severe muscle atrophy of the muscles of mastication in a Doberman Pincher with MM. (Courtesy of Dr. David Lipsitz.)

DIAGNOSTIC TESTS

Initial diagnostic tests for any myopathy should always include complete blood count and serum chemistry profile including creatinine kinase (CK) level. Biochemical changes in patients with MM are generally nonspecific but may include elevated CK during the acute phase, hyperglobulinemia, anemia, proteinuria, and leukocytosis[1,3,9]. An ELISA test for circulating antibodies in the serum against type 2M muscle fibers is available and is highly specific[10]. A positive result of this test in conjunction with clinical signs confirms the diagnosis of MM. A false negative may occur in patients in the end-stage of the disease where the muscle fibers are mostly lost and replaced by fibrotic tissue, and also in patients that have received corticosteroids before testing[1].

Electromyelography (EMG) of the muscles of mastication shows abnormal spontaneous activity such as fibrillation potentials, positive sharp waves, and complex repetitive charges[1,3]. EMG cannot differentiate between neuropathic and myopathic causes and results may be normal in patients in the end-stage of the disease. Muscle biopsy is very important for determining the stage of the disease and the long-term prognosis by documenting the severity of fiber loss and degree of fibrosis[1]. Care must be taken to biopsy a muscle of mastication such as the temporalis, and avoid biopsy of muscles not involved in mastication such as the frontalis muscle. Biopsy of muscles during the acute phase shows sites of necrosis and phagocytosis of type 2M fibers with perivascular infiltration of mononucleate cells[1,3]. The chronic and end-stages show loss of myofibers, minimal cellular infiltrate, and endomysial and perimysial fibrosis[8]. If signs of systemic illness are present, infectious diseases and other autoimmune disorders should be ruled out via antibody titers[1].

MANAGEMENT

Early diagnosis and treatment with immunosuppressive doses of corticosteroids are essential for the best long-term prognosis. Treatment with corticosteroids should be initiated during the acute phase. Administration during the end-stage of the disease is generally not beneficial. Therapy is usually not effective in dogs that have experienced multiple episodes of inflammation and show signs of muscle fibrosis[3]. Prednisone can be administered at 2 mg/kg and maintained until maximum jaw function has been regained and CK levels have returned to normal[1]. Tapering of the prednisone dose should occur over 4–6 months with no more than a 50% dose decrease per month. The patient should be maintained on the lowest every other day dose that controls clinical signs. It may be possible to discontinue steroid therapy if clinical signs do not return, but many patients will need to be administered steroids for life. Early discontinuation of steroids often leads to relapse of the disease and progression to the chronic phase. Azathioprine can also be used in patients that do not tolerate, or are refractory, to steroid administration. The initial dose is 2–4 mg/kg once daily or EOD while prednisone is tapered to a maintenance dose or discontinued. Side-effects of steroids include polyuria, polydypsia, polyphagia, and gastric ulceration. Side-effects of azathioprine can include bone marrow suppression and hepatotoxicity. Cyclosporine can also be used, but requires extensive therapeutic monitoring.

Without early recognition and aggressive treatment, myofiber loss and muscle fibrosis may result in irreversible jaw dysfunction and severe muscle atrophy[1]. Patients in the chronic and end-stages of the disease may have extensive fibrosis causing trismus. However, forcible manual retraction of the jaw as a treatment is contraindicated due to risk of mandibular fracture, TMJ fracture or luxation, and tearing of fibrotic tissue with subsequent production of more fibrous tissue[9]. Exercises with objects such as rubber balls can help increase the range of jaw motion.

KEY POINTS

- Clinical signs such as masticatory muscle enlargement, oral pain, and trismus in combination with a positive 2M antibody test is diagnostic for MM.
- Early diagnosis and aggressive corticosteroid therapy will provide the best prognosis for recovery and long-term function.
- Biopsy of the muscles of mastication (most commonly the temporalis) can provide valuable information on the stage of the disease and help determine long-term prognosis.
- The end-stage of the disease is characterized by near complete loss of myofibers, scant cellular infiltration, and fibrosis of the muscles of mastication.

Craniomandibular osteopathy

DEFINITION
Craniomandibular osteopathy (CMO) is a non-neoplastic, noninflammatory proliferative bone disease of immature dogs involving the occipital bones, tympanic bulla, zygomatic portions of the temporal bone, and mandibular rami[11–13].

ETIOLOGY AND PATHOGENESIS
Onset of the disease generally occurs between 4–8 months of age. Bilateral irregular new bone formation occurs on the mandible, tympanic bullae, temporal bone, and occipital bone. Certain breeds are overrepresented, including the West Highland white terrier, Cairn terrier, and Scottish terrier. An autosomal recessive inheritance pattern is suspected based on a retrospective study of West Highland white terriers[14]. The osseous lesions are the result of complex and varied pathological changes. This includes osteoclastic resorption of lamellar bone, replacement of lamellar bone by primitive coarse bone, loss of normal bone marrow spaces, replacement of marrow by a highly vascular fibrous stroma, and formation of new coarse trabecular bone with a pattern of irregular cement lines indicating the sporadic and rapid deposition and resorption of the abnormal bone[11]. Inflammatory cells may also be present. The bony proliferation ceases once the dog is skeletally mature and endochondral ossification ends, around 9–11 months of age[11–13]. The proliferative bone may then regress to some degree, although in severe cases the dog may no longer be able to open the mouth[11–13].

CLINICAL FEATURES
Presenting signs are mandibular pain, pyrexia, inability to open the mouth, difficulty in prehension, mastication and swallowing, and thickening of the mandibular rami. There are acute stages and remission stages[15]. Restricted jaw movement and atrophy of masticatory muscles may be obvious in severely affected dogs. Mandibular swelling without pain or eating difficulties occurs in some dogs, especially of larger breeds (329). Radiographic changes are generally bilateral but often asymmetric, with irregular bony proliferation involving the mandible and TMJ in about 50% of cases[12,15] (330). Changes can be confined to the mandible or less frequently confined to the tympanic bulla-petrous temporal region. The calvarium and tentorium ossium are often thickened and other skull bones may be affected[12]. Bony proliferation is less detectable around the alveoli and interalveolar spaces of the mandibular teeth. The angular process and enlarging tympanic bulla can fuse, mechanically obstructing the motion of the jaw and forming a solid bar of abnormal bone between the two structures[11]. Concurrent long bone lesions resembling later stages of metaphyseal osteopathy have been observed in a few terriers with craniomandibular osteopathy[11,12].

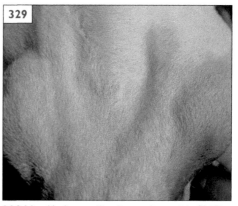

329 Mandibular swelling in a patient with CMO.

DIFFERENTIAL DIAGNOSIS
- Neoplasia.
- Osteomyelitis.
- Periostitis from trauma.
- MM (trismus and atrophy of muscles of mastication).

DIAGNOSTIC TESTS
Diagnosis of CMO is confirmed by radiographs and presence of clinical signs. Bone biopsy may be helpful in atypical cases. The histopathology demonstrates resorption of existing lamellae, proliferation of coarse trabecular bone beyond normal periosteal boundaries, replacement of marrow spaces by vascular fibrous stroma, and infiltration at the periphery of new bone by inflammatory cells. Irregular cement lines are present in the new irregular bone[11,12].

MANAGEMENT
CMO is self-limiting. Abnormal bone proliferation eventually slows and becomes static at about 1 year of age, once the physes have closed[12,13,15]. Lesions may then regress completely or near completely. In severe cases, prehension and mastication are still impaired even after the cessation of the disease[2,12,13,15]. Surgical excision of exostoses is usually unrewarding, and euthanasia may be elected. The prognosis is guarded when extensive changes affect the tympanic–petrous temporal areas and adjacent mandible. Ankylosis and adhesions may then develop, permanently restricting jaw movements and eating. Rostral mandibulectomy can be a useful salvage procedure in these cases[12]. Anti-inflammatory drug treatment can reduce pain and discomfort, but the effect on lesions is unknown.

KEY POINTS
- CMO is a disease of juvenile dogs and certain terrier breeds are overrepresented.
- The disease process will cease and even partially regress once the animal reaches skeletal maturity.
- Treatment involves nutritional support and pain management until the lesions regress.
- Surgical excision of exostoses may be performed, but is often unrewarding in severe cases.
- The prognosis is poor in severe cases where movement of the TMJ is significantly restricted.

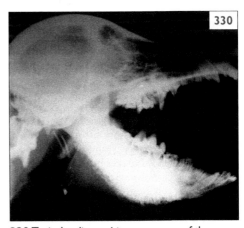

330 Typical radiographic appearance of the bony proliferation on the ventral mandible of a dog with CMO. (Courtesy of University of Pennsylvania Dental Department.)

Idiopathic trigeminal neuritis

DEFINITION
Idiopathic trigeminal neuritis is characterized by acute onset of bilateral trigeminal motor paralysis causing an inability to close the mouth.

ETIOLOGY AND PATHOGENESIS
The cause of this disorder is unknown. Neuritis can be caused by trauma, neoplastic infiltration, or infectious causes. Horner's syndrome may be present due to involvement of the postganglionic sympathetic axons coursing in the ophthalmic nerve. Demyelination of the trigeminal nerve may occur, but the brainstem is unaffected. Recovery is assumed to follow remyelination[2,16,17].

CLINICAL FEATURES
There is no predilection for breed, age, or sex and it can occur in dogs and cats. Dogs with this disorder present with a laxity of the jaw and the inability to close the mouth (**331**). The mouth can be manually closed but then immediately drops open[2]. Facial sensation is usually intact. Horner's syndrome may also be present[16,18]. Swallowing is typically normal but prehending food is not possible. Spontaneous recovery usually occurs in 2–3 weeks but may take months to completely resolve. Occasionally mandibular neuropraxia can occur from stretching of the branches of the masticatory muscle motor nerves when the animal attempts to open its mouth too far, or to carry heavy weights (rocks or branches) in the mouth[2,17].

DIFFERENTIAL DIAGNOSES
- Neoplasia (infiltrative or intracranial).
- TMJ luxation/fracture.
- Botulism.
- Infectious.
- Brainstem injury.
- Rabies.
- Hypothyroidism.

DIAGNOSTIC TESTS
The diagnosis of idiopathic trigeminal neuritis is reached by the presence of clinical signs, exclusion of differential diagnoses, and spontaneous recovery. Biopsy of the muscles of mastication reveals denervation atrophy.

Histopathology of the nerve is not generally performed, but has been shown to demonstrate a nonsuppurative inflammation of the trigeminal nerve and ganglion[16,18].

MANAGEMENT
Spontaneous recovery generally occurs within 2–3 weeks, but complete resolution of clinical signs may not occur for several months. Corticosteroid therapy does not appear to alter the course of the disease[2,16–18].

KEY POINTS
- Laxity of the jaw and inability to close the mouth are the prominent features of this disorder.
- Facial sensation is intact.
- Spontaneous recovery generally occurs within 2–3 weeks.
- No pharmacologic agent or therapy has been shown to alter the course of the disease.

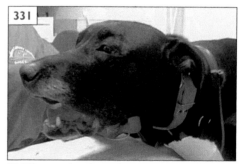

331 'Dropped jaw' in a dog with idiopathic trigeminal neuritis. (Courtesy of Dr. Brook Niemiec.)

Temporomandibular joint luxation

DEFINITION
Temporomandibular joint (TMJ) luxation is a result of separation of the mandibular condyles from the articular surfaces of the temporal bone and mandibular fossae[19].

ETIOLOGY AND PATHOGENESIS
The cause of TMJ luxations is often related to head trauma. It may occur as an isolated injury or be associated with other maxillofacial injuries, such as fractures[20]. Generally the condylar process displaces rostrodorsally[19,20]. The mandibular condyle can also be displaced caudally, which is typically associated with fracture of the retroarticular process[20].

CLINICAL FEATURES
The animal may present with an inability to close the mouth and/or the mandible may be deviated to the side opposite the luxated joint (**332**). Other maxillofacial injuries may be present simultaneously.

DIFFERENTIAL DIAGNOSES
- TMJ dysplasia.
- Foreign body.
- CMO.
- Mandibular fracture.
- Maxillary fracture.
- Idiopathic trigeminal neuritis.

DIAGNOSTIC TESTS
Radiographs or computed tomography (CT) are useful in confirming the diagnosis as well as evaluating for concurrent injuries[19,20]. The most reliable radiographic sign is increased TMJ space, which can be most evident on a dorsoventral projection[19].

MANAGEMENT
Closed reduction of TMJ luxations should be attempted with the patient under general anesthesia. The condyle is forced ventrally by using a fulcrum in between the maxillary and mandibular molar teeth, and closing the mouth to lever the condylar process in a ventrocaudal direction back into the mandibular fossa[19-21]. The occlusion should be checked carefully, as this is a strong indicator that the luxation has been properly reduced. After reduction, the joint should be stabilized with a tape muzzle or interarcade wiring for 1–2 weeks to prevent luxation from recurring[19,21]. Refractory luxations can be treated with open reduction and suture imbrication of the joint capsule or, more commonly, with mandibular condylectomy[20]. Mandibular condylectomy can also be performed in cases where the joint becomes fibrosed or ankylosed from injury[19].

KEY POINTS
- TMJ luxations are usually caused by trauma.
- The patient should be carefully evaluated for other injuries such as maxillofacial fractures and neurologic signs.
- Closed reduction should be performed under anesthesia and the joint should be stabilized with a loose fitting nylon muzzle or interarcade wiring for 1–2 weeks after reduction.
- Chronic luxations or ankylosed joints can be managed with open reduction or mandibular condylectomy.

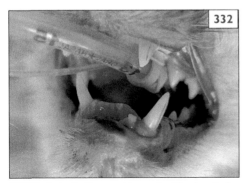

332 Typical misalignment in a cat with a luxated TMJ. (Courtesy of Dr. Brook Niemiec.)

Temporomandibular joint dysplasia

DEFINITION

TMJ dysplasia is characterized by degeneration of the joint components resulting in subluxation and recurrent locking of the mandible in an open-mouthed position.

ETIOLOGY AND PATHOGENESIS

The etiology of TMJ dysplasia is unknown. Irish setters, Bassett hounds, and some spaniel breeds have been represented, and the age of onset is early adulthood[2,19,22]. The mandibular condyloid processes and mandibular fossa become deformed (**333**) which allows subluxation of the joint, and locking of the joint in an open-mouthed position often occurs. Joint instability leads to osteoarthritis, pain, and locking of the jaw. Mandibular symphyseal laxity can also allow independent movement of the mandibles, which results in malpositioning of coronoid processes lateral to the zygomatic arch[19]. A similar process can also occur after trauma to the TMJ, causing fibrotic changes which limit the range of motion or allows locking of the mouth in the open position[20].

CLINICAL FEATURES

The dog may present with the jaw locked in an open position, or the owner may describe episodes where the jaw is locked open and the dog paws at the mouth. The dog may be able to manually release the locked jaw.

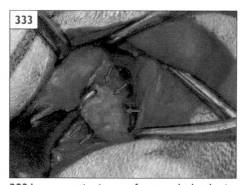

333 Intraoperative image of a severely dysplastic TMJ. Arrows indicate the enlarged and misshapen condyloid process of the mandible.

DIFFERENTIAL DIAGNOSES

- CMO.
- TMJ luxation.
- MM.
- Foreign body.
- Idiopathic trigeminal neuropathy.
- Botulism.

DIAGNOSTIC TESTS

A skull radiograph series under general anesthesia, or heavy sedation, is needed for diagnosis. Closed and open mouth views can confirm the diagnosis. Degenerative changes such as increased or irregular joint spaces, shallow mandibular fossae, and osteoarthritis may be noticed in a lateral projection. An open-mouthed ventrodorsal projection can demonstrate the coronoid process positioned lateral to the zygomatic arch[19]. CT may also demonstrate degenerative changes of the TMJ.

MANAGEMENT

Manual reduction can be attempted in an awake animal, but the problem often recurs. Surgical treatment of the disease is accomplished with either partial zygomatic arch resection, or mandibular condylectomy[2,19,20,22].

KEY POINTS

- TMJ dysplasia is a degenerative joint disease of unknown etiology.
- Dogs may present with the jaw locked in an open-mouthed position.
- Surgical treatment involves removal of a portion of the zygomatic arch or mandibular condylectomy to prevent the jaw from locking open.

Fractures

DEFINITION

Oromaxillofacial fractures can provide unique challenges for treatment. In the case of trauma, multiple injuries may be present at the same time, and may be compounded by serious complications such as neurologic damage. Treatment of traumatic oromaxillofacial fractures should be performed once the patient has been fully assessed for existing diseases and is stable to undergo anesthesia and surgical repair. Pathological fractures can be difficult to repair because of reduced healing properties secondary to an underlying cause such as neoplasia or infection.

ETIOLOGY AND PATHOGENESIS

There are many different types of oromaxillofacial fractures that can occur because of trauma or pathological process. Some occur more commonly than others, and each type may need to be approached differently. Some examples of oromaxillofacial fractures include:

- Mandibular symphyseal separation (**334, 335**).
- Mandibular body (**336, 337**).

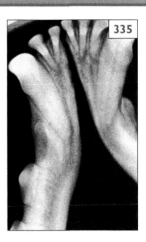

335 Dental radiographs revealing a widened symphysis, consistent with a symphyseal separation.

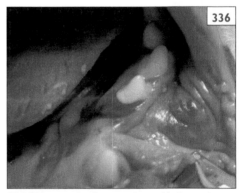

336 Photograph of a typical mandibular mid-body fracture in a dog. (Courtesy of Dr. Brook Niemiec.)

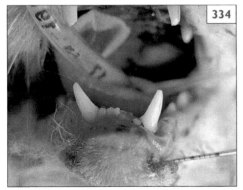

334 Typical presentation of a cat with a symphyseal separation. (Courtesy of Dr. Brook Niemiec.)

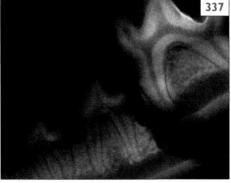

337 Radiograph of a typical mandibular mid-body fracture in a dog. (Courtesy of Dr. Brook Niemiec.)

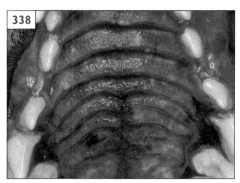

338 Photograph of a typical maxillary fracture in a dog.

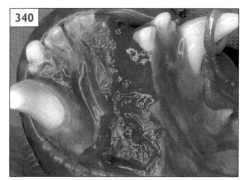

340 Obvious rostral mandibular fracture in a dog.

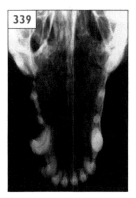

339 Radiograph of the patient in **338**.

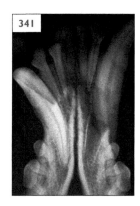

341 Radiograph of the patient in figure **340**.

- Mandibular ramus.
- Maxillary (including zygomatic, palatine, frontal, nasal, and maxillary bones) (**338, 339**).

Oral fractures have special considerations such as limited access, sterility, and maintenance of proper occlusion. Concurrent diseases such as periodontal disease and viability of the bone structure can also affect treatment of oral fractures[22]. The muscular forces acting on the oromaxillofacial structures are also important to consider during treatment of mandibular body fractures. The temporal, masseter, and medial pterygoid muscles are responsible for closing the mouth and can generate tremendous occlusal forces on the mandible[20]. Fractures of the mandible are more common than maxillary fractures, and are generally more obvious due to greater mobility and dropped jaw appearance or obvious malocclusion (**340, 341**). Symphyseal separation is the most common oral fracture seen in the cat[20,22,23]. Circumferential wiring is often sufficient for repair of these fractures.

Mandibular body fractures are the most common fractures seen in the dog[2,22,24]. Favorable mandibular fractures are those with fracture lines that run caudodorsally (**342**), because the masseter, temporal, and pterygoid muscles insert on the caudal end of the mandible, and therefore cause compression of the fracture fragments. Conversely, unfavorable fracture lines run caudoventrally (**343**). These are unfavorable due to the fact that the muscles of mastication exert force upward on the distal

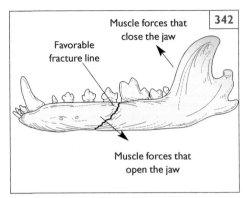

342 Medical illustration of a favorable mandibular fracture.

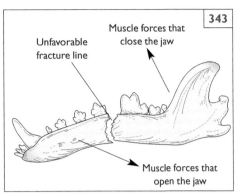

343 Medical illustration of an unfavorable mandibular fracture.

segment and the digastric muscles tend to pull the rostral segment down and caudally, displacing the fragments[2,20,22]. For these reasons, favorable fractures tend to maintain their alignment and generally require less fixation than do unfavorable (or comminuted) fractures.

Mandibular ramus fractures are less common than mandibular body or symphyseal fractures, accounting for about 12% of mandibular fractures in dogs[23]. Repair can be difficult due to the large muscle mass present. If displacement is minimal, internal fixation may not be needed due to the supportive effect of the surrounding musculature. Unilateral fractures dorsal to the condylar process can generally be managed with a loose nylon muzzle over a 2–3 week period, but fractures below that level may require up to 4–5 weeks[22]. Callous formation that may interfere with normal jaw movements is a concern with fractures in this region. Fracture cases with obvious malocclusions should be checked for concurrent fractures or luxations of the TMJ[22]. Internal repair is difficult except in large dogs, and therefore these fractures are usually managed conservatively. Fractures of the coronoid and angular processes are rare and also generally treated conservatively[20].

TMJ fractures are uncommon. Severely comminuted fractures may progress to arthrosis, which can be treated with condylectomy if the range of motion is significantly decreased or chronic pain is present[2,20–22]. Simple nondisplaced fractures may be treated with conservative therapy such as a tape muzzle. Fixation of other fractures with interarcade fixation or an orthodontic device such as a masel chain, can reduce movement of the TMJ to facilitate healing[22].

Maxillary fractures often do not require stabilization and may be more difficult to detect. Displacement is often minimal. Loose nylon muzzles can be used for conservative treatment. Digital reduction and soft tissue repair are adequate in most cases[20]. More severely comminuted fractures can be treated with interdental fixation and/or wiring the mouth shut, in which case an esophagostomy tube should be used for feeding. Miniplates can be used in the maxilla, or external fixation can be considered[20,22].

Midline palatal fractures are often a result of high-rise syndrome in cats (**344**) and are rare in dogs[20]. The injury is a separation of the interincisive suture, or the median palatine sutures of the palatine processes of the maxillary and palatine bones, rather than a true fracture[25]. These fractures are generally treated via reduction with gentle digital pressure and suturing of soft tissue defects. Separations which are not treated can progress to oronasal fistulas if severe[20].

CLINICAL FEATURES

Fractures may be obvious in some patients because of malocclusion, swelling, or tissue trauma. Other fractures or injuries may not be as obvious on initial examination because of nondisplacement or covering with large muscle masses. Patients may have concurrent injuries due to severe trauma such as neurologic damage from head trauma, pneumothorax, long bone fractures, and significant soft tissue or internal injuries. Pathological fractures can result from severe periodontal disease, neoplasia, or metabolic disorders affecting the integrity of the bone. Clinical signs consistent with these pathological processes should be noted and considered as a cause for fracture, especially with a history of mild trauma or no trauma at all.

DIFFERENTIAL DIAGNOSES

- Trauma.
- Severe periodontal disease.
- Neoplasia.
- TMJ luxation from dysplastic process.
- Osteomyelitis.
- Hypoparathyroidism.

DIAGNOSTIC TESTS

- Thorough examination under sedation or general anesthesia in the stable patient.
- Skull and/or dental radiographs in the anesthetized patient.
- Serum chemistry, complete blood count, and parathyroid hormone level.
- Thoracic +/– abdominal radiographs.
- Histopathology.
- Bacterial culture and sensitivity.

MANAGEMENT

Fractures of the maxilla and mandible are often concurrent with injuries to the head and other parts of the body. Malocclusion is a serious complication that can be associated with maxillofacial fractures[2,20–22]. Improper occlusion can lead to abnormal wear of teeth, trauma to periodontal tissues, and difficulty with mastication (**345**). Certain methods of repair, especially those involving implants, often iatrogenically damage the structures of the oral cavity, most notably the teeth and tooth roots. Fracture fixation with pins, plates, or screws is rarely necessary and generally contraindicated in the oral cavity. There are many other superior methods for fixation that should not cause iatrogenic damage to structures of the oral cavity. The injuries themselves often damage the vitality of the teeth which should be monitored radiographically for complications. Pharyngostomy tube placement is helpful for maintaining proper occlusion during oral fracture repair[22]. Extracting periodontally healthy and/or stable teeth in the fracture line at the time of fracture is not currently recommended. Teeth may provide stability to the fracture repair and can always be extracted at a later date if causing a problem[2].

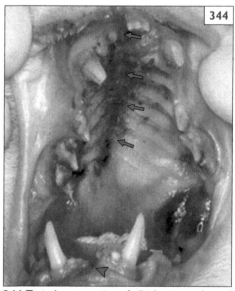

344 Typical presentation of a 'high-rise syndrome' midline palatal fracture in a cat (arrows). Note also the step defect indicative of a mandibular symphyseal separation (arrowhead).

Fractures caused by a pathological process such as periodontal disease or neoplasia can be difficult to treat successfully (**346, 347**). Therefore, a guarded prognosis for complete healing should always be given. In these cases, diseased teeth should be extracted before fracture stabilization (**348**). Neoplastic pathological fractures are generally not repaired, rather the affected portions excised by mandibulectomy or maxillectomy[19,22]. In all cases of pathological fractures, the underlying cause should be addressed before attempting fixation.

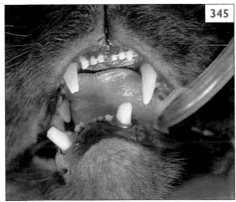

345 Traumatic malocclusion in a cat secondary to improper fracture fixation. (Courtesy of Dr. Brook Niemiec.)

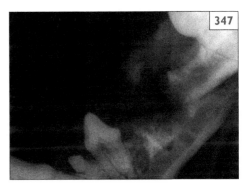

347 Pathological fracture secondary to a melanoma in a dog. (Courtesy of Dr. Brook Niemiec.)

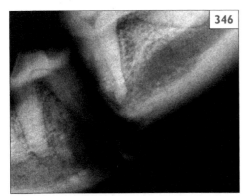

346 Pathological fracture secondary to severe periodontal and secondary endodontic disease of a mandibular fourth premolar in a dog. (Courtesy of Dr. Brook Niemiec.)

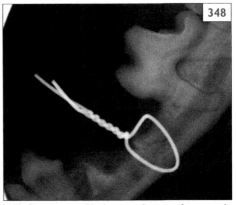

348 Circum-mandibular wire fracture fixation of a pathological fracture following extraction of the diseased teeth. (Courtesy of Dr. Brook Niemiec.)

Possible stabilization techniques for maxillofacial fractures include: acrylic intraoral splinting (**349**), loose fitting nylon muzzle (**350**), interfragmentary wiring (**351**), interarcade wiring with or without acrylic (**352–354**), and external fixation (**355**). Techniques such as pinning or plating are not recommended, or should be used sparingly in the oral cavity, due to the high risk of damaging vital structures such as vessels, nerves, and tooth roots (**356**). Bone plates must be contoured perfectly for proper occlusion and the plates should be placed ventrally to avoid the tooth roots[2,20–22]. Again, there is risk for entering mandibular canal and damaging the neurovascular structures. Use of external fixation, pins, or plates are rarely necessary except in severely comminuted fractures and should be avoided except under special circumstances. Often, the clinician must customize the repair using multiple techniques to achieve the successful outcome of functional occlusion and movement. For example, a loose fitting nylon muzzle can provide excellent adjunct stabilization of maxillofacial fractures.

KEY POINTS

- Successful treatment of maxillofacial fractures includes thorough assessment of the whole patient, as concurrent injuries or diseases are often present.
- Multiple fixation techniques exist, and customization or use of more than one technique may be necessary.
- Care must be taken to avoid vital structures such as neurovascular structures and tooth roots.
- Maintenance of proper occlusion is essential when repairing maxillofacial fractures.

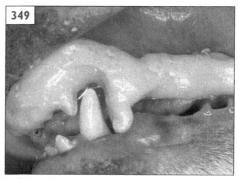

349 Acrylic splint applied to the maxillary teeth of a dog.

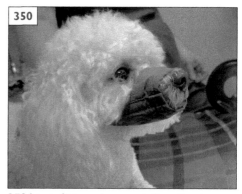

350 Loose fitting nylon muzzle for adjunct stabilization of a mandibular fracture. (Courtesy of Dr. Brook Niemiec.)

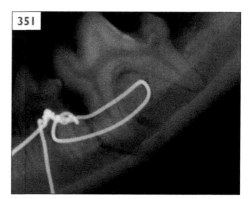

351 Interosseus wiring of a mandibular fracture (two wires provide superior stabilization and should be performed if possible). (Courtesy of Dr. Brook Niemiec.)

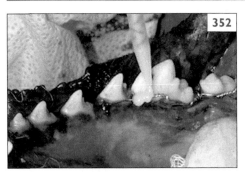

352 Interarcade wiring in a dog for mandibular fracture repair. In this case it is being used as a base for an acrylic splint.

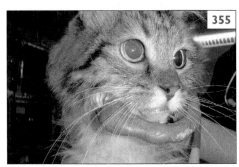

355 External fixator on the mandible of a cat. This type of fixation is rarely indicated. (Courtesy of Dan Frankel.)

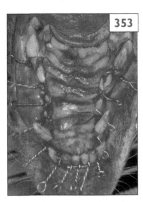

353 Interarcade wiring in a dog for maxillary fracture repair.

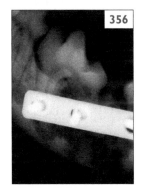

356 Bone plate improperly applied to the mandible of a dog. Note the screw through the mesial root of the first molar as well as the nonunion fracture (secondary to infection).

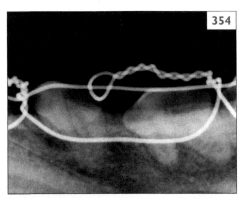

354 Dental radiograph of the patient in **352** revealing excellent reduction of the fracture line.

Traumatic tooth avulsion and luxation

DEFINITION
Avulsion is the tearing away of a body part accidentally or surgically. Luxation is misplacement or misalignment of a joint or organ. Teeth can be traumatically avulsed or luxated from the alveolus.

ETIOLOGY AND PATHOGENESIS
Tooth avulsion and luxation injuries are usually a result of trauma and the maxillary canine and incisor teeth are most often affected[22,26,27]. Many times the tooth becomes caught on a rigid object and is avulsed or luxated as the animal attempts to pull away. Other causes of tooth avulsion and luxation are falls, dog fights, or automobile trauma[26,28].

CLINICAL FEATURES
Animals may present with a true avulsion injury, where the tooth is completely separated from the alveolus (**357**). With luxation injuries the tooth may still be partially attached to alveolar bone but deviated from its normal position (**358, 359**). The tooth may be luxated in coronal direction, which is termed extrusive luxation. The tooth may also be displaced into the alveolus, which is termed intrusive luxation[28]. There may be a history of trauma or an unsupervised period. There are often traumatic injuries to the periodontal tissues, including alveolar fractures, gingival lacerations, and mucosal tears.

DIFFERENTIAL DIAGNOSES
- Fractured root.
- Maxillary or mandibular fracture.
- Severe periodontal disease.
- Neoplasia.

DIAGNOSTIC TESTS
- Dental radiographs.
- Skull radiographs.

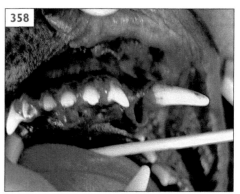

358 Luxated maxillary left canine (204) in a dog. (Courtesy of Dr. Brook Niemiec.)

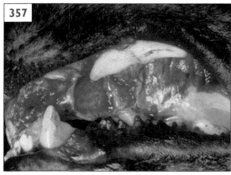

357 Avulsed maxillary canine in a dog. (Courtesy of Dr. Brook Niemiec.)

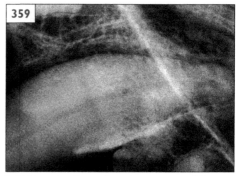

359 Dental radiograph of the patient in **358**. (Courtesy of Dr. Brook Niemiec.)

MANAGEMENT

A completely avulsed tooth should be immediately placed in milk and should be reimplanted as soon as possible. Best results occur when the tooth can be reimplanted within 30 minutes[26]. The tooth should not be scrubbed or sterilized or the periodontal ligament cells may be destroyed. If there is significant debris on the tooth it should be cleaned with great care to avoid damage to cells that can repair the periodontal ligament. Gentle lavage with saline can be used to remove gross debris[26]. For luxated teeth, management includes stabilization and care of fractured alveolar bone and damaged mucosal tissue. After reimplantation, the tooth is often stabilized with orthopedic wire and an acrylic splint (**360**). The fixation should not be completely rigid or root resorption or ankylosis may occur[22,28]. Endodontic therapy must be performed on avulsed and luxated teeth, as the blood supply to the tooth is almost always disrupted by the trauma (**361**). The endodontic therapy is typically performed after the splint has been in place for 2 weeks[22,26-28]. The splint may be left in place for 4–12 weeks depending on the severity of the injury and presence of alveolar fractures.

KEY POINTS

- Avulsed teeth should be kept moist in milk until reimplantation.
- Reimplantation should take place as soon as possible.
- Radiographs should be taken to identify root fractures, severe periodontal disease, or neoplasia that would require exodontic therapy of the avulsed tooth.
- The tooth should be stabilized with an acrylic and wire splint, with normal tooth movement possible to prevent resorption or ankylosis.
- Endodontic therapy of the avulsed tooth must be performed, even with successful reimplantation, due to the inevitable loss of blood supply to the tooth.

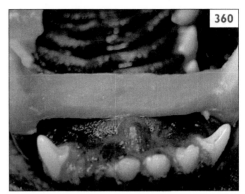

360 Postoperative stabilization of the patient in **358**. (Courtesy of Dr. Brook Niemiec.)

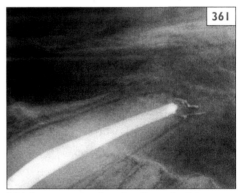

361 Postoperative dental radiograph of the patient in **358** revealing excellent obturation of the root canal system and healed bone. (Courtesy of Dr. Brook Niemiec.)

Root fractures

DEFINITION
Root fractures are fractures of the tooth structure below the cementoenamel junction.

ETIOLOGY AND PATHOGENESIS
In contrast to crown fractures, which are typically caused by hard objects, flexible or malleable objects may cause root fractures and spare the crown[22,29]. Root fractures are clinically detected only if the coronal segment is displaced or mobile. They are typically diagnosed radiographically, although nondisplaced fractures may go undetected.

CLINICAL FEATURES
Typically, the only obvious clinical sign is tooth mobility. However, if the tooth becomes nonvital, intrinsic staining may result. The level at which the root is fractured determines the mobility of the crown segment. Fractures close to the neck of the tooth are usually more mobile and have a greater risk of bacterial contamination from the oral cavity[22] (**362**).

DIFFERENTIAL DIAGNOSES
- Tooth avulsion or luxation.
- Crown fracture.
- Alveolar bone fracture.
- Advanced periodontal disease.

DIAGNOSTIC TESTS
- Dental radiographs (**363**).

MANAGEMENT
If the root fracture is stable and the pulp is vital and uncontaminated, it may heal without complication. Repair occurs as new cementum is laid down on the external root surface and reparative dentin is formed internally[22,30]. If mobility of the tooth fragments is present and the tooth is vital, acrylic splints can be used for stabilization during the healing period (**360**). Salvage procedures include root resection in conjunction with endodontic treatment. Teeth which are both mobile and nonvital are best treated by extraction.

KEY POINTS
- Root fractures may be difficult to detect clinically and radiographically.
- Stable root fractures can heal without intervention.
- Stabilization of mobile fracture fragments is essential.
- Salvage procedures involve root resection and endodontic therapy.

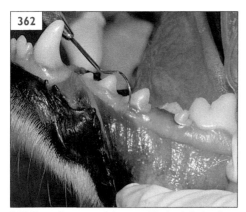

362 Root fracture of the mandibular left third premolar (307) in a dog with mobility and periodontal loss.

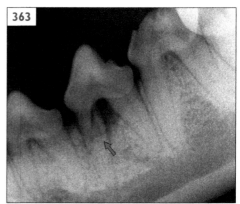

363 Dental radiograph of the patient in **362** revealing a root fracture on the mesial root and associated periodontal disease (arrow).

Osteomyelitis

DEFINITION
Osteomyelitis is defined as inflammation of bony tissues such as bone marrow, cortical bone, and periosteum.

ETIOLOGY AND PATHOGENESIS
The mandible of cats and dogs in one study was the third most common site for anaerobic osteomyelitis[31]. Fractures and tooth infections are common causes of osteomyelitis in the oral cavity. Penetrating wounds and hematogenous spread are also routes for infection and inflammation of bone to occur[22]. Bacterial and fungal osteomyelitis can occur, with fungal infections occurring less commonly. Sequestrum formation and osteomyelitis can also occur as a complication of radiation therapy for neoplasia. Radiation necrosis of bone can occur several weeks after radiation therapy[32].

CLINICAL FEATURES
Animals may present with fever, malaise, oral pain, soft tissue swelling, or draining tracts[2]. A history of infection or periodontal disease may also support the diagnosis. Nonhealing wounds, incisions, or nonunion of fractures can be causes and complications of osteomyelitis (**364, 365**). Osteomyelitis of the jaw is seen radiographically as a proliferative reaction of the periosteum at the periphery of the lesion with lysis of the associated cortical and alveolar bone (**366**). The bone lysis may give the appearance that teeth are supported primarily by soft tissue, but seldom are teeth displaced[22].

DIFFERENTIAL DIAGNOSES
- Neoplasia.
- Severe periodontal disease.
- Periosteal reaction.
- Hypoparathyroidism.
- Radiation necrosis.

DIAGNOSTIC TESTS
- Skull and/or dental radiographs.
- Histopathology.
- Cytology.
- Bacterial culture and sensitivity.
- Fungal culture.
- Fungal serology.

MANAGEMENT
Conservative management of osteomyelitis is generally unsuccessful. Aggressive surgical curettage and resection to normal bone is often required for resolution of the syndrome[20,22]. Tissue from these lesions should be submitted for histopathology, especially those that do not respond to aggressive surgical debridement and long-term antibiotic therapy. A broad-spectrum bactericidal antimicrobial should be administered until the bacterial culture and sensitivity results are known[20].

KEY POINTS
- Osteomyelitis can occur from hematogenous spread or introduction of bacteria from surgical procedures or severe periodontal disease.
- Successful treatment of osteomyelitis often involves aggressive surgical debridement and long-term antibiotic therapy.
- Any nonhealing lesion or nonunion should be biopsied to rule-out neoplastic processes.

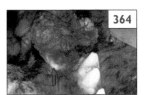

364 Osteomyelitis in the mandible of a dog near the first molar (arrow).

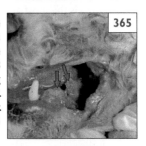

365 Severe osteomyelitis (arrows) in the mandible of a dog 8 months following extractions. (Courtesy of Dr. Brook Niemiec.)

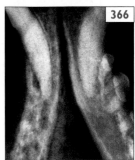

366 Dental radiograph of the patient in **365** revealing typical bone mottling and periosteal reaction. (Courtesy of Dr. Brook Niemiec.)

Tumors and cysts

- Osteosarcoma.
- Fibrosarcoma.
- Osteochondroma.
- Chondrosarcoma.
- Multiple myeloma.
- Epulids.
- Squamous cell carcinoma.
- Melanoma.
- Odontoma.
- Multilobular osteoma.
- Transmissible venereal tumor (TVT).

DEFINITION
Neoplasia means new growth, and includes benign and malignant masses. Neoplastic masses can be metastatic or nonmetastatic, and are characterized based on the tissue of origin.

ETIOLOGY AND PATHOGENESIS
The oral cavity is the fourth most common site for malignant neoplasia with oral malignancies accounting for 5.3% of all malignancies found in the dog and 6.7% in the cat[2,22]. The most common malignant oral tumor found in dogs is melanosarcoma (**367**), followed by squamous cell carcinoma (**368**), and fibrosarcoma (**369**)[22,33,34]. In cats, squamous cell carcinoma (**370**) is most common, followed by fibrosarcoma and melanosarcoma[2,22,33]. Melanoma is the most aggressive with invasion and recurrence as well as a high rate of early metastasis to the lungs, lymph nodes, and bones. It affects males more than females, and small breed dogs may be overrepresented[22,34]. Squamous cell carcinoma can invade bone, and

the tonsillar form generally carries a worse prognosis. Many fibrosarcomas are invasive to bone and have a high local recurrence rate with late metastasis. The maxilla and mandible each represent 3% of all osteosarcoma sites. These

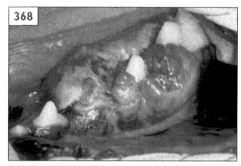

368 Squamous cell carcinoma of the mandible of a dog with secondary necrosis.

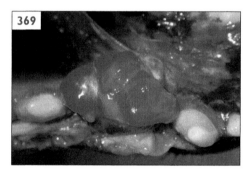

369 Fibrosarcoma of the mandibular attached gingiva in a dog.

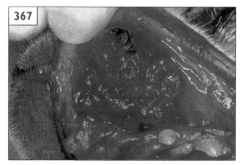

367 Melanoma on the maxilla of a dog.

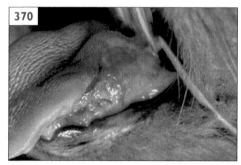

370 Sublingual squamous cell carcinoma in a cat.

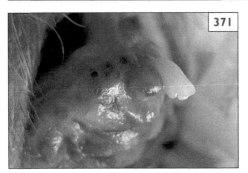

371 Fibromatous epulis on the maxilla of a dog.

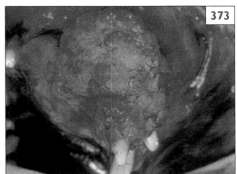

373 Acanthomatous ameloblastoma (epulis) on the maxilla of a dog.

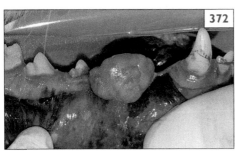

372 Ossifying epulis on the mandible of a dog.

axial osteosarcomas carry a slightly better prognosis than appendicular, as they are slower to metastasize[22,35]. (See Chapter 9 for a more in depth discussion of oral neoplasia.)

Benign tumors do not destroy the tissues from which they arise, and do not metastasize. Complete surgical excision is usually curative. In the oral cavity, papillomas and odontogenic tumors are most common. Oral papillomas are caused by a canine virus in the dog, and may occur on the oral mucosa, lips, tongue, and esophagus. Odontogenic tumors arise from cellular components of the developing tooth structure[22]. Epulids are considered epithelial odontogenic tumors and the main types are fibrous (371), ossifying (372), giant cell, and acanthomatous ameloblastoma (373). (See Chapter 6 for a more in depth discussion of epulids.)

Cysts can be classified as primordial, dentigerous (follicular and eruption), periodontal ligament, and gingival (newborn and adult odontogenic). Mesenchymal tumors are represented by cementoma, cementoblastoma, and benign odontogenic mesenchymal tumors. Odontomas are mixed tumors and can be described as compound or complex. Compound odontomas may contain multiple tooth-like structures called denticles. Complex odontomas are disorganized masses with no tooth-like structures[22]. (See Chapter 4 for a more in depth discussion of odontogenic cysts and tumors.)

CLINICAL FEATURES

Oral cavity neoplasms can be difficult to detect by the owner until they have dramatically increased in size. They can also be misdiagnosed as abscesses, gingivitis, stomatitis, gingival hyperplasia, cheilitis, tonsillitis, sialadentitis, salivary mucoceles, ranulas, or osteomyelitis. The owner may notice halitosis, dysphagia, oral pain, excessive salivation, oral bleeding, facial swelling and asymmetry, mobile or displaced teeth, lethargy, weight loss, or respiratory distress[2,22].

DIFFERENTIAL DIAGNOSES

- Osteomyelitis.
- Cysts.
- Gingival enlargement.
- Lymphocytic-plasmacytic gingivitis/stomatitis.
- Eosinophilic granuloma.
- Glossitis.

DIAGNOSTIC TESTS
- Complete blood count and serum chemistries.
- Three-view thoracic radiographs.
- Skull and/or dental radiographs (**374**).
- Histopathology.
- Cytology.
- Culture and sensitivities (bacterial and fungal).
- Regional lymph node excisional biopsies.
- Computed tomography (CT).
- Magnetic resonance imaging (MRI).

MANAGEMENT
Work-up for oral masses should include blood panel, dental radiographs, chest radiographs, cytology, biopsy with normal tissue included, +/– culture/sensitivity. Advanced diagnostic imaging, such as CT or MRI, can be used to develop a plan for surgical excision and examine the patient for metastatic disease. Regional lymph nodes should also be examined if a malignancy is suspected or confirmed, by excisional biopsy of the parotid, medial retropharyngeal, and mandibular lymph nodes[36,37]. Cytologic examination of the regional lymph nodes is limited to the mandibular lymphocentrum, and as many as 45% of cases with metastasis to the parotid or medial retropharyngeal node did not have metastasis to the mandibular node[37]. Wide surgical excision is indicated for malignant tumors followed by appropriate treatment with radiation, chemotherapy, immunotherapy, or combination. Benign tumors can be cured with complete surgical excision. Radiation therapy can also be used to shrink tumors before surgery, or used after surgical excision has left microscopic disease. The prognosis for malignant tumors varies according to the biologic behavior of the tumor, size at time of diagnosis, and evidence of distant metastasis.

KEY POINTS
- Oral neoplasms can be confined locally or metastasize to distant locations.
- A complete patient work-up is imperative for staging the neoplasm and ruling out non-neoplastic disorders.
- Treatment and prognosis varies according to the biologic behavior of the specific tumor.
- Surgical excision can be curative for benign tumors.
- Malignant tumors are generally treated with wide surgical excision when feasible, followed by radiation, chemotherapy, or immunotherapy.

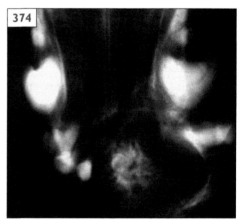

374 Dental radiograph of the patient in **373** revealing significant bony reaction.

Hyperparathyroidism

DEFINITION
Hyperparathyroidism can be either primary or secondary. Primary hyperparathyroidism is an abnormal, excessive secretion of parathyroid hormone from the parathyroid glands. Secondary hyperparathyroidism is a result of another disorder such as nutritional deficiency or chronic renal disease, which causes disruption of calcium and phosphorus homeostasis.

ETIOLOGY AND PATHOGENESIS
An excessive amount of circulating parathyroid hormone (PTH) results in resorption of calcium from the bones in an attempt to maintain calcium homeostasis. The first bone affected is the mandible, followed by the maxilla, other skull bones, and then the axial skeleton. The bones of the jaw can become severely demineralized and soft. Primary hyperparathyroidism is usually due to a parathyroid adenoma. An inverse linear relationship exists between serum calcium and PTH concentrations. This negative feedback system is disrupted during primary hyperparathyroidism. PTH is continuously secreted and calcium is continuously resorbed from the bone, resulting in severe demineralization. With secondary hyperparathyroidism, decreased serum calcium from poor nutrition or loss from chronic renal disease causes an increase in PTH secretion and subsequent resorption of calcium from bone occurs. Both of these disease processes can cause the syndrome commonly known as 'rubber jaw'[15,38].

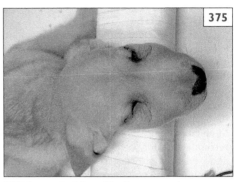

375 Severe facial swelling in a young dog secondary to renal secondary hyperparathyroidism. The patient was subsequently diagnosed with congenital polycystic renal disease. (Courtesy of Dr. Brook Niemiec.)

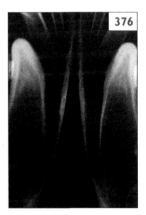

376 Dental radiograph of the patient in **375**; note the severe osteoporosis. (Courtesy of Dr. Brook Niemiec.)

CLINICAL FEATURES
Dogs affected with hyperparathyroidism can have an array of clinical signs such as polyuria, polydipsia, depression, weakness, muscle wasting, inappetence, muscle twitching, and seizures. Dogs may present with a urinary tract infection or uroliths. Most clinical signs are related to hypercalcemia[38]. Animals with severely demineralized bone may present with facial swelling and deformity (**375**).

DIFFERENTIAL DIAGNOSES
- Lymphoma.
- Anal sac adenocarcinoma.
- Chronic renal failure.
- Hypoadrenocorticism.
- Nutritional secondary hyperparathyroidism.
- Carcinomatosis.

DIAGNOSTIC TESTS
- Ionized calcium.
- PTH.
- Serum chemistry.
- Complete blood count.
- Urinalysis.
- Radiography: skull, thoracic, lumbar, dental (**376**).
- Ultrasonography: neck, abdomen.
- Radionuclide scan.

MANAGEMENT

The underlying cause of the hyperparathyroidism must be determined in order to initiate the appropriate treatment. Surgical excision of the parathyroid glands is the treatment of choice for parathyroid gland adenomas. The animal must be carefully monitored for several days postoperatively for hypocalcemia[38]. Supplementation of calcium is usually recommended for several weeks postoperatively, and serial monitoring of serum calcium is required for successful management. Secondary hyperparathyroidism due to renal failure can be difficult to treat due to the poor prognosis for reversing kidney damage. Treatment of other secondary causes of hyperparathyroidism can have varying prognoses depending on the disease.

KEY POINTS

- Hyperparathyroidism can be primary or secondary.
- Primary hyperparathyroidism is generally caused by a parathyroid adenoma hypersecreting PTH.
- Determining the underlying cause of hyperparathyroidism is paramount when initiating treatment.
- Severe demineralization of bone may occur due to hyperparathyroidism, resulting in a condition known as rubber jaw.

Tetanus

DEFINITION

Tetanus is caused by a potent neurotoxin formed in the body by *Clostridium tetani*; a motile, gram-positive, nonencapsulated, obligate anaerobic, spore-forming bacterium.

ETIOLOGY AND PATHOGENESIS

C. tetani spores are introduced into an existing wound or by penetrating injuries. Introduction of spores can also occur during ovariohysterectomy or parturition[39,40]. The spores are ubiquitous and can survive for years in soil without direct sunlight. Clinical signs occur typically 5–10 days after injury, but due to increased resistance to the disease in dogs and cats, the onset can be delayed for up to 3 weeks. Two toxins have been identified from C. *tetani*, tetanolepsin and tetanospasmin. Tetanospasmin is more clinically significant and has marked effects on neurologic function. It can be transported by the bloodstream to distant sites or it may enter the axons of the nearest motor nerves and migrate through motor axons to the neuronal cell bodies in the spinal cord or brainstem. Tetanospasmin blocks inhibitory transmission to motor neurons. It inhibits release of glycine and GABA of inhibitory neurons of the brain and spinal cord, causing increased extensor activity due to the dominance of extensor muscles in muscular activity[41]. Tetanus can also exhibit localized effects, which is often the case in cats that are more resistant to the toxin[42].

CLINICAL FEATURES

Patients with generalized tetanus present with a stiff gait (sawhorse stance), extensor rigidity of the limbs, elevated tail, and trismus (which is caused by contraction of masticatory muscles). Animals often have an elevated rectal temperature due to excessive muscular activity. The ears are erect, the lips are drawn back and the forehead is often wrinkled as a result of facial spasm. The contraction of these muscles is often described as smiling or sneering and is termed risus sardonicus. Affected animals are very sensitive to external stimuli, and severe muscle spasms and seizure-like activity can be induced. Severely affected animals die from the respiratory or cardiovascular dysfunction of uncontrollable muscle spasms. In mildly affected animals, normal function usually returns within 3 weeks of initiation of treatment.

DIFFERENTIAL DIAGNOSES
- Lead poisoning.
- Strychnine poisoning.
- MM.
- CMO.

DIAGNOSTIC TESTS
There is no specific test for tetanus. Diagnosis is confirmed on the basis of classic clinical signs and the presence or history of a wound. Tetanospasmin antibody titers can be measured in the serum, but this test is generally not performed. Serum chemistry may reveal elevated CK levels[42].

MANAGEMENT
Surgical debridement of the wound can reduce the number of organisms present, and reduce the amount of toxin produced. In addition, flushing the wound with hydrogen peroxide may produce an aerobic environment unfavorable to the organisms. Antitoxin can be given but it will only neutralize circulating unbound toxin. The dose for antitoxin is 100–1000 U/kg, given slowly intravenously. The patient should be tested for hypersensitivity to the antitoxin prior to administration. Antibiotics (such as penicillin G and metronidazole) do not neutralize circulating toxin or affect bound toxin. However, they have been shown to reduce significantly the amount of toxin released in experimental tetanus by killing the *C. tetani* organism[41]. Penicillin G should be administered subcutaneously or intramuscularly at a high dose, 20,000–50,000 IU/kg TID–QID for 10 days. The intramuscular injection can also be given in close proximity to the wound. Metronidazole may be more effective because of its bactericidal action against most anaerobes. The dose for metronidazole is 10 mg/kg TID for 10 days, with care being taken to avoid toxicity[42]. Supportive treatment is critical for successful recovery. The patient may require manual assistance to eat and drink, or placement of a feeding tube. Keeping the patient in a dark and quiet area can reduce hypersensitivity to external stimuli, and in some cases sedation with phenothiazines, barbiturates, or benzodiazapenes may be required. Muscle relaxants, such as methocarbamol, can help with muscle spasms. In severe cases, tracheostomy for laryngeal spasm or mechanical ventilation for respiratory paralysis is needed until new axon terminals are created and the animal recovers. Many severely affected animals are euthanized due to the extremely time consuming and expensive nursing care that is required[41,42].

KEY POINTS
- Tetanus is caused by a toxin produced by the anaerobic bacterium, *Clostridium tetani*.
- Diagnosis is based on classic clinical signs of muscle rigidity, risus sardonicus, and presence of a wound.
- Treatment is mostly supportive, with antibiotic therapy for reduction of bacterial numbers and toxin production.
- Severely affected animals are often euthanized due to onset of respiratory compromise, laryngeal spasms, and severe muscle spasms.

Botulism

DEFINITION
Clostridium botulinum is a gram-positive, spore-forming, saprophytic, anaerobic rod that is distributed in soil worldwide. Botulism is an intoxication caused by the neurotoxin produced by this organism, which results in neuromuscular paralysis.

ETIOLOGY AND PATHOGENESIS
Ingestion of preformed type C botulism toxin is the method of intoxication. Botulism in dogs can be attributed to eating carrion or raw meat. The toxin is absorbed from the gastrointestinal tract and enters the lymphatic system. The incubation period can range from hours to several days after ingestion. The toxin then binds to the neuromuscular junction of cholinergic nerves. The botulinum toxin prevents the presynaptic release of acetylcholine at the neuromuscular junction; both the spontaneous release of acetylcholine and its release caused by a nerve action potential are inhibited. Binding of the toxin occurs very quickly and is irreversible[43]. Blockage of acetylcholine release results in generalized lower motor neuron and parasympathetic dysfunction. The earlier the signs appear, the more serious the disease. The duration of illness, in dogs that recover, ranges from 14–24 days.

CLINICAL FEATURES
Clinical signs are characterized by a symmetric ascending weakness from the rear to the forelimbs that can result in quadriplegia. Cranial nerve motor responses are affected, causing mydriasis, decreased jaw tone, decreased gag reflexes, and excess salivation. Megaesophagus may be present. If recovery occurs, it results from the development of new terminal axons with functional neuromuscular junctions. Cranial nerve, neck, and forelimb functions tend to return first[42].

DIFFERENTIAL DIAGNOSES
- Myasthenia gravis.
- Tick bite paralysis.
- Coon hound paralysis.
- Protozoal myoneuritis.

DIAGNOSTIC TESTS
Diagnosis is usually based on clinical signs and history. The diagnosis is confirmed by presence of the botulism toxin in the serum, feces, vomitus, or samples of the suspected food source. The isolated toxin is then injected into mice to determine if they develop clinical signs of botulism. Culture of tissues and feces can sometimes isolate and identify *C. botulinum*.

MANAGEMENT
Antitoxin is not effective after the toxin has penetrated the nerve endings, but it may prevent further toxin binding if intestinal absorption and circulation are still occurring. The use of antibiotics such as Penicillin G and metronidazole are controversial since the disease is usually caused by ingestion of preformed toxin and not bacterial infection. Bacterial lysis may also occur and release more toxin. Antibiotics are generally only used to treat secondary infections such as aspiration pneumonia. Supportive care is the most important part of treatment[42].

KEY POINTS
- Botulism is an intoxication caused by ingestion of a preformed toxin produced by *Clostridium botulinum*.
- Animals that eat raw meat or carrion can be at increased risk for ingesting the toxin.
- Binding of the toxin to the neuromuscular junction is irreversible, and recovery only occurs after the axons have regenerated.
- Treatment involves mostly supportive care; antibiotics are only helpful in treating secondary bacterial infections, such as aspiration pneumonia.

Malignant Oral Neoplasia

Ravinder S. Dhaliwal

- **Introduction**

- **Malignant melanoma**

- **Fibrosarcoma**

- **Squamous cell carcinoma**

- **Histologically low-grade, biologically high-grade, fibrosarcoma**

- **Osteosarcoma**

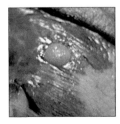
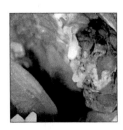
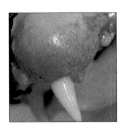
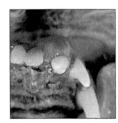

Introduction

Oral tumors represent the fourth most common malignancy in dogs and cats. Neoplasms of the oral cavity include both odontogenic and nonodontogenic tumor types. Laryngeal and oropharyngeal tumors are often classified under head and neck cancer by some clinicians and are not discussed in this chapter. The current review discusses the biologic behavior, clinical presentations, and therapeutics of the most common oral malignancies in dogs and cats. A variety of histologic types of oral tumors has been described in the literature[1-4].

Because of the histologic diversity noted with odontogenic tumors, there has been confusion and disagreement on the terminology and classification of these lesions[2,5-8]. The nomenclature is complex. However, most tumor types are treated either with surgery or radiation therapy. The reader is advised to refer to a veterinary pathology book for descriptive details of specific odontogenic tumor types. The so-called calcifying odontogenic cyst (COC) represents a heterogeneous group of lesions that exhibit a variety of clinicopathological and behavioral features. It is beyond the scope of this chapter to discuss each odontogenic tumor in detail. Dentigerous cysts are discussed in Chapter 4.

ETIOLOGY AND PATHOGENESIS

A true etiology is not known in most cases. Some investigators suggest that flea control products, diet, and perhaps environmental tobacco smoke might be associated with risk of oral squamous cell carcinoma in cats[9,10]. Papillomavirus DNA is frequently associated with canine oral squamous cell carcinomas[11,12].

CLINICAL FEATURES

Clinical signs seen in both canine and feline patients with oral tumors include the presence of an erosive fleshy oral mass, halitosis, hemorrhage, dysphagia, anorexia, loss of teeth, facial swelling, thickening of the mandible or maxilla, sneezing, pain, dyspnea, voice change, pawing at the mouth, or weight loss. Unfortunately, oral tumors frequently go unnoticed by the owner until the clinical signs reach a fairly advanced stage.

DIFFERENTIAL DIAGNOSES
- Granuloma or benign oral growths such as nodular fasciitis, fibromatosis.
- Epulids.
- Eosinophilic granuloma.
- Dentigerous cysts.
- Abscess.

DIAGNOSTIC TESTS AND CLINICAL STAGING

After obtaining a complete history and performing a general physical examination, a thorough oral examination (oftentimes general anesthesia is required) should be performed and all results should be documented. The first step in oral examination is careful inspection and palpation of the mass for:
- Size and site.
- Presence of ulceration and/or necrosis.
- Fixation to the underlying tissues.
- Abnormal mobility of teeth.

Regional lymph nodes should routinely be palpated for size, shape, consistency, and fixation to the surrounding tissues. If lymphadenopathy is noted, cytologic or histologic evaluation must be performed. In a retrospective study evaluating the regional lymph nodes of dogs and cats with oral or maxillofacial neoplasms, 17% had metastatic disease histologically[13].

General physical examination may give indications of distant metastasis. Three-view thoracic radiographs are indicated in all cases of suspected malignancy. Radiographic examination (preferably dental) of the affected jaw is mandatory. With the increased availability of computed tomography (CT) and magnetic resonance imaging (MRI) these advanced imaging techniques are now more frequently used at referral institutions. These techniques are much more sensitive and provide detailed information about the extent of the mass[14]. The same images can also be used for radiation treatment planning.

A fine-needle aspirate is usually of limited value in diagnosing intraoral lesions. However, based on aspiration cytology, differentiation between inflammation and malignancy may be established. An incisional or excisional biopsy is strongly recommended to confirm the histopathological diagnosis. Care should be taken to avoid severely inflamed or necrotic parts of the lesion.

Oral tumours can be staged using the TNM-classification (primary tumor, regional lymph node, distant metastasis), which has been introduced by the WHO[15]. Using this system, patients can be classified into one of four clinical stages. It has been demonstrated that prognosis worsens as the tumor stage increases from I to IV.

MANAGEMENT

Curative intent therapy means *en bloc* surgical excision or full course radiation therapy such as 12–16 or more fractions based on 3–5 fractions delivered in a week. The goal of curative intent therapy is to achieve a long-term remission or tumor control. Palliative therapy is indicated for patients where a curative intent therapy can not be performed, either because of concurrent medical conditions, advanced clinical stage, or financial concerns.

Complete *en bloc* surgical excision with 1.5–2 cm margins of 'normal' tissue is the treatment of choice for the majority of the oral tumors, especially those located in the rostral oral cavity[16,17].

Radiation therapy should be considered in cases where complete excision is not feasible, or if the tumor is located in the caudal oral cavity. Orthovoltage machines capable of delivering low energy external beam radiation are not optimal for treating oral malignancies in most cases. Megavoltage radiation therapy is currently the standard of care for dogs with oral tumors. Acute effects of oral radiation such as oral mucositis, alopecia, local moist dermatitis, and desquamation occur in almost every case. However, these effects are not dose limiting. These effects are reversible, medically manageable, and resolve over 2–3 weeks after completion of radiation therapy. The late effects of radiation such as bone or muscle necrosis are less likely to occur. These late effects, if they occur, are irreversible and are dose limiting factors. In one retrospective study, 2 out of 57 dogs (3.5%) irradiated for oral acanthomatous epulis, developed a secondary malignancy at the irradiated site at 5.2 and 8.7 years after completion of radiation therapy. The authors revealed that the risk of radiation-induced carcinogenesis is relatively low and an event that occurs years after radiation therapy. This late effect of radiation is more of a problem in younger dogs[18].

Chemotherapy is indicated for patients with a diagnosis of oral lymphoma, melanoma, osteosarcoma, or other high-grade malignancies which carry a metastatic potential[1,19].

KEY POINTS
- All oral malignancies are locally aggressive.
- With the exception of oral melanoma, the majority of oral malignancies are slow to metastasize.
- Wide surgical excision and/or radiation therapy should be considered early in the course of the disease.
- In the future, molecular techniques may be used to aid in prognosis and clinical staging of oral tumors. This will also help to predict the precise targeted therapy.

Malignant melanoma

DEFINITION
Oral malignant melanoma (OMM) is the most frequent malignant neoplasm of the oral cavity in dogs. OMM typically occurs in older dogs with a reported mean age of 11 years. Cocker spaniels, German Shepherds and dogs with heavily pigmented oral mucosa may be predisposed[20–23].

BIOLOGIC BEHAVIOR, ETIOLOGY, AND PATHOGENESIS
Melanomas arising from nonsun-exposed sites such as the oral cavity, exhibit different biologic behavior and distinct mechanisms of molecular transformation from those which have direct sun exposure (i.e. on skin)[24]. The usual behavior of OMM is focal infiltration, recurrence, and metastasis to regional lymph nodes, and less frequently to lungs and other organs. Therefore, nearly all oral melanomas are considered malignant. The most important prognostic factors of canine OMM are:
- Tumor stage.
- Size.
- Mitotic activity.
- Evidence of tumor recurrence after a prior treatment[25].

Favorable prognostic factor for OMM include:
- Rostral tumor sublocation.
- Lack of bone lysis.
- Microscopic tumor burden[26].

CLINICAL FEATURES
Malignant melanoma can be located in any part of the oral cavity, but occurs most often on the gingiva, followed by the buccal or labial mucosa, palate, and dorsal surface of the tongue. They are classically dark pigmented (**377**); however, amelanotic melanoma will be pink to red (**378**). In gingival lesions, dental disruption is common and bone involvement is frequently seen. These tumors can grow quite rapidly resulting in large masses prior to therapy (**379**).

DIFFERENTIAL DIAGNOSES
- Other round cell tumors such as lymphomas, mast cell tumor, histiocytoma, and plasmacytoma.
- Carcinomas.
- Sarcomas.
- Osteogenic tumors.

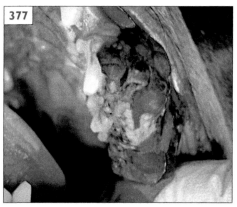

377 Large melanoma on the left maxilla of a dog. (Courtesy of Dr. Brook Niemiec.)

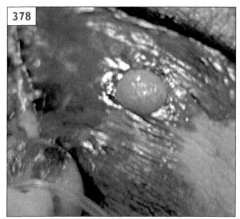

378 Early amelanotic melanoma on the buccal mucosa of a dog. (Courtesy of Dr. Brook Niemiec.)

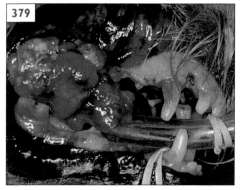

379 Very large melanoma on the maxilla of a dog. (Courtesy of Dr. Brook Niemiec.)

DIAGNOSTIC TESTS

Cytologically, the diagnosis of OMM may be challenging due to the variation in the degree of pigmentation: some tumors may even be completely unpigmented. Another complicating factor is that the microscopic features can resemble carcinomas, sarcomas, lymphomas, and osteogenic tumors. Thus, immunohistochemical confirmation[23,27] of the diagnosis of melanoma is frequently necessary to establish a prognosis and therapeutic plan. Biopsy of the oral mass is taken to confirm the diagnosis. This should be performed with any suspect area, no matter how small (**380**) due to the severity of the disease and rapidity of growth and metastasis.

Obtain intraoral dental radiographs to determine the extent of bony involvement (**381**, **382**). Regional lymph nodes, if palpable, should be aspirated or biopsied to rule out metastasis. After diagnosis is confirmed, routine clinical staging consisting of 3-view thoracic radiographs, complete blood panel, urinalysis, and abdominal ultrasound should be performed.

MANAGEMENT

Treatment options for OMM include:
- Surgery.
- Chemotherapy.
- Immunotherapy.
- Radiation therapy.

Complete *en bloc* surgical excision with 1.5–2 cm margins of 'normal' tissue is the treatment of choice for the majority of oral tumors, especially those located in the rostral oral cavity[16,17]. Radiation therapy should be considered in cases where complete excision is not feasible, or if the tumor is located in the caudal oral cavity.

Regardless of treatment protocol, local recurrence and distant dissemination are still frequent[28]. External beam radiation therapy is effective in local disease control of canine OMM[26]. Hypofractionated radiation therapy (such as: once a week in 8 Gy fractions to a total cumulative dose of 32 Gy; or twice a week in 6 Gy to a total cumulative dose of 36 Gy) is the treatment of choice for OMM[29,30]. A combination of cisplatin and piroxicam has shown antitumor activity against canine OMM[19]. An overall median survival time of 363 days has been reported in dogs treated with

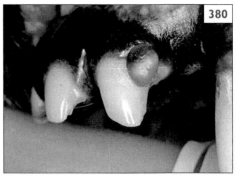

380 Very small and inconspicuous melanoma on the maxillary gingiva of a dog. Early detection and therapy resulted in a positive outcome. (Courtesy of Dr. Brook Niemiec.)

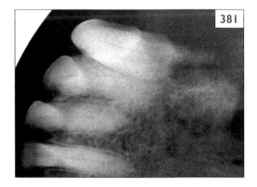

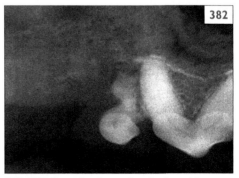

381, 382 Dental radiographs of a dog with melanoma of the maxilla. Note the significant bony destruction. (Courtesy of Dr. Brook Niemiec.)

hypofractionated radiation therapy and platinum-containing chemotherapy[30]. We currently administer carboplatin either in adjunctive or adjuvant settings for dogs with OMM.

Cancer vaccines are intended either to treat existing cancers (therapeutic vaccines) or to prevent the development of cancer (prophylactic vaccines). The therapeutic vaccines are designed to treat cancer by stimulating the immune system to recognize and attack cancer cells without harming normal cells. Canine melanoma xenogenic DNA vaccine contains human tyrosinase, which is a melanosomal glycoprotein, essential in melanin synthesis. Canine tyrosinase on melanocytes is considered by the immune system as 'self' and not foreign, therefore an immune response is not generated. However, using a xenogenic (other species) tyrosinase, an antitumor response is initiated.

Canine melanoma xenogenic DNA vaccine can aid in prolonging overall survival when administered to patients in whom complete local control has been achieved. The vaccine is indicated for the treatment of dogs with stage II or stage III OMM for which good local control has been achieved. The injection is administered intramuscularly with a transdermal device into the medial thigh region. Initial treatment requires administration of four doses of vaccine at 2-week intervals followed by booster dose at 6-month intervals[31,32].

KEY POINTS

- Radiation therapy can provide good long-term, local tumor control for oral malignant melanoma.
- Paraneoplastic syndromes, such as hypercalcemia of malignancy, are rare in dogs with malignant melanoma[33].

Fibrosarcoma

DEFINITION

Fibrosarcoma (FSA) or fibroblastic sarcoma is a malignant mesenchymal tumor derived from fibrous connective tissue and characterized by immature proliferating fibroblasts or undifferentiated anaplastic spindle cells. Canine oral FSA occurs at a young age in large breed dogs, with a mean age of 4–5 years. In small breed dogs it occurs at about 8 years of age.

BIOLOGIC BEHAVIOR, ETIOLOGY, AND PATHOGENESIS

FSAs are locally invasive and have a high recurrence rate after surgical excision. They seldom metastasize except late in the clinical course. Prognosis is variable depending on location, histologic grade, and size or clinical stage at time of diagnosis. Histologically, the tumor may present three different degrees of differentiation: low grade (differentiated), intermediate malignancy, and high malignancy (anaplastic).

CLINICAL FEATURES

The maxilla is the most common location for these tumors to occur. Initially, oral FSA may present as a clinically innocuous, lobulated, sessile, painless and nonhemorrhagic submucosal mass of normal coloration (**383**). Alternatively, it may be a rapidly enlarging, hemorrhagic mass with severe ulceration (**384**). Most often, it appears as a protruberant mass at the dental margins and palate (**385**). It may also originate from the nasal cartilages, the lateral surface of the maxilla or palate, as a smooth mass with an intact epithelial covering. Finally, FSAs have been diagnosed on the tongue (**386**).

DIFFERENTIAL DIAGNOSES

- Other mesenchymal tumors such as osteosarcoma, mast cell tumor, malignant fibrous histiocytoma, benign fibromas, nodular fasciitis, fibromatosis.
- Carcinomas.
- Osteogenic tumors.

DIAGNOSTIC TESTS

Dental radiographs (**387**) and biopsy of the oral mass will confirm the diagnosis.

Regional lymph nodes, if palpable, should be aspirated or biopsied to rule out metastasis.

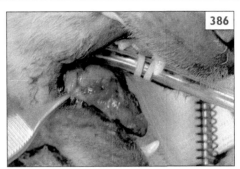

383 Early fibrosarcoma on the palate of a cat. (Courtesy of Dr. Brook Niemiec.)

386 Aggressive fibrosarcoma of the tongue of a dog. (Courtesy of Dr. Brook Niemiec.)

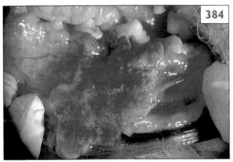

384 Large, invasive fibrosarcoma on the mandible of a dog. (Courtesy of Dr. Brook Niemiec.)

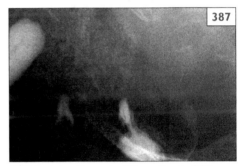

387 Dental radiograph of the patient in **385**. Note the complete bony destruction.

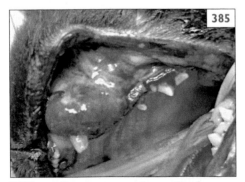

385 Large fibrosarcoma on the maxilla of a cat. (Courtesy of Dr. Brook Niemiec.)

As previously described, routine clinical staging with 3-view of thoracic radiographs, complete blood work, urinalysis, and abdominal ultrasound should be performed as well.

MANAGEMENT

Well-differentiated FSA is treated by wide local excision. More poorly differentiated tumors require radical surgery, including removal of potentially invaded muscle and bone. Radiotherapy may be used to treat microscopic disease postoperatively, or as salvage for recurrences. In one retrospective study, time-to-progression for curatively-treated dogs with oral soft tissue sarcoma was 333 days versus 180 days for the palliatively-treated dogs, with an overall survival of 331 days[34]. Efficacy of adjunctive chemotherapy is not known. However, some clinicians consider chemotherapy for tumors with high histologic grades.

KEY POINTS

- Wide surgical excision is the treatment of choice.
- FSA is most commonly seen in young, large breed dogs.

Squamous cell carcinoma

DEFINITION

Squamous cell carcinoma (SCC) is the most common oral malignancy in cats and second most common in dogs[35]. The gingiva is the most common site for canine SCC. It occurs in older dogs with a mean age of approximately 9 years, and there is no reported sex predilection. Papillary SCC has been reported in very young dogs. Lingual and tonsillar SCC are less common[36]. In cats with oral SCC, lesions are most often located in the premolar/molar region of the maxilla, premolar region of the mandible, and the sublingual region.

BIOLOGIC BEHAVIOR, ETIOLOGY, AND PATHOGENESIS

These neoplasms are locally aggressive, and distant metastasis to the regional lymph nodes and lungs have been reported late in the disease process. Tonsillar SCC are much more aggressive with early metastasis to the regional lymph nodes. It appears that feline maxillary and tongue SCC have a poor prognosis, responding only rarely to any kind of therapy. Mandibular SCC is more amenable to therapy and carries a little better prognosis then maxillary and lingual region SCC. A rostral mandibular location in the cat has a fair prognosis. Cure is possible with very early lesions and wide surgical excision. Papillomavirus DNA is frequently associated with canine oral SCC (**388, 389**).

CLINICAL FEATURES

Oral gingival lesions are generally erosive and fleshy (**390**). Dental disruption with local bone invasion is common. On the skin of the maxillofacial and mandibular region, SCC can present as a chronic nonhealing ulcer without proliferation (**391**). Feline oral SCC is oftentimes diagnosed at an advanced clinical stage. A firm mass can be palpated in the mandibular or maxillary region (**392**). In more advanced cases of maxillary SCC, exophthalmos and facial distortion is also evident. Sublingual lesions can be palpated in the ventral body caudal to the frenulum (**393**).

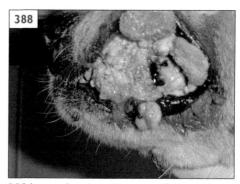

388 Inverted viral papilloma in a 13-year-old mixed breed dog. These lesions are atypical in old age and often do not regress spontaneously. In this case, these lesions did not respond to local immunotherapy.

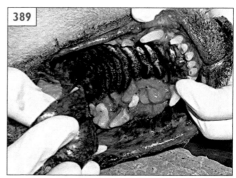

389 The same dog as in **388** after completion of a 4-week course of external beam radiation therapy. A complete remission was observed and the dog remained symptom free for the remainder of its life.

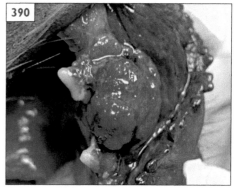

390 Large SCC on the mandible of a dog. (Courtesy of Dr. Brook Niemiec.)

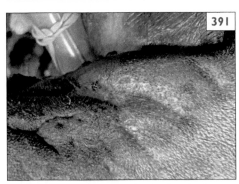

391 Early SCC on the mandibular lip of a dog. (Courtesy of Dr. Brook Niemiec.)

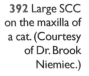

392 Large SCC on the maxilla of a cat. (Courtesy of Dr. Brook Niemiec.)

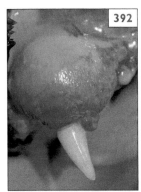

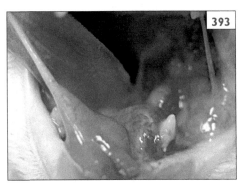

393 Sublingual SCC in a cat. (Courtesy of Dr. Brook Niemiec.)

DIFFERENTIAL DIAGNOSES

- Other tumor types such as amelanotic melanoma, epulids, sarcomas.
- Foreign body trapped under the tongue, especially in cats.
- Eosinophilic granuloma complex.

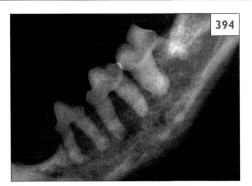

394 Radiographic appearance of SCC in the mandible of a cat. (Courtesy of Dr. Brook Niemiec.)

DIAGNOSTIC TESTS

Dental radiographs (**394**) and biopsy of the oral mass will confirm the diagnosis.

Regional lymph nodes, if palpable, should be aspirated or biopsied to rule out metastasis. After the diagnosis is confirmed, routine clinical staging consisting of 3-view thoracic radiographs, complete blood work, urinalysis, and abdominal ultrasound should be performed.

MANAGEMENT

Wide local excision is often curative in early cases with rostral location. Canine lingual SCC are best managed with partial glossectomy. Radiation therapy should be considered for local control, or palliative reasons in cases where surgical excision is not possible[37]. SCC appears to be radiosensitive but not radiocurable. Photodynamic therapy has also been reported to be effective in canine oral SCC[38.] A combination of cisplatin and piroxicam has shown antitumor activity against canine oral SCC[19]. Similarly, in an another retrospective study Schmidt *et al.*[39] reported that piroxicam at a dosage of 0.3 mg/kg (0.14 mg/lb) PO every 24 hours has a response rate similar to the other cytotoxic therapies in the treatment of canine oral SCC.

KEY POINTS

- Radiation therapy can provide local disease control in dogs with oral SCC[29].
- Radiation therapy in cats with sublingual or caudal oral cavity SCC has been disappointing. However, for palliative reasons local irradiation in cats with oral SCC can be considered.

Histologically low-grade, biologically high-grade, fibrosarcoma

DEFINITION
The histologically low-grade, biologically high-grade fibrosarcoma is another distinct histologic entity of oral FSA. It has been reported in large-breed dogs (primarily Golden Retrievers)[40].

BIOLOGIC BEHAVIOR, ETIOLOGY, AND PATHOGENESIS
Biologically, these tumors exhibit rapid growth, invasion, and metastatic potential. The histopathological findings are suggestive of a fibroma or a well-differentiated FSA.

CLINICAL FEATURES
Most dogs are presented with a rapidly enlarging swelling of the maxillofacial region, with a nonerosive gingival mass covered by intact epithelium (**395**).

DIFFERENTIAL DIAGNOSES
- FSA.
- Fibroma.
- Nodular fasciitis.
- Other nonodontogenic tumors.

DIAGNOSTIC TESTS
Biopsy of the oral mass should be taken to confirm the diagnosis. After the diagnosis is confirmed, routine clinical staging with 3-view thoracic radiographs, complete blood work, urinalysis and abdominal ultrasound should be performed.

Dental radiographs may provide clues to the aggressive nature of this lesion (**396**).
CT scan or MRI are often required for local staging and treatment planning.

MANAGEMENT
The treatment approach for this tumor type has not yet been optimized. Different treatment modalities including surgical excision in combination with radiation therapy, surgery alone, radiation therapy alone, and radiation therapy used adjunctly with localized hyperthermia, all seem to have prolonged the survival times in some dogs[40].

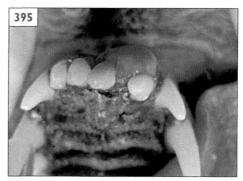

395 Early histologically low-grade, biologically high-grade, fibrosarcoma on the maxillary gingiva of a dog. (Courtesy of Dr. Brook Niemiec.)

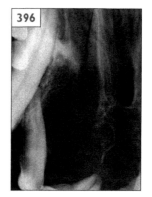

396 Dental radiograph of the patient in **395**. (Courtesy of Dr. Brook Niemiec.)

KEY POINTS
- This tumor has typically been reported in large breed dogs.
- Local recurrence is extremely common with this type of tumor.

Osteosarcoma

DEFINITION
Osteosarcoma (OSA) of the mandible or maxilla is variably reported in the oral cavity in dogs. Medium and large-sized breeds, middle-aged to older dogs, and females seem to be more commonly affected[41]. Feline oral OSA is much less common accounting for 2.4% of all oral tumors[42].

BIOLOGIC BEHAVIOR, ETIOLOGY, AND PATHOGENESIS
Oral OSA appears to be locally aggressive. The rate of metastasis of oral OSA is lower than appendicular OSA. Older literature suggests that mandibular OSA has a poor prognosis with a median survival of 1.5 months after mandibulectomy[43]. Newer studies, however, reflect mandibular OSA as prognostically favorable with a median survival of 7 months[44].

CLINICAL FEATURES
Clinically, the lesion can appear as a gross, fleshy mass. In early stages, the mass may or may not appear ulcerative (**397**). Local bony invasion causes significant facial swelling (**398**).

DIFFERENTIAL DIAGNOSES
- Other nonodontogenic tumors.
- Epulids.

DIAGNOSTIC TESTS
Dental radiographs and biopsy of the oral mass will confirm the diagnosis. Regional lymph nodes, if palpable, should be aspirated or biopsied to rule out metastasis. After the diagnosis is confirmed, routine clinical staging with 3-view thoracic radiographs, complete blood work, urinalysis, and abdominal ultrasound should be performed.

MANAGEMENT
The treatment of choice for oral OSA is wide or radical excision. A median survival time of 5 and 7 months has been reported for maxillary and mandibular OSA, respectively[45]. Local recurrence following incomplete excision, or distant metastasis, caused most therapeutic failures. Radiation therapy should be considered for microscopic disease if the surgical margins are not clean. Radiation therapy can also be used for palliative reasons in very advanced cases.

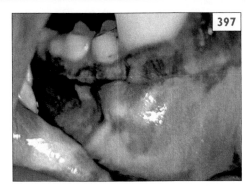

397 Early mandibular osteosarcoma in a dog. (Courtesy of Dr. Brook Niemiec.)

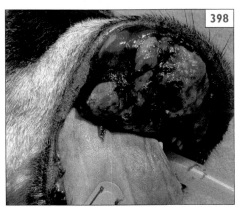

398 Large maxillary osteosarcoma in a dog resulting in facial deformity. (Courtesy of Dr. Brook Niemiec.)

Adjuvant or adjunctive chemotherapy with carboplatin or doxorubicin as a single agent, or as an alternate regimen, should be considered.

KEY POINTS
- Aggressive surgical excision should be considered early in the course of the disease.
- Feline oral OSA is uncommon.

Pathologies of the Salivary System

Brook A. Niemiec

- **Sialoceles**

- **Salivary gland tumors**

- **Sialoliths (salivary stones)**

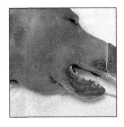 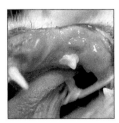 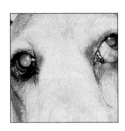 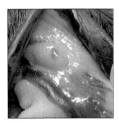

Sialoceles

DEFINITION

Sialoceles are retention cysts (pseudocysts) of salivary fluids[1]. They are not true cysts as they lack an epithelial lining[2]. Ranulas are sialoceles which are typically found under the tongue[3] or on the floor of the mouth[1]. Sialoceles are the most common problem associated with the salivary gland in dogs and cats[4].

ETIOLOGY AND PATHOGENESIS

These lesions occur secondary to a rupture of a salivary duct resulting in the spillage of mucin into the surrounding soft tissue[1]. The most common cause of the rupture is trauma[1,5,6]. Trauma can be blunt (e.g. hit by a car), sharp (e.g. gunshot), or foreign body (e.g. foxtail) in origin. In addition, it is not uncommon for these to occur after oral surgery (extraction, oral fracture repair, or neoplastic excision) due to transection of a salivary duct[7]. There are numerous cases however, in humans and animals with no history of trauma[1,6]. Sialoceles can also result from blockage of the duct by mucin, sialoliths, or inflammation[3]. Finally, there is one report in which dirofilariasis was the suspected cause[8]. The spilled mucin elicits an inflammatory reaction in the surrounding tissue and creates increased swelling. In general, the mucin pools ventral to the site of rupture.

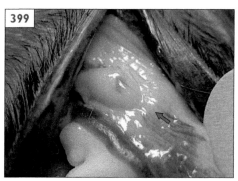

399 Small zygomatic mucocele in a dog (arrow).

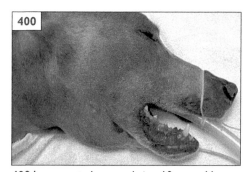

400 Large ventral mucocele in a 10-year-old Weimaraner. Note the swelling under the mandible.

CLINICAL FEATURES

Sialoceles appear as a dome-shaped mucosal swelling, and can range from a few millimeters to several centimeters in diameter[1] (**399**). If they are superficial, the mucin imparts a bluish hue, but if deeper they are normal in color[1]. Sialoceles are generally soft and fluctuant, but some can feel firm[1]. Typically they are nonpainful; however, if significant inflammation or secondary infection is present, there may be pain associated with the lesion. Dachshunds, Poodles, and Australian Silky Terriers appear over represented[2]. A recent history of maxillofacial trauma or surgery is supportive but not definitive, as this also increases the possibility for hematoma or abscess.

The presenting complaint is usually a swelling that may wax and wane. The duration can be from days to months depending on size, location, and owner level of scrutiny. On occasion, the swelling will increase at mealtimes and decrease slowly thereafter. In some cases, dysphagia or ptyalism may be the presenting sign[6]. Finally, these swellings may rupture on their own and then refill over time[1]. The location depends on the salivary gland that is involved. The most common clinically evident mucoceles seen in veterinary dentistry are the ranula, which are found in the floor of the mouth[2]. These may extend through the ventral neck musculature and may be seen externally below the level of the ventral mandible (**400**). In human medicine, this is called a plunging ranula[9]. Ranulas are produced by drainage from the sublingual glands and ducts[2].

DIFFERENTIAL DIAGNOSES

- Abscess/granuloma.
- Neoplasia.
- Hematoma.
- Sialolith.

DIAGNOSTIC TESTS

Dental radiographs should be exposed to evaluate for possible etiologic agents (sialolith, bullet, fracture) as well as bone loss secondary to neoplasia or infection.

Diagnosis is supported by fluid analysis and cytology. The typical cytologic finding is the presence of foamy histiocytes (macrophages)[1]. If any question remains, histopathology should be performed. Histologically, these appear as an area of spilled mucin surrounded with granulation tissue[1].

If the identity of the supplying gland is not obvious (which is often the case in the sublingual type or ranula) the surgeon has two options. The first is to image the area in question, in attempt to isolate the offending duct. The classic method is a contrast sialogram; however this is very technically difficult and invasive[6]. A newer method of magnetic resonance (MR) sialography has shown promise as a noninvasive means of imaging the salivary system, and may be preferable to sialogram[10,11]. The other option for surgical cure the first time, is to resect both of the sublingual and mandibular glands (see below)[6]. Prior to definitive surgery, a complete work-up including bleeding times should be performed to ensure patient safety.

MANAGEMENT

On rare occasions, these lesions may be short lived, and will rupture and heal by themselves[1]. This appears to be the case most often with the comparatively rare parotid gland mucoceles[12]. In addition, this would only be expected in the smallest of mucoceles, which are unlikely to be diagnosed in the veterinary field. The vast majority of the time, they persist unless definitive therapy is performed.

Surgery is indicated in all cases that persist past a few weeks or recur following the initial rupture.

There are several techniques that have been advocated for these lesions. The surgical technique of choice for large mucoceles (especially the plunging ranula) is surgical excision of the cyst along with the salivary gland(s) that are feeding the lesion[1,4,5,13,14]. This method has been shown to be vastly superior to any other surgical technique in several human studies[13,15] and is the technique of choice because it has the best chance of cure with the first surgery. Due to the fact that the

mandibular gland and its ducts are intimately related to the sublingual, it is recommended to remove both of them[6]. This does not appear to affect the salivary flow negatively[6].

In cases of very large mucoceles, drainage of the remaining fluid-filled cavity rather than *en bloc* removal is preferred. Following excision of the gland and ligation of the duct, ventral drainage is established. In some instances, this can be performed by making a stab incision and suturing a Penrose into the surgically created defect[6]. With large lesions however, especially ranulas, marsupialization is recommended[6].

Marsupialization of the lesion is performed via the following steps[6]. First, an elliptical incision is created in the overlying mucosa. Following drainage of the mucin, the epithelial lining is sutured to the adjacent connective tissue on either side of the cyst to allow long-term drainage. Marsupialization, without gland removal, may be effective in rare cases, especially smaller ones[16,17]. However, due to the lack of success with this method, it is not recommended. In addition, simple drainage of the cyst with a needle and syringe is not recommended as swelling will recur within 48 hours in 42% of patients[2], and will eventually recur in almost all patients.

Recently, some nonsurgical remedies have been developed in the human field. These consist of draining the cyst and then injecting a sclerosing agent into the space. Examples of medications which have been tested with success include nickel gluconate-mercurius heel-potentized swine organ preparations[18] and OK-432[19,20].

KEY POINTS

- Sialoceles/mucoceles occur most commonly secondary to trauma.
- These lesions are nonpainful, soft, and occasionally wax and wane.
- Removal of the salivary gland which is supplying the mucin is generally required for cure, especially in large lesions.
- New medications may allow for successful nonsurgical therapy.

Salivary gland tumors

DEFINITION
Salivary gland neoplasia is defined as a primary tumor of a salivary gland[1]. However, other soft tissue tumors (especially lymphoma) have been reported in the salivary glands, and it is also possible for the salivary gland to be a point of metastasis for other tumors[1,3].

ETIOLOGY AND PATHOGENESIS
The vast majority of salivary cancers are malignant. The most commonly reported type is an adenocarcinoma, but there is wide variation of the histologic type[21]. The mandibular is the most commonly involved gland, followed by the parotid[22]. Metastasis to regional lymph nodes is common, but distant spread is less likely[23].

CLINICAL FEATURES
Salivary neoplasia is rare in small animal medicine, and is typically diagnosed in older dogs and cats. In the general population, there does not appear to be a breed or sex predilection[24]. However, one report suggests a higher incidence in Siamese cats, particularly males of the breed[23].

Historical signs are most commonly nonspecific and may include ptyalism, quidding, dysphagia, partial to complete anorexia, and halitosis. External physical findings include a firm, nonpainful swelling with location depending on the gland involved[3,25] (**401**). Sublingual, mandibular, and molar gland involvement usually results in a submandibular or ventral neck swelling. Involvement of the parotid gland generally results in swelling at the base of the ear. Maxillary swelling is seen in cases of zygomatic gland tumors. Finally, swelling of the upper lip can result from cancer of the accessory salivary tissue.

Occasionally, zygomatic or parotid gland neoplasia can result in exophthalmus (**402**) or eye metastasis and secondary complications[26,27]. In addition, the tumor may also cause a salivary mucocele, which may be the presenting sign[25].

DIFFERENTIAL DIAGNOSES[21,22]
- Abscess/granuloma.
- Mucoceles.
- Salivary gland infarction.
- Sialadenitis.
- Sialolith.
- Lymphoma.
- Reactive lymphadenopathy.

DIAGNOSTIC TESTS
The first step toward diagnosis is fine-needle aspiration cytology which should differentiate inflammatory/infectious disease from neoplasia[25]. Radiographs (dental if possible) should be exposed to evaluate for other possible etiologic agents (sialolith) as well as periosteal reaction. Definitive diagnosis usually requires histopathology. This can be performed via a wedge or core needle sample, or submitted following definitive surgery. A complete work-up including bleeding times should be performed prior to definitive surgery, to ensure patient safety.

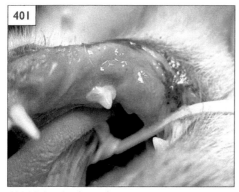

401 Molar gland neoplasia in a cat.

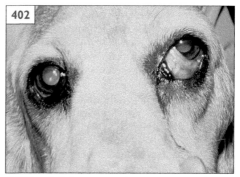

402 Exophthalmus secondary to a zygomatic gland carcinoma. (Courtesy of Dr. Barbara Steele.)

MANAGEMENT

Aggressive *en bloc* surgical removal is the preferred method of therapy when possible[1,3,25]. In cases where the tumor has remained within the gland capsule, complete salivary gland excision can prove curative[1]. Excision of the sublingual and mandibular glands is technical but fairly straightforward. However, parotid and zygomatic gland removal is very technically demanding[6]. These surgeries should only be attempted by an experienced surgeon.

Unfortunately, the majority of cases are extracapsular at the time of diagnosis[3]. This requires a much more aggressive surgery and removal of a significant amount of 'normal' tissue to ensure a surgical cure. This often involves removal of numerous vital tissues due to the location of the glands. Fortunately, veterinary patients tend to be very resilient, even with surgery which requires extirpation of the ipsilateral neck[25].

Postoperative radiation therapy has proven beneficial in cases of salivary gland tumors and is considered the gold standard of care by some in the human field[28–30]. If complete surgical cure is not possible, radiation therapy for microscopic disease can achieve acceptable results[25]. In fact, radiation therapy alone has produced favorable results in human studies[29,31,32].

While the mainstays of management for salivary gland tumors are surgery and radiation therapy, recent advances in chemotherapy within the human field are showing some promise[33–35]. Chemotherapy however, is generally only used in advanced, inoperable, recurrent, or metastatic disease. It should not be the first line of treatment, although some may use it as an adjunct or induction therapy[35–37].

KEY POINTS

- Typical presentations mimic benign lesions (such as ranula and abscess) and therefore may be misdiagnosed originally.
- Cytology can often differentiate from inflammation, but biopsy is required for definitive diagnosis.
- Surgical excision +/– radiation therapy is the key to management.
- Chemotherapy should be considered in cases of inoperable, recurrent, or metastasized disease. It may also be of use in initial therapy.

Sialoliths (salivary stones)

DEFINITION

Sialoliths are calcifications found in salivary glands or ducts[3].

ETIOLOGY AND PATHOGENESIS

Sialoliths are believed to arise due to the deposition of calcium around a nidus of debris within the duct lumen[1]. The debris may be mucus, epithelial cells, bacteria, or foreign bodies. One study has implicated that mitochondria and lysosomal bodies from the ductal system of the submandibular gland are an etiological source for calcification in the gland[38]. An additional study suggests that they may occur in individuals with a deficit of crystallization inhibitors, such as myoinositol hexaphosphate[39]. Finally, at least one paper reports that they may occur secondary to sialadenitis[40]. The true etiology is unclear, but they do not appear to be related to any problem with calcium/phosphorus metabolism[1].

CLINICAL FEATURES

The most common clinical sign of a sialolith is facial or oral swelling[1] (**403**). If this is due to a large stone, the swelling will be very hard. However, if a small stone has caused salivary back-up or a sialocele, the swelling may be soft, and wax and wane with mealtimes. Pain is variable depending on location and severity.

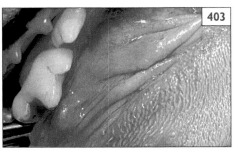

403 A small sialolith in the sublingual salivary duct.

DIFFERENTIAL DIAGNOSES
- Abscess/granuloma.
- Neoplasia.
- Hematoma.
- Sialocele.

DIAGNOSTIC TESTS
Radiographs (skull and dental) should be exposed to evaluate size and location of the stone (**404**). Some stones may not be visible on radiographs due to variability of calcification[1]. In addition, a small stone may be missed or misdiagnosed as an intrabony lesion, due to superimposition of the alveolar bone[1]. Sialography, ultrasound, computed tomography, MRI, and sialendoscopy may be useful in difficult cases[1,41]. The stones are round or oval in shape, and typically yellow in color, although white and yellowish-brown colorations are possible[1]. Stone analysis is generally not indicated.

MANAGEMENT
Small stones in major ducts can occasionally be gently massaged into the duct orifice[3]. For large stones (or small ones that cannot be moved) surgical removal is often necessary[1]. If the stone has created significant inflammation of the salivary duct or gland, removal of the gland should be considered.

Recent advances in diagnosis and therapy have opened up newer less invasive techniques for treating this disease process. One of these alternative therapies is removal of the stone utilizing salivary gland endoscopy (sialendoscopy)[1,41]. However, lithotripsy (internal or external) has been proven as an effective and noninvasive method for treating this condition, especially in the parotid gland or duct[1,42,43]. It is still effective, but less so, with submandibular stones[44]. Lithotripsy (+/− sialendoscopy) appears to be the current first line therapy in human medicine, especially with parotid or smaller submandibular stones[42,45,46].

KEY POINTS
- This condition is not associated with calcium/phosphorus metabolism.
- Sialoliths may cause a sialocele.
- Meticulous evaluation of radiographs is critical in cases of small stones.
- Massaging the stone forward is the first line of therapy.
- Lithotripsy and/or sialendoscopy should be attempted as a noninvasive technique.
- In nonresponsive cases, or with very large stones, surgical excision is also an option.

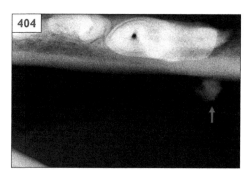

404 Intraoral dental radiograph of the patient in **403**. The sialolith is visible lingual to the first molar (arrow).

Appendices

AVDC-approved abbreviations

	Definition
AB	abrasion
APG	apexogenesis
APX	apexification
AT	attrition
B	biopsy
B/E	biopsy excisional
B/I	biopsy incisional
BG	bone graft (includes placement of bone substitute or bone stimulant material)
C	canine
CA	caries
CBU	core build up
CFL	cleft lip
CFL/R	cleft lip repair
CFP	cleft palate
CFP/R	cleft palate repair
CMO	craniomandibular osteopathy
CR	crown
CRA	crown amputation
CR/M	crown metal
CRL	crown lengthening
CR/PFM	crown porcelain fused to metal
CR/P	crown preparation
CRR	crown reduction
CS	culture/susceptibility
DT	deciduous (primary) tooth
DTC	dentigerous cyst
E	enamel
E/D	enamel defect
E/H	enamel hypocalcification or hypoplasia
FB	foreign body
F	flap
F/AR	apically repositioned periodontal flap
F/CR	coronally repositioned periodontal flap
F/L	lateral sliding periodontal flap
FGG	free gingival graft
FRE	frenoplasty (frenotomy, frenectomy)
FX	fracture (tooth or jaw)
	For tooth fracture abbreviations, see under T/FX

FX/R	repair of jaw fracture
FX/R/P	pin repair of jaw fracture
FX/R/PL	plate repair of jaw fracture
FX/R/S	screw repair of jaw fracture
FX/R/WIR	wire repair of jaw fracture
FX/R/WIR/C	cerclage wire repair of jaw fracture
FX/R/WIR/ID	interdental wire repair of jaw fracture
FX/R/WIR/OS	osseous wire repair of jaw fracture
G	granuloma
G/B	buccal granuloma (cheek chewing lesion)
G/L	sublingual granuloma (tongue chewing lesion)
G/E/L	eosinophilic granuloma – lip
G/E/P	eosinophilic granuloma – palate
G/E/T	eosinophilic granuloma – tongue
GH	gingival hyperplasia/hypertrophy
GR	gingival recession
GTR	guided tissue regeneration
GV	gingivoplasty (gingivectomy)
IM	impression and model
IMP	implant
I1,2,3	Incisor teeth
IO	interceptive (extraction) orthodontics
IO/D	deciduous (primary) tooth interceptive orthodontics
IO/P	permanent (secondary) tooth interceptive orthodontics
IP	inclined plane
IP/AC	acrylic inclined plane
IP/C	composite inclined plane
IP/M	metal (i.e. lab produced) inclined plane
LAC	laceration
LAC/B	laceration buccal (cheek)
LAC/L	laceration lip
LAC/T	laceration tongue
M1,2,3	molar teeth
MAL	malocclusion – see web page
MAL/1	class I malocclusion (normal jaw relationship, specific teeth are incorrectly positioned)
MAL/2	class II malocclusion (mandible shorter than maxilla)
MAL/3	class III malocclusion (maxilla shorter than mandible)
MAL/1 or 2 or 3/BN	base narrow mandibular canine tooth
MAL/1 or 2 or 3/RXB	rostral crossbite
MAL/1 or 2 or 3/CXB	caudal crossbite
MAL/1 or 2 or 4/WRY	wry bite
MN	mandible or mandibular
MN/FX	mandibular fracture
MX	maxilla or maxillary
MX/FX	maxillary fracture
OA	orthodontic appliance
OAA	adjust orthodontic appliance
OA/BKT	bracket orthodontic appliance
OA/BU	button orthodontic appliance
OA/EC	elastic (power chain) orthodontic appliance
OA/WIR	wire orthodontic appliance
OAI	install orthodontic appliance
OAR	remove orthodontic appliance
OC	orthodontic/genetic consultation

OM	oral mass
OM/AD	adenocarcinoma
OM/EPA	acanthomatous ameloblastoma (epulis)
OM/EPF	fibromatous epulis
OM/EPO	osseifying epulis
OM/FS	fibrosarcoma
OM/LS	lymphosarcoma
OM/MM	malignant melanoma
OM/OS	osteosarcoma
OM/PAP	papillomatosis
OM/SCC	squamous cell carcinoma
ONF	oronasal fistula
ONF/R	oronasal fistula repair
OR	orthodontic recheck
OST	osteomyelitis
PC	pulp capping
PC/D	direct pulp capping
PC/I	indirect pulp capping
PDI	periodontal disease index
PD0	normal periodontium
PD1	gingivitis only
PD2	<25% attachment loss
PD3	25–50% attachment loss
PD4	>50% attachment loss
PE	pulp exposure
PM1,2,3,4	premolar teeth
PRO	periodontal prophylaxis (examination, scaling, polishing, irrigation)
R	restoration of tooth
R/A	restoration with amalgam
R/C	restoration with composite
R/CP	restoration with compomer
R/I	restoration with glass ionomer
RAD	radiograph
RC	root canal therapy
RC/S	surgical root canal therapy
RD	retained deciduous (primary) tooth

RL is no longer used for resorptive lesion. See TR for tooth resorption.

RPC	root planing – closed
RPO	root planing – open
RRX	root resection (crown left intact)
RR	internal root resorption
RRT	retained root tip
RTR	retained tooth root
S	surgery
S/M	mandibulectomy
S/P	palate surgery
S/X	maxillectomy
SC	subgingival curettage
SN	supernumerary
SPL	splint
SPL/AC	acrylic splint
SPL/C	composite splint
SPL/WIR	wire reinforced splint
ST	stomatitis
ST/CU	stomatitis – contact ulcers
ST/FFS	stomatitis – feline faucitis-stomatitis

SYM	symphysis
SYM/S	symphyseal separation
SYM/WIR	wire repair of symphyseal separation
T	tooth
T/A	avulsed tooth
T/FX	fractured tooth (see next seven listings for fracture types)
T/FX/EI	enamel infraction
T/FX/EF	enamel fracture
T/FX/UCF	uncomplicated crown fracture
T/FX/CCF	complicated crown fracture
T/FX/UCRF	uncomplicated crown-root facture
T/FX/CCRF	complicated crown-root fracture
T/FX/RF	root fracture
	For further information on the tooth fracture definitions, see the Tooth Fracture section in the Nomenclature web page.
T/I	impacted tooth
T/LUX	luxated tooth
T/NE	near pulp exposure
T/NV	nonvital tooth
T/PE	pulp exposure
T/V	vital tooth
TMJ	temporomandibular joint
TMJ/C	temporomandibular joint condylectomy
TMJ/D	TMJ dysplasia
TMJ/FX	TMJ fracture
TMJ/LUX	TMJ luxation
TMJ/R	reduction of TMJ luxation
TP	treatment plan
TR	tooth resorption
TR1	TR Stage 1: mild dental hard tissue loss (cementum or cementum and enamel)
TR2	TR Stage 2: moderate dental hard tissue loss (cementum or cementum and enamel with loss of dentin that does not extend to the pulp cavity)
TR3	TR Stage 3: deep dental hard tissue loss (cementum or cementum and enamel with loss of dentin that extends to the pulp cavity); most of the tooth retains its integrity
TR4	TR Stage 4: extensive dental hard tissue loss (cementum or cementum and enamel with loss of dentin that extends to the pulp cavity); most of the tooth has lost its integrity (TR4a) Crown and root are equally affected (TR4b) Crown is more severely affected than the root (TR4c) Root is more severely affected than the crown
TR5	TR Stage 5: remnants of dental hard tissue are visible only as irregular radiopacities, and gingival covering is complete
TRX	tooth partial resection (e.g. hemisection)
VP	vital pulp therapy
X	simple closed extraction of a tooth
XS	extraction with tooth sectioning, nonsurgical
XSS	surgical (open) extraction of a tooth

Southern California Veterinary Dental Specialties
Brook Niemiec, DVM, Dip. AVDC, Fellow AVD

Name:_____ Date:_____

Anesthetic protocol:

Pre-medication
Atropine_____
Buprenorphine___
Butorphanol_____
Morphine_____

Induction
Valium _____
Propoflo_____
O Sevoflorane/O$_2$

Maintenance
O Oxygen
O Isoflurane
O Sevoflurane

Diagnostic
O Biopsy
O Culture

Skull type
O Brachycephalic
O Mesocephalic
O Dolichocephalic

Mandibular symphysis
O Intact
O Luxated

Occlusion
O Scissors
O Brachygnathic
O Even
O Anterior crossbite
O Posterior crossbite
O Prognathic
O Wry
O Endentulous

Temporomandibular palpation
O Normal
O Pain
O Crepitus
O Clicking
O Inhibited
O Luxated

Prophylaxis:

Crown scaling
O Hand
O Ultrasonic

Subgingival
O Exploration
O Subgingival curettage
O Root planing
O Doxirobe

Polishing
O Chlorhexidine + pumice
O Fluoride Tx regeneration

Exodontia
O Crown amputation
O Routine extraction
O Sectioning
O Buccal cortical bone removal
O Alveoloplasty
O Suture
  O Chromic gut___
  O Monocryl___

Restoration
O Fillings
  O Composite
  O Glass ionomer

	110	109	108	107	106	105	104	103	102	101	201	202	203	204	205	206	207	208	209	210
Mobility/furcation																				
Perio pocket																				
Attachment loss																				

Right

Buccal ⟶

Palatal ⟶

Lingual ⟶

Buccal ⟶

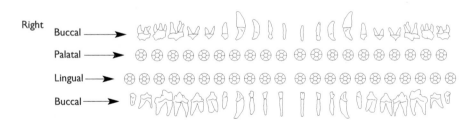

	411	410	409	408	407	406	405	404	403	402	401	301	302	303	304	305	306	307	308	309	310	311
M/F																						
P																						
AL																						

CA- Caries
CWD- Crowding
ED- Enamel defect
F- Furcation exposure
Fx- Fractured tooth
GH- Gingival hyperplasia
GR- Gingival recession

GV- Gingivectomy
M- Mobility
O- Missing tooth
PD- Persistent deciduous
PE- Pulp exposure
R- Rotated tooth
R/C- Restoration/composite

RPC- Root plane closed
RPO- Root plane open
RR- Retained root
S/E- Extrinsic staining
S/I- Intrinsic staining
W- Worn
X- Extracted

Southern California Veterinary Dental Specialties
Brook Niemiec, DVM, Dip. AVDC, Fellow AVD

Name:_____ Date:_____

Anesthetic protocol:

Pre-medication
Atropine_____
Buprenorphine___

Induction
Valium _____
Propoflo_____
O Sevoflorane/O$_2$

Maintenance
O Oxygen
O Isoflurane
O Sevoflurane

Diagnostic
O Biopsy
O Culture

Skull type
O Brachycephalic
O Mesocephalic
O Doliococephalic

Mandibular symphysis
O Intact
O Luxated

Occlusion
O Scissors
O Brachygnathic
O Even
O Anterior crossbite
O Posterior crossbite
O Prognathic
O Wry
O Endentulous

Temporomandibular palpation
O Normal
O Pain
O Crepitus
O Clicking
O Inhibited
O Luxated

Prophylaxis:

Crown scaling
O Hand
O Ultrasonic

Subgingival
O Exploration
O Subgingival curettage
O Root planing
O Gingivectomy

Polishing
O Chlorhexidine + pumice
O Fluoride Tx

Exodontia
O Crown amputation
O Routine extraction
O Sectioning
O Buccal cortical bone removal
O Alveoloplasty
O Suture
  O Chromic gut___
  O Monocryl___

Restoration
O Fillings
O Composite
O Glass ionomer

	109	108	107	106	104	103	102	101	201	202	203	204	206	207	208	209
Mobility/furcation																
Perio pocket																
Attachment loss																

Right   Left

Buccal ➤

Palatal ➤

Lingual ➤

Buccal ➤

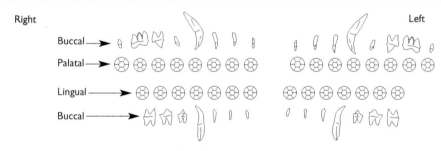

	409	408	407	404	403	402	402	401	301	302	303	304	307	308	309
M/F															
P															
AL															

AT- Attrition
CA- Crown amputation
ED- Enamel defect
F- Furcation exposure
Fx- Fractured tooth
GH- Gingival hyperplasia
GR- Gingival recession
GV- Gingivectomy

M- Mobility
O- Missing tooth
P- Periodontal pocket
PE- Pulp exposure
PD- Persistent deciduous
R- Rotated tooth
RPC- Root planing closed

RPO- Root planing open
SI- Staining/intrinsic
S/E- Staining extrinsic
TR- Tooth resorptive lesion
X- Extracted

References

Chapter 1

1 Harvey, CE (1985). Anatomy of the oral cavity in the dog and cat. In: Harvey CE (ed), *Veterinary Dentistry*. WB Saunders, Philadelphia.

2 Floyd MR (1991). The modified Triadan system: nomenclature for veterinary dentistry. *Journal of Veterinary Dentistry* **8**(4):18–19.

3 Verstraete FJM (1997). Anatomical variations in the dentition of the domestic cat. *Journal of Veterinary Dentistry* **14**(4):137–40.

4 Crossley DA (1995). Clinical aspects of rodent dental anatomy. *Journal of Veterinary Dentistry* **12**:131–135.

5 Capello V, Gracis M (2005). *Rabbit and Rodent Dentistry Handbook*. Zoological Education Network Inc, Lake Worth, pp. 3–42.

6 Kertesz P (1993). *A Colour Atlas of Veterinary Dentistry and Oral Surgery*. Wolfe Publishing, Aylesbury.

7 Crossley DA (1995). Clinical aspects of lagomorph dental anatomy: the rabbit (*Oryctolagus cuniculus*). *Journal of Veterinary Dentistry* **12**:137–140.

8 Bellows JE, Dumais Y, Gioso MA, Reiter AM, Verstraete FJ (2005). Clarification of veterinary dental nomenclature. *Journal of Veterinary Dentistry* **22**(4):272–9.

9 Orsini P, Hennet P (1992). Anatomy of the mouth and teeth of the cat. *Veterinary Clinics of North America* **22**(6):1265–77.

10 Wheeler RC (1969). *A Textbook of Dental Anatomy and Physiology*. WB Saunders, Philadelphia.

11 Wiggs RB, Lobprise HB (1997). *Veterinary Dentistry: Principles and Practice*. Lippincott–Raven, Philadelphia.

12 Verstraete FJM (1999). *Colour Self-Assessment Review of Veterinary Dentistry*. Manson, London.

13 Avery JK (1992). *Essentials of Oral Histology and Embryology: a Clinical Approach*. Mosby Year Book, St. Louis.

14 Harvey CE, Emily PP (1993). *Small Animal Dentistry*. Mosby Year Book, St. Louis.

15 Nanci, A (2003). *Ten Cate's Oral Histology: Development, Structure, and Function*. Mosby, St. Louis.

16 Gorrel C, Penman S, Emily P (1993). *Handbook of Small Animal Oral Emergencies*. Pergammon, Oxford, New York.

17 Crossley DA (1995). Tooth enamel thickness in the mature dentition of domestic dogs and cats: preliminary study. *Journal of Veterinary Dentistry* **12**(3):111–3.

18 Evans HE (1993). *Miller's Anatomy of the Dog*, 3rd edn. WB Saunders, Philadelphia.

19 Hudson LC, Hamilton WP (1993). *Atlas of Feline Anatomy for Veterinarians*. WB Saunders, Philadelphia.

20 Bubb WJ, Sims MH (1986). Fiber type composition of rostral and caudal portions of the digastric muscle in the dog. *American Journal of Veterinary Research* **47**(8):1834–42.

21 Scapino RP (1965). The third joint of the canine jaw. *Journal of Morphology* **116**:23–50.

22 Rawlinson J (2004). Tackling the canine and feline temporomandibular joint. *Proceedings of the 18th Annual Veterinary Dental Forum*, pp. 7–11.

23 Reiter AM (2004). Symphysiotomy, symphysiectomy, and intermandibular arthrodesis in a cat with open-mouth jaw locking: case report and literature review. *Journal of Veterinary Dentistry* **21**: 147–158.

24 Gioso MA, Carvalho VGG (2005). Oral anatomy of the dog and cat in veterinary dentistry practice. *Veterinary Clinics of North America, Small Animal Practice* **35**:763–780.

25 Harvey CE (1987). Palate defects in dogs and cats. *Compendium on Continuing Education for the Practicing Veterinarian* **9**:404–418.

26 Rosenzweig LJ (1993). *Anatomy of the Cat*. Brown Publishers, Dubuque, p. 181.

27 Okuda A, Inoue E, Asari M (1996). The membranous bulge lingual to the mandibular molar tooth of a cat contains a small salivary gland. *Journal of Veterinary Dentistry* **13**:61–64.

28 Rumph PF, Garret PD, Gray BW (1980). Facial lymph nodes in dogs. *Journal of the American Veterinary Medical Association* **176**:342–344.

29 Shelton ME, Forsythe WB (1979). Buccal lymph node in the dog. *American Journal of Veterinary Research* **40**(11):1638–9.

30 Smith MM (1995). Surgical approach for lymph node staging of oral and maxillofacial neoplasms in dogs. *Journal of the American Animal Hospital Association* **31**(6):514–8.

31 Herring ES, Smith MM, Robertson JL (2002). Lymph node staging of oral and maxillofacial neoplasms in 31 dogs and cats. *Journal of Veterinary Dentistry* **19**:122–6.

Chapter 2

1 Wiggs RB, Lobprise HB (1997). *Veterinary Dentistry: Principles and Practice.* Lippincott–Raven, Philadelphia.

2 Cohen S, Liewehr F (2002). Diagnostic procedures. In: Burns RC, Cohen S (eds). *Pathways of the Pulp.* Mosby, St. Louis.

3 Dupont G (2005). Diseases of the mouth in small animals. In: Kahn CM (ed). *The Merck Veterinary Manual,* 9th edn. Merck & Co, Inc, Whitehouse Station, p. 283.

4 Poffenbarger EM (1991). Lymphatic system. In: McCurnin DM, Poffenberger FM (eds). *Small Animal Physical Diagnosis and Clinical Procedures.* WB Saunders, Philadelphia, p. 123.

5 Poffenbarger EM (1991). Head and neck. In: McCurnin DM, Poffenberger FM (eds). *Small Animal Physical Diagnosis and Clinical Procedures.* WB Saunders, Philadelphia, p. 30.

6 Done SH, Evans SA, Goody PC, Stickland NC (1996). *Color Atlas of Veterinary Anatomy.* The Dog & Cat. Mosby, London. Volume 3, pp. 1.14–15.

7 dos Anjos MN (1970). Labial edema in hypothyroidism. *New England Journal of Medicine* **283**(2):101.

8 Gorani A, Oriani A, Cambiaghi S (2005). Seborrheic dermatitis-like tinea faciei. *Pediatric Dermatology* **22**(3):243–4.

9 McIntyre GT, Millett DT (2006). Lip shape and position in Class II division 2 malocclusion. *The Angle Orthodontist* **76**(5):739–44.

10 Feldman EC, Greco DS, Hodges CM, Peterson ME, Shipman LW, Turner JL (1991). Congenital hypothyroid dwarfism in a family of giant Schnauzers. *Journal of Veterinary Internal Medicine* **5**(2):57–65.

11 Harvey CE, Emily PP (1993). *Small Animal Dentistry.* Mosby, Philadelphia.

12 Blood DC, Studdert VP (eds). (1996). *Baillière's Comprehensive Veterinary Dictionary.* Baillière Tindall, London.

13 Agnihotri A, Marwah N, Dutta SJ (2006). Dilacerated unerupted central incisor: A case report. *Journal of the Indian Society of Pedodontics and Preventive Dentistry* **24**(3):152–4.

14 Regezi JA, Sciubba JJ, Jordan RCK (2003). Abnormalities of teeth. In: Regezi JA, Sciubba JJ, Jordan RCK (eds). *Oral Pathology: Clinical Pathological Correlations,* 4th edn. Elsevier Science, St. Louis.

15 Jafarzadeh H, Abbott PV (2007). Dilaceration: review of an endodontic challenge. *Journal of Endodontics* **33**(9):1025–30.

16 Ligh RQ (1981). Coronal dilaceration. *Oral Surgery, Oral Medicine, & Oral Pathology* **51**(5):567.

17 Pavlica Z., V. Erjavec, M. Petelin (2001). Teeth abnormalities in the dog. *Acta Veterinaria* **70**: 65–72.

18 Hamasha AA, Al-Khateeb T, Darwazeh (2002). A prevalence of dilaceration in Jordanian adults. *International Endodontic Journal* **35**(11): 910–12.

19 Kronfeld R (1934). Dens in dente. *Journal of Dental Research* **14**(1):49–66.

20 Silberman A, Cohenca N, Simon JH (2006). Anatomical redesign for the treatment of dens invaginatus type III with open apexes: a literature review and case presentation. *Journal of the American Dental Association* **137**(2):180–5.

21 Pandey SC, Pandey RK (2005). Radicular dens invaginatus: a case report. *Journal of the Indian Society of Pedodontics and Preventative Dentistry* **23**:151–2.

22 DeForge DH (1992). Dens in dente in a six-year-old Doberman Pinscher. *Journal of Veterinary Dentistry* **9**(3):9.

23 Moskow BS, Canut PM (1990). Studies on root enamel. (2) Enamel pearls. A review of their morphology, localization, nomenclature, occurrence, classification, histogenesis, and incidence. *Journal of Clinical Periodontology* **17**(5):275–81.

24 Bundzman ER, Modesto A (1999). Hypomaturation amelogenesis imperfecta: account of a family with an X-linked inheritance pattern. *Brazilian Dental Journal* **10**(2): 111–16.

25 Crawford PJ, Aldred M, Bloch-Zupan A (2007). Amelogenesis imperfecta. *Orphanet Journal of Rare Diseases* **2**(17):1–11.

26 Seedorf H, Springer IN, Grundner-Culemann E, Albers HK, Reiss A, Fuch H, Hrabe de Angelis M, Acil Y (2004). Amelogenesis imperfecta in a new animal model – a mutation in chromosome 5 (human 4q21). *Journal of Dental Research* **83**(8):608–12.

27 Kamboj M, Chandra A (2007). Dentinogenesis imperfecta type II: an affected family saga. *Journal of Oral Science* **49**(3):241–4.

28 Eickhoff M, Seeliger F, Simon D, Fehr M (2002). Erupted bilateral compound odontomas in a dog. *Journal of Veterinary Dentistry* **19**(3):137–43.

29 Dunfee BL, Sakai O, Pistey R, and Gohel A (2006). Radiologic and pathological characteristics of benign and malignant lesions of the mandible. *Radiographics* **26**:1751–1768.

30 Vengal M, Arora H, Ghosh S, Pai KM (2007). Large erupting complex odontoma: a case report. *Journal of the Canadian Dental Association* **73**(2):169–73.

31 Mulligan TW, Aller MS, Williams CA (1998). *Atlas of Canine & Feline Dental Radiography.* Veterinary Learning Systems, Trenton.

32 Verstraete FJ, Terpak CH (1997). Anatomical variations in the dentition of the domestic cat. *Journal of Veterinary Dentistry* **14**(4):137–40.

33 Verstraete FJ, van Aarde RJ, Nieuwoudt BA, Mauer E, Kass PH (1996). The dental pathology of feral cats on Marion Island, part I: congenital, developmental and traumatic abnormalities. *Journal of Veterinary Dentistry* **115**(3):265–82.

34 Dole RS, Spurgeon TL (1998). Frequency of supernumerary teeth in a dolichocephalic canine breed, the Greyhound. *American Journal of Veterinary Research* **59**(1):16–17.

35 Kannan SK, Suganya, Santharam H (2002). Supernumerary roots. *Indian Journal of Dental Research* **13**(2):116–19.

36 Koleoso DC, Shaba OP, Isiekwe MC (2004). Prevalence of intrinsic tooth discolouration among 11–16 year-old Nigerians. *Odonto-stomatologie tropicale* **27**(106):35–9.

37 Lindner DL, Marretta SM, Pijanowski GJ, Johnson AL, Smith CW (1995). Measurement of bite force in dogs: a pilot study. *Journal of Veterinary Dentistry* **12**(2):49–52.

38 de Lahunta A, Lobprise HB, Wiggs RB (1994). Microglossia in three littermate puppies. *Journal of Veterinary Dentistry* **11**(4):129–33.

39 Lobprise HB, Wiggs RB (1993). Anatomy, diagnosis and management of disorders of the tongue. *Journal of Veterinary Dentistry* **10**(1):16–23.

40 Madewell BR, Stannard AA, Pulley LT, Nelson VG (1980). Oral eosinophilic granuloma in Siberian husky dogs. *Journal of the American Veterinary Medical Association* **177**(8):701–3.

41 Ochs DL, Irving GW 3rd, Casey HW (1978). Eosinophilic granuloma in the cat: two cases involving the tongue. *Veterinary Medicine, Small Animal Clinician* **73**(10):1275–7.

42 Natori J, Shimizu K, Nagahama M, Tanaka S (1999). The influence of hypothyroidism on wound healing. An experimental study. *Journal of Nippon Medical School* = Nihon Ika Daigaku zasshi **66**(3):176–80.

43 Osman F, Franklyn JA, Holder RL, Sheppard MC, Gammage MD (2007). Cardiovascular manifestations of hyperthyroidism before and after antithyroid therapy: a matched case-control study. *Journal of the American College of Cardiology* **49**(1):71–81. Epub 2006 Dec 13.

44 Epstein M, Kuehn NF, Landsberg G, Lascelles DX, Marks SL, Schaedler JM, Tuzio H (2005). AAHA Senior care guidelines for dogs and cats. *Journal of the American Animal Hospital Association* **41**:81–91.

45 Anderson JG, Harvey CE (1993). Masticatory muscle myositis. *Journal of Veterinary Dentistry* **10**(1):6–8.

46 Jensen L, Setser C, Simone A, Smith M, Suelzer M (1994). Assessment of oral malodor in dogs. *Journal of Veterinary Dentistry* **11**(2):71–4.

47 Davot JL, Delille B, Hennet P (1995). Oral malodor in dogs: measurement using a sulfide monitor. *Journal of Veterinary Dentistry* **12**(3):101–3.

48 Floyd MR (1991). The modified Triadan system: nomenclature for veterinary dentistry. *Journal of Veterinary Dentistry* **8**(4):18–19.

49 Verstraete F (1999). *Self-Assessment Color Review of Veterinary Dentistry.* Iowa State University Press, Ames, p. 9.

50 Holmstrom SE, Frost P, Eisner ER (1992). *Veterinary Dental Techniques for the Small Animal Practitioner,* 2nd edn. WB Saunders, Philadelphia, pp. 246, 248.

51 Carranza, FA, Takei HH (2006). Radiographic aids in the diagnosis of periodontal disease. In: Carranza FA, Takei HH, Newman MG (eds). *Carranza's Clinical Periodontology,* 9th edn. WB Saunders, Philadelphia, pp. 456–7.

52 Ammons WF, Harrington GW (2006). Furcation: the problem and its management. In: Carranza FA, Takei HH, Newman MG (eds). *Carranza's Clinical Periodontology,* 9th edn. WB Saunders, Philadelphia, p. 827.

53 Koch WM, Bhatti N, Williams MF, Eisele DW (2001). Oncologic rationale for bilateral tonsillectomy in head and neck squamous cell carcinoma of unknown primary source. *Otolaryngology and Head and Neck Surgery* **124**(3):331–3.

54 Evans HE (1993). The digestive apparatus and abdomen. In: Evans HE (ed). *Miller's Anatomy of the Dog*, 3rd edn. WB Saunders, Philadelphia, pp. 388, 397.

55 Hennet PR, Harvey CE (1992). Craniofacial development and growth in the dog. *Journal of Veterinary Dentistry* **9**(2):11–18.

Further information
www.avdc.org
www.EVDC.org
www.vasg.org

Chapter 3

1 Niemiec BA, Sabitino D, Gilbert T (2004). Equipment and basic geometry of dental radiography. *Journal of Veterinary Dentistry* **21**(1):48–52.

2 Mulligan TW, Aller MS, Williams CA (1998). In: *Atlas of Canine and Feline Dental Radiology*. Veterinary Learning Systems, Trenton.

3 Holmstrom SE, Frost P, Eisner ER (1998). In: *Veterinary Dental Techniques*, 2nd edn. WB Saunders, Philadelphia.

4 Wiggs RB, Lobprise HB (1997). In: *Veterinary Dentistry: Principles and Practice.* Lippincott–Raven, Philadelphia.

5 Oakes A (2000). In: Deforge DH, Colmery BH (eds). *An Atlas of Veterinary Dental Radiology.* Iowa State University Press, Ames.

6 Niemiec BA, Sabitino D, Gilbert T (2004). Developing dental radiographs. *Journal of Veterinary Dentistry* **21**(2):116–21

7 Eisner ER (2000). In: Deforge DH, Colmery BH (eds). *An Atlas of Veterinary Dental Radiology.* Iowa State University Press, Ames.

8 Niemiec BA, Furman R (2004). Feline dental radiology. *Journal of Veterinary Dentistry* **21**(4):252–7.

9 Niemiec BA, Furman R (2004). Canine dental radiology. *Journal of Veterinary Dentistry* **21**(3):186–90.

10 Gracis M (1999). Radiographic study of the maxillary canine tooth of four mesaticephalic cats. *Journal of Veterinary Dentistry* **16**(3):115–128.

11 Gracis M, Harvey CE (1998). Radiographic study of the maxillary canine tooth in mesaticephalic dogs. *Journal of Veterinary Dentistry* **15**(2):73–8.

12 Niemiec BA (2005) Dental radiographic interpretation. *Journal of Veterinary Dentistry* **22**(1):53–9.

13 Verstraete FJ (1999). *Self-Assessment Color Review of Veterinary Dentistry.* Iowa State University Press, Ames.

14 DeBowes LJ, DeForge DH, Kesel L, Hawkins BJ (2000). In: Deforge DH, Colmery BH (eds). *An Atlas of Veterinary Dental Radiology.* Iowa State University Press, Ames.

15 Aller MS (2000). In: Deforge DH, Colmery BH (eds). *An Atlas of Veterinary Dental Radiology.* Iowa State University Press, Ames.

16 Glickman GN, Pileggi R (2002). In: Cohen S, Burns RC (eds). *Pathways of the Pulp*, 8th edn. Mosby, St. Louis.

17 Niemiec BA (2005). Fundamentals of endodontics. *Veterinary Clinics of North America, Small Animal Practice* **35**(4): 837–68.

18 Hennet PR, Bellows J (2000). In: Deforge DH, Colmery BH (eds). *An Atlas of Veterinary Dental Radiology.* Iowa State University Press, Ames.

19 Lyon KF, Visser CJ, Okuda A, Anthony JMG (2000). In: Deforge DH, Colmery BH (eds). *An Atlas of Veterinary Dental Radiology.* Iowa State University Press, Ames.

20 Trowbridge H, Kim S, Suda H (2002). In: Cohen S, Burns RC (eds). *Pathways of the Pulp*, 8th edn. Mosby, St. Louis.

21 Cohen AS, Brown DC (2002). In: Cohen S, Burns RC (eds). *Pathways of the Pulp,* 8th edn. Mosby, St. Louis.

22 Marretta SM, Anthony JMG (2000). In: Deforge DH, Colmery BH (eds). *An Atlas of Veterinary Dental Radiology.* Iowa State University Press, Ames.

23 Anthony JMG, Marretta SM, Okuda A (2000). In: Deforge DH, Colmery BH (eds). *An Atlas of Veterinary Dental Radiology.* Iowa State University Press, Ames.

24 Rosenberg P (2002). In: Cohen S, Burns RC (eds). *Pathways of the Pulp*, 8th edn. Mosby, St. Louis.

25 DuPont GA, DeBowes LJ (2002). Comparison of periodontitis and root replacement in cat teeth with resorbtive lesions. *Journal of Veterinary Dentistry* **19**(2):71–5.

26 Reiter AM, Mendoza KA (2002). Feline odontoclastic resorptive lesions. An unsolved enigma in veterinary dentistry. *Veterinary Clinics of North America, Small Animal Practice* **32**:791–837.

27 Dupont GA (2005). Radiographic evaluation and treatment of feline dental resorptive lesions. *Veterinary Clinics of North America, Small Animal Practice* **35**(4):943–62.

28 DuPont GA (2002). Crown amputation with intentional root retention for dental resorbtive lesions in cats. *Journal of Veterinary Dentistry* **19**(2):107–10.

29 Ogilvie GK, Moore AS (2006). *Managing the Canine Cancer Patient, a Practical Guide to Compassionate Care.* Veterinary Learning Systems, Yardley.

30 Anderson JG, Revenaugh AF (2000). In: Deforge DH, Colmery BH (eds). *An Atlas of Veterinary Dental Radiology.* Iowa State University Press, Ames.

Chapter 4

1 Hobson P (2005). Extraction of retained primary canine teeth in the dog. *Journal of Veterinary Dentistry* **22**(2):132–7.

2 Harvey CE, Emily PP (1993). In: *Small Animal Dentistry.* Mosby, St. Louis.

3 Wheeler RC (1974). *Dental Anatomy, Physiology, and Occlusion.* WB Saunders, Philadelphia, p. 24.

4 Wiggs RB, Lobprise HB (1997). *Veterinary Dentistry, Principles and Practice.* Lippincott–Raven, Philadelphia.

5 Hale FA (2005). Juvenile veterinary dentistry. *Veterinary Clinics of North America, Small Animal Practice* **35**:789–817.

6 Ulbricht RD, Marretta SM, Klippert LS (2003). Surgical extraction of a fractured, nonvital deciduous tooth in a tiger. *Journal of Veterinary Dentistry* **20**(4): 209–12.

7 Holmstrom SE, Frost P, Eisner ER (1998). In: *Veterinary Dental Techniques*, 2nd edn. WB Saunders, Philadelphia.

8 Cohen, AS, Brown DC (2002). Orofacial dental pain emergencies: endodontic diagnosis and management. In: Cohen AS and Burns RC (eds). *Pathways of the Pulp*, 8th edn. Mosby, St. Louis, pp. 31–76.

9 Golden AL, Stoller NS, Harvey CE (1982). A survey of oral and dental diseases in dogs anesthetized at a veterinary hospital. *Journal of the American Animal Hospital Association* **18**:891–9.

10 Neville BW, Damm DD, Allen CM, Bouquot JE (2002). In: *Oral & Maxillofacial Pathology*, 2nd edn. WB Saunders, Philadelphia.

11 Trope M, Chivian N, Sigurdsson A, Vann WF (2002). Traumatic injuries. In: Cohen S and RC Burns (eds). *Pathways of the Pulp*, 8th edn. Mosby, St. Louis, pp. 603–50.

12 Stockard CR, Johnson AL (1941). *Genetic and Endocrine basis for Differences in Form and Behavior.* Wistar Institute of Anatomy and Biology, Philadelphia, p. 149.

13 Shipp AD, Fahrenkrug P (1992). *Practitioner's Guide to Veterinary Dentistry.* Dr. Shipps Laboratories, Beverly Hills.

14 De Simoi A (2006). Complications of mandibular brachygnathism in a North African leopard. *Journal of Veterinary Dentistry* **23**(2):89–95.

15 Harris EF, Johnson MG (1991). Heritability of craniometric and occlusal variables: a longitudinal sib analysis. *American Journal of Orthodontics & Dentofacial Orthopedics* **99**:258–68.

16 Bellows J (2004). *Atlas of Canine Dentistry: Malocclusions and Breed Standards.* Waltham publication, Gaithersburg.

17 Brine EJ (1999). Endodontic disease of the mandibular first molar tooth secondary to caudal cross bite in a young Shetland sheepdog. *Journal of Veterinary Dentistry* **16**(1):15–18.

18 Angle EH (1900). Treatment of malocclusion of the teeth and fractures of the maxillae. *Angle's System*, 6th edn. S White Manufacturing Co, Philadelphia.

19 Profit WR (2000). In: *Contemporary Orthodontics.* Mosby, St. Louis.

20 Niemiec BA (1998). Unerupted, supernumary P1 causing lingual deviation of the lower left canine (304). *Veterinary Dental Forum Proceedings*, New Orleans.

21 Verhaert L (1999). A removable orthodontic device for the treatment of lingually displaced mandibular canine teeth in dogs. *Journal of Veterinary Dentistry* **16**(2):69–75.

22 Amimoto A, Iwamoto S, Taura Y, Nakama S, Yamanouchi T (1993). Effects of surgical orthodontic treatment for malalignment due to the prolonged retention of deciduous canines in young dogs. *Journal of Veterinary Medical Science* **55**(1):73–9.

23 Niemiec BA, Mulligan TM (2001). Assessment of vital pulp therapy for nine complicated crown fractures and fiftyfour crown reductions in dogs and cats. *Journal of Veterinary Dentistry* **18**(3):122–5.

24 Niemiec BA (2005). Fundamentals of endodontics. *Veterinary Clinics of North America, Small Animal Practice* **35**(4):837–68.

25 Litton SF, Ackerman LV, Isaacson RJ, Shapiro B (1970). A genetic study of class III malocclusion. *American Journal of Orthodontics* **58**:565–77.

26 Rossman LE, Garber DADA, Harvey CE (1985). Disorders of teeth. In: Harvey CE (ed). *Veterinary Dentistry.* WB Saunders, Philadelphia, p. 79.

27 Bhaskor SN (1961). *Synopsis of Oral Pathology.* Mosby, St Louis, p. 129.

28 Stapleton BL, Clarke LL (1999). Mandibular canine tooth impaction in a young dog. Treatment and subsequent eruption: a case report. *Journal of Veterinary Dentistry* 16(3):105–8.

29 Bryan RA, Cole BO, Welbury RR (2005). Retrospective analysis of factors influencing the eruption of delayed permanent incisors after supernumerary tooth removal. *European Journal of Pediatric Dentistry* 6(2):84–9.

30 Taney KG, Smith MM (2006). Surgical extraction of impacted teeth in a dog. *Journal of Veterinary Dentistry* 23(3):168–77.

31 Raghoebar GM, Boering G, Vissink A (1991). Clinical, radiographic, and histological characteristics of secondary retention of permanent molars. *Journal of Dentistry* 19:164–70.

32 Surgeon TW (2000). Surgical exposure and orthodontic extrusion of an impacted canine tooth in a cat: a case report. *Journal of Veterinary Dentistry* 17(2):81–5.

33 Niemiec BA (2006). Dentigerous cyst in a 10-year-old dog. *Veterinary Dental Forum Proceedings.*

34 Kramek BA, O'Brien TD, Smith FO (1996). Diagnosis and removal of a dentigerous cyst complicated by an ameloblastic fibro-odontoma in a dog. *Journal of Veterinary Dentistry* 13(1):9–11.

35 Anderson JG, Harvey CE (1993). Odontogenic cysts. *Journal of Veterinary Dentistry* 4:5–9.

36 Eikhoff M, Seeliger F, Simon D, Fehr M (2002). Erupted bilateral compound odontomas in a dog. *Journal of Veterinary Dentistry* 19(3):137–43.

37 Hale FA, Wilcock BP (1996). Compound odontoma in a dog. *Journal of Veterinary Dentistry* 13(3):93–5.

38 Regezi JA, Kerr DA, Courtney RM (1978). Odontogenic tumors: analysis of 706 cases. *Journal of Oral Surgery* 36(10):771–8.

39 Poulet FM, Valentine BA, Summers BA (1992). A survey of epithelial odontogenic tumors and cysts in dogs and cats. *Veterinary Pathology* 29(5):369–80.

40 Head KW, Else RW, Dubielzig RR (2002). Tumors of the alimentary tract. In: Mutin DJ (ed). *Tumors in Domestic Animals.* Iowa State Press, Ames, pp. 406–7.

41 Brody RS, Morris AL (1960). Odontoma associated with an undifferentiated carcinoma in the maxilla of a dog. *Journal of the American Veterinary Medical Association* 137:553–9.

42 Mani NJ (1974). Odontoma syndrome: report of an unusual case with multiple multiform odontomas of both jaws. *Journal of Dentistry* 2(4):149–52.

43 Al-Sahhar WF, Putrus ST (1985). Erupted odontoma. *Oral Surgery, Oral Medicine, & Oral Pathology* 59(2): 225–6.

44 Yuka K, Calka O, Kiroglu AF, Akdeniz N, Cankaya H (2004). Hairy tongue: a case report. *Acta Otorhinolaryngologica Belgica* 58(4): 161–3.

45 Heymann WR (2000). Psychotropic agent-induced black hairy tongue. *Cutis* 66(1):25–6.

46 Tamam L, Annagur BB (2006). Black hairy tongue associated with olanzapine treatment: a case report. *The Mount Sinai Journal of Medicine* 73(6):891–4.

47 Crossley DA (1995). Tooth enamel thickness in the mature dentition of domestic dogs and cats, preliminary study. *Journal of Veterinary Dentistry* 12(3):111–13.

48 Trowbridge HO, Syngcuk K, Hideaki S (2002). Structure and functions of the dentin–pulp complex In: Cohen S and Burns RC (eds). *Pathways of the Pulp*, 8th edn. Mosby, St. Louis, pp 411–56.

49 Trowbridge HO (1985). Intradental sensory units: physiological and clinical aspects. *Journal of Endodontics* 11:489–98.

50 Nair R (2002). Pathobiology of the periapex. In: Cohen A and Burns RC (eds). *Pathways of the Pulp*, 8th edn. Mosby, St. Louis, pp. 457–500.

51 Stanley HR, White CL, McCray L (1966). The rate of tertiary (reparative) dentin formation in the human tooth. *Oral Surgery* 21:180–9.

52 Harvey RG, McKeever PJ (1998). Nodular dermatoses. In: *A Colour Handbook of Skin Diseases of the Dog and Cat.* Manson Publishing, London, pp. 57–80.

53 Gross TL, Ihrke PJ, Walden EJ (1992). Epidermal Tumors. In: *Veterinary Dermatopathology.* Mosby Year Book, pp. 334–6.

54 Scott DW, Miller WM, Griffin CE (1995). Neoplastic and non-neoplastic tumors. In: *Small Animal Dermatology.* WB Saunders, Philadelphia, pp. 994–7.

55 Watrach AM, Small E, Case MY (1970). Canine papillomas: progression of oral papilloma to carcinoma. *Journal of the National Cancer Institute* 45:915–20.

56 Bregman CL, Hirth RS, Sundburg JP, Christensen EF (1987). Cutaneous neoplasms in dogs associated with canine oral papillomavirus vaccine. *Veterinary Pathology* **24**:477–87.

Chapter 5

1 Ozcelik B, Kuraner T, Kendir B, Asan E (2000). Histopathological evaluation of the dental pulps in crown-fractured teeth. *Journal of Endodontics* **26**(3):271–3.

2 Baysan A, Lynch E (2003). Treatment of cervical sensitivity with a root sealant. *American Journal of Dentistry* **16**(2):135–8.

3 Ricucci D, Pascon EA, Ford TR, Langeland K (2006). Epithelium and bacteria in periapical lesions. *Oral Surgery, Oral Medicine, Oral Pathology, Oral Radiology, & Endodontics* **101**(2):241–51.

4 Verstraete FJM (2003). Oral pathology. In: Slatter D (ed). *Textbook of Small Animal Surgery*, 3rd edn. WB Saunders. Volume 2, pp. 2638–51.

5 Hale FA (1998). Dental caries in the dog. *Journal of Veterinary Dentistry* **15**(2):79–83.

6 Marsh PD (1999). Microbiologic aspects of dental plaque and dental caries. *Dental Clinics of North America Cariology* **43**(4):599–614.

7 Zero DT (1999). Dental caries process. *Dental Clinics of North America Cariology* **43**(4):635–61.

8 Wiggs RB, Lobprise HB (1997). *Veterinary Dentistry, Principles and Practice.* Lippincott–Raven.

9 DuPont GA, DeBowes LJ (2002). Comparison of periodontitis and root replacement in cats with resorptive lesions. *Journal of Veterinary Dentistry* **19**(2):71–5.

10 Burke FJ, Johnston N, Wiggs RB, Hall AF (2000). An alternative hypothesis from veterinary science for the pathogenesis of noncarious cervical lesions. *Quintessence International* **31**(7):475–82.

11 Gorrel C, Larsson A (2002). Feline odontoclastic resorptive lesions: unveiling the early lesion. *Journal of Small Animal Practice* **43**(11):482–8.

12 Reiter AM, Lewis JR, Okuda A (2005). Update on the etiology of tooth resorption in domestic cats. *Veterinary Clinics of North America, Small Animal Practice* **35**(4):913–42.

13 Trope M, Chivian N, Sigurdsson A, Vann WF (2002). Traumatic injuries. In: Cohen S and Burns RC (eds). *Pathways of the Pulp*, 8th edn. Mosby, St. Louis, pp. 103–44.

14 DuPont G (1995). Crown amputation with intentional root retention for advanced feline resorptive lesions: a clinical study. *Journal of Veterinary Dentistry* **12**:9–13.

15 Lommer MJ, Verstraete FJ (2000). Prevalence of odontoclastic resorption lesions and periapical radiographic lucencies in cats: 265 cases (1995–1998). *Journal of the American Veterinary Medical Association* **217**(12):1866–9.

16 Neville BW, Damm DD, Allen CM, Bouquot JE (2002). Abnormalities of teeth. In: *Oral and Maxillofacial Pathology*, 2nd edn. WB Saunders, Philadelphia, pp. 49–106.

17 Neville BW, Damm DD, White DK, Waldron CA (1991). *Color Atlas of Clinical Oral Pathology.* Lea and Febiger, Philadelphia, pp. 60–4.

18 Regezi JA, Sciubba J (1993). *Oral Pathology Clinical-Pathological Correlations*, 2nd edn. WB Saunders, Philadelphia, p. 508.

19 Trowbridge HO (1985). Intradental sensory units: physiological and clinical aspects. *Journal of Endodontics* **11**:489–98.

20 Litonjua LA, Andreana S, Cohen RF (2005). Toothbrush abrasions and noncarious cervical lesions: evolving concepts. *Compendium of Continuing Education in Dentistry* **26**(11):767–8.

21 Casanova-Rosado JF, Medina-Solis CE, Vellejos-Sanchez AA, Casanova-Rosado AJ, Avila-Burgos L (2005). Dental attrition and associated factors in adolescents 14 to 19 years: a pilot study. *International Journal of Prosthodontics* **18**(6):516–19.

22 Bakland LK (1992). Root resorption. *Dental Clinics of North America* **36**:491–507.

23 Trope M (1998). Root resorption of dental origin: classification based on etiology. *Practical Periodontology and Aesthetic Dentistry* **10**:515–22.

24 Trope M, Chivian N (2002). Root resorption. In: Cohen S, Burns RC (eds). *Pathways of the Pulp*, 8th edn. Mosby, St. Louis, pp. 603–50.

25 Tredwin CJ, Scully C, Bagan-Sebastian JV (2005). Drug-induced disorders of teeth. *Journal of Dental Research* **84**(7):596–602.

26 Hale FA (2001). Localized intrinsic staining of teeth due to pulpitis and pulp necrosis in dogs. *Journal of Veterinary Dentistry* **18**(1):14–20.

27 Wang HL, Glickman GN (2002). Endodontic and periodontic interrelationships. In: Cohen S, Burns RC (eds). *Pathways of the Pulp*, 8th edn. Mosby, St. Louis, pp. 651–64.

28 Coyle M, Toner M, Barry H (2006). Multiple teeth showing invasive cervical resorption – an entity with little known histological features. *Journal of Oral Pathology and Medicine* **35**(1):55–7.

29 Liang H, Burkes EJ, Frederiksen NL (2003). Multiple idiopathic cervical root resorption: systematic review and report of four cases. *Dento-Maxillo Facial Radiology* **32**(3):150–5.

Chapter 6

1 Quirynen M, Teughels W, Kinder Haake S, Newman MG (2006). Microbiology of periodontal diseases. In: *Carranza's Clinical Periodontology*. WB Saunders, St. Louis, pp. 134–69.

2 Nisengard RJ, Kinder Haake S, Newman MG, Miyasaki KT (2006). Microbial interactions with the host in periodontal diseases. In: *Carranza's Clinical Periodontology*. WB Saunders, St. Louis, pp. 228–50.

3 Merin RL (2006). Results of periodontal treatment. In: *Carranza's Clinical Periodontology*. WB Saunders, St. Louis, pp. 1206–14.

4 Wiggs RB, Lobprise HB (1997). Oral exam and diagnosis. In: *Veterinary Dentistry, Principles and Practice*. Lippincott–Raven, Philadelphia.

5 Holmstrom SE, Frost Fritch P, Eisner ER (2004). *Veterinary Dental Techniques for the Small Animal Practitioner*. WB Saunders, Philadelphia, pp. 188–91.

6 Lea SC, Landini G, Walmsley AD (2006). The effect of wear on ultrasonic scaler tip displacement amplitude. *Journal of Clinical Periodontology* 33(1):37–41.

7 Arabaci T, Çiçek Y, Canakçi CF (2007). Sonic and ultrasonic scalers in periodontal treatment: a review. *International Journal of Dental Hygiene* 5(1):2–12.

8 Kozlovsky A, Artzi Z, Nemcovsky CE, et al. (2005). Effect of air-polishing devices on the gingiva: a histologic study in the canine. *Journal of Clinical Periodontology* 32:329–34.

9 Gengler WR, Kunkle BN, Romano D, et al. (2005). Evaluation of a barrier dental sealant in dogs. *Journal of Veterinary Dentistry* 22(3):157–9.

10 Hardham J, Dreier K, Wong J, Sfintescu C (2005). Pigmented-anaerobic bacteria associated with canine periodontitis. *Veterinary Microbiology* 106(1-2):119–28.

11 Gustafsson A, Ito H, Asman B, et al. (2006). Hyper-reactive mononuclear cells and neutrophils in chronic periodontitis. *Journal of Clinical Periodontology* 33:126–9.

12 Barendregt DS, Van der Velden U, Timmerman MF, et al. (2006). Comparison of two automated periodontal probes and two probes with a conventional readout in periodontal maintenance patients. *Journal of Clinical Periodontology* 33:276–82.

13 Pattison AM, Pattison GL (2006). Scaling and root planing. In: *Carranza's Clinical Periodontology*. WB Saunders, St. Louis, pp. 749–97.

14 Zetner K, Rothmueller G (2002). Treatment of periodontal pockets with doxycycline in Beagles. *Veterinary Therapeutics* 3(4):441–52.

15 Ryan ME (2005). Nonsurgical approaches for the treatment of periodontal disease. *Dental Clinics of North America* 49:611–36.

16 Carranza FA, Takei HH (2006). Phase II periodontal therapy. In: *Carranza's Clinical Periodontology*. WB Saunders, St. Louis, pp. 881–6.

17 Perry DA, Schmid MO, Takei HH (2006). Phase I periodontal therapy. In: *Carranza's Clinical Periodontology*. WB Saunders, St. Louis, pp. 722–7.

18 Caffesse RG, Sweeney PL, Smith BA (1986). Scaling and root planing with and without periodontal flap surgery. *Journal of Clinical Periodontology* 13(3):205–10.

19 DeBowes LJ (2005). Simple and surgical exodontia. *Veterinary Clinics of Small Animals* 35:963–84.

20 Haffajee AD (2006). Systemic antibiotics: to use or not to use in the treatment of periodontal infections. That is the question. *Journal of Clinical Periodontology* 33:359–61.

21 Hardham J, Reed M, Wong J, et al. (2005). Evaluation of a monovalent companion animal periodontal disease vaccine in an experimental mouse periodontitis model. *Vaccine* 23(24):3148–56.

22 Persson GR (2005). Immune responses and vaccination against periodontal infections. *Journal of Clinical Periodontology* 32;Suppl 6:54–6.

23 Lafzi A, Farahani RM, Shoja MA (2007). Phenobarbitol-induced gingival hyperplasia. *Journal of Contemporary Dental Practice* 8(6):50–6.

24 Eggerath J, English H, Leichter JW (2005). Drug-associated gingival enlargement: case report and review of aetiology, management and evidence-based outcomes of treatment. *Journal of New Zealand Society of Periodontology* 88:7–14.

25 Lewis JR, Reiter AM (2005). Management of generalized gingival enlargement in a dog: case report and literature review. *Journal of Veterinary Dentistry* 23:160–9.

26 Yanai YK, Iwasaki T, Sakai H, et al. (1999). Clinicopathological study of canine oral epulides. *Journal of Veterinary Medical Science* 61(8):897–902.

27 Verstraete Frank JM (2003). Oral pathological. In: Slatter D (ed). *Textbook of Small Animal Surgery*, pp. 2648–49.

28 McEntee MC, Page RL, Theon A, *et al.* (2004). Malignant tumor formation in dogs previously irradiated for acanthomatous epulis. *Veterinary Radiology & Ultrasound* **45**(4):357–61.

29 Zwemer TJ (1993). In: *Boucher's Clinical Dental Terminology:* a glossary of accepted terms in disciples of dentistry. Mosby, Philadelphia, p. 116.

30 Lyon KF (2005). Gingivostomatitis. In: *Veterinary Clinics of North America, Small Animal Practice* **35**(4):891–911.

31 Lommer MJ, Verstraete FJM (2003). Concurrent oral shedding of feline calicivirus and feline herpesvirus 1 in cats with chronic gingivostomatitis. *Oral Microbiology & Immunology* **18**:131–4.

32 Hardy WD, Zuckerman E, Corbishley J (2002). Serological evidence that *Bartonella* cause gingivitis and stomatitis in cats. In: *Proceedings of the 16th Annual Veterinary Dental Forum,* pp. 79–82.

33 Harley R, Gruffydd-Jones TJ, Day MJ (1998). Determination of salivary and serum immunoglobulin concentrations in the cat. *Veterinary Immunology & Immunopathology* **65**:99–112.

34 Hennet P (1997). Chronic gingiva-stomatitis in cats: long-term follow-up on 30 cases treated by dental extractions. *Journal of Veterinary Dentistry* **14**(1):15–21.

35 Plumb DC (2005). *Plumb's Veterinary Drug Handbook,* 5th edn. Blackwell Professional Publishing, Ames.

36 Sato R, Inanami O, Tanaka Y, Takase M, Naito Y (1996). Oral administration of bovine lactoferrin for treatment of intractable stomatitis in feline immunodeficiency virus (FIV)-positive and FIV-negative cats. *American Journal of Veterinary Research* **57**(10):1443–6.

37 Southerden P, Gorrel C (2007). Treatment of a case of refractory feline chronic gingivostomatitis with feline recombinant interferon omega. *Journal of Small Animal Practice* **48**(2):104–6.

Chapter 7

1 Wiggs RB, Lobprise HB (1997). In: *Veterinary Dentistry, Principles and Practice.* Lippincott–Raven, Philadelphia.

2 Verstraete FJ (1999). *Self-Assessment Colour Review of Veterinary Dentistry.* Manson Publishing, London, p. 78.

3 Smith MM (2000). Oronasal fistula repair. *Clinical Techniques, Small Animal Practice* **15**(4):243–50.

4 De Simoi A (2006). Complications of mandibular brachygnathism in a North African leopard. *Journal of Veterinary Dentistry* **23**(2):89–95.

5 Hale FA (2005). Juvenile veterinary dentistry. *Veterinary Clinics of North America, Small Animal Practice.* **35**(4):789–817.

6 Woodward TM (2006). Greater palatine island axial pattern flap for repair of oronasal fistula related to eosinophilic granuloma. *Journal of Veterinary Dentistry* **23**(3):161–6.

7 Dib GC, Tangerina RP, Abreu CE, Santos Rde P, Gregorio LC (2005). Rhinolithiasis as cause of oronasal fistula. *Revista Brasileira de Otorrinolaringologia* **71**(1):101–3.

8 Marretta SM (2001). Palatal surgery. *Atlantic Coast Veterinary Conference Proceedings.*

9 Marretta SM, Smith MM (2005). Single mucoperiosteal flap for oronasal fistula repair. *Journal of Veterinary Dentistry* **22** (3):200–5.

10 Holmstrom SE, Frost P, Eisner ER (1998). Exodontics. In: *Veterinary Dental Techniques,* 2nd edn. WB Saunders, Philadelphia, pp. 215–54.

11 Harvey CE, Emily PP (1993). In: *Small Animal Dentistry.* Mosby, St. Louis.

12 Hennet P (2001). Oronasal fistula and palatal repair. *Proceedings of the World Small Animal Veterinary Association.*

13 Marretta SM, Grove TK, Grillo TK (1991). Split palatal U-flap: a new technique for repair of caudal hard palate defects. *Journal of Veterinary Dentistry* **8**(1):5–8.

14 De Souza HJ, Amorim FV, Corgozinho KB, Tavares RR (2005). Management of the traumatic oronasal fistula in the cat with a conical silastic prosthetic device. *Journal of Feline Medicine and Surgery* **7**(2):129–33.

15 Robertson JJ, Dean PW (1987). Repair of a traumatically induced oronasal fistula in a cat with a rostral tongue flap. *Veterinary Surgery* **16**(2):164–6.

16 Bredal WP, Gunnes G, Vollset I, Ulstein TL (1996). Oral eosinophilic granuloma in three Cavalier King Charles spaniels. *Journal of Small Animal Practice* **37**:499–504.

17 Madewell BR, Stannard AA, Pully LT, Nelson VG (1980). Oral eosinophilic granuloma in Siberian Husky dogs. *Journal of the American Veterinary Medical Association* **177**:701–3.

18 Leiferman KM (1991). A current perspective on the role of eosinophils in dermatologic diseases. *Journal of the American Academy of Dermatology* **24**:1101–12.

19 Harvey RG, McKeever PJ (1998). Ulcerative dermatoses. In: *A Colour Handbook of Skin Diseases of the Dog and Cat.* Manson Publishing, London, pp. 81–106.

20 Wilkenson GT, Bate MJ (1984). A possible further manifestation of feline eosinophilic granuloma complex. *Journal of the American Animal Hospital Association* 20:519–26.

21 Hirshberg A, Amariglio N, Akrish S, *et al.* (2006). Traumatic ulcerative granuloma with stromal eosinophilia: a reactive lesion of the oral mucosa. *American Journal of Clinical Pathology* 126(4):522–9.

22 Garcia M, Pagerois X, Curco N, Tarroch X, Vives P (2002). Eosinophilic ulcer of the oral mucosa: 11 cases. *Annales de Dermatologie et de Vénéréologie* 129(6–7):871–3.

23 Leistra WH, van Oost BA, Willemse T (2005). Nonpruritic granuloma in Norwegian forest cats. *Veterinary Record* 156(18):575–7.

24 Frost P, Williams CA (1986). Feline dental disease. *Veterinary Clinics of North America, Small Animal Practice* 16:851.

25 Manfra-Marreta S, Matheissen D, Matus R, Patniak A (1990). Surgical management of oral neoplasia. In: Bojrab MJ, Tholen M (eds). S*mall Animal Oral Medicine and Surgery.* Lea & Febiger, Philadelphia, p. 108.

26 Silvestros SS, Mamalis AA, Sklavounou AD, Tzerbos FX, Rontogianni DD (2006). Eosinophilic granuloma masquerading as aggressive periodontitis. *Journal of Periodontology* 77(5):917–21.

27 Holzhauer AM, Abdelsayed RA, Sutley SH (1999). Eosinophilic granuloma: a case report with pathological fracture. *Oral Surgery, Oral Medicine, Oral Pathololology, Oral Radiology, Endodontics* 87(6):756–9.

28 Mezei MM, Tron VA, Stewart WD, Rivers JK (1995). Eosinophilic ulcer of the oral mucosa. *Journal of the American Academy of Dermatology* 33(5):734–40.

29 Withrow ST, Norris AM, Dubielzig RR (1985). Oropharyngeal neoplasms. In: Harvey CE (ed). *Veterinary Dentistry.* WB Saunders, Philadelphia, p. 123.

30 Reedy LM (1982). Results of allergy testing and hyposensitization in selected feline skin diseases. *Journal of the American Animal Hospital Association* 18:618–23.

31 Rosencrantz WS (1993). Feline eosinophilic granuloma complex. In: Griffin CE, Kwochka KW, MacDonald JM (eds). *Current Veterinary Dermatology.* Mosby Year Book, St. Louis, pp. 319–24.

32 Gruffydd-Jones TJ, Evan RJ, Gaskel CJ (1983). The alimentary system. In: Pratt PW (ed). *Feline Medicine.* American Veterinary Publishers, Santa Barbara, p. 201.

33 MacEwan EG, Hess PW (1987). Evaluation of effect of immunomodulation of the feline eosinophilic granuloma complex. *Journal of the American Animal Hospital Association* 23:519–26.

34 Olivry T, Rivierre C, Jackson HA, Murphy KM, Davidson G, Sousa CA (2002). Cyclosporine decreases skin lesions and pruritis in dogs with atopic dermatitis: a blinded randomized prednisolone-controlled trial. *Veterinary Dermatology* 13(2):77–87.

35 Steffan J, Favrot C, Mueller R (2006). A systematic review and meta-analysis of the efficacy and safety of cyclosporine for the treatment of atopic dermatitis in dogs. *Veterinary Dermatology* 17(1):3–16.

36 Steffan J, Parks C, Seewald W, *et al.* (2005). Clinical trial evaluating the efficacy and safety of cyclosporine in dogs with atopic dermatitis. *Journal of the American Veterinary Medical Association* 226(11):1855–63.

37 Noli C, Scarampella F (2006). Prospective open pilot study on the use of cyclosporine for feline allergic skin disease. *Journal of Small Animal Practice* 47(8):434–8.

38 Vercelli A, Raviri G, Cornegliani L (2006). The use of cyclosporine to treat feline dermatosis: a retrospective analysis of 23 cases. *Veterinary Dermatology* 17(3):201–6.

39 Last RD, Suzuki Y, Manning T, Lindsay D, Galipeau L, Whitbred TJ (2004). A case of fatal systemic toxoplasmosis in a cat being treated with cyclosporine A for feline atopy. *Veterinary Dermatology* 15(3):194–8.

40 O'Neill T, Edwards GA, Holloway SA (2001). Clinical use of cyclosporine A and ketoconazole in the treatment of perianal fistula. *Proceedings of the WSAVA World Congress.*

41 Zain R, Abdul Hamid J, Awang MN (1986). Traumatic granuloma/eosinophilic ulcer. *Annals of the Academy of Medicine,* Singapore 15(3):451–3.

42 Carmichael DT (2004). Diagnosing and treating chronic ulcerative paradental stomatitis. *Veterinary Medicine* 99(12):1008–11.

43 Smith MM (1995). Oral and salivary gland disorders. In: Ettinger SJ, Feldman EC (eds). *Textbook of Veterinary Internal Medicine,* 4th edn. WB Saunders, Philadelphia, pp. 1084–97.

44 Scott DW, Miller Jr WH, Griffin CE (2001). Immune-mediated disorders. In: *Muller and Kirk's Small Animal Dermatology*, 6th edn. WB Saunders, Philadelphia, pp. 667–799.

45 Noli C, Koeman JP, Willemse T (1995). A retrospective evaluation of adverse reactions to trimethoprim-sulphonamide combinations in dogs and cats. *Veterinary Quarterly* 17(4):123–8.

46 Ndiritu CG, Enos LR (1977). Adverse reactions to drugs in a veterinary hospital. *Journal of the American Veterinary Medical Association* 171(4):335–9.

47 Frank AA, Ross JL, Sawvell BK (1992). Toxic epidermal necrolysis associated with flea dips. *Veterinary and Human Toxicology* 34(1): 57–61.

48 Lee JA, Budjin JB, Mauldin EA (2002). Acute necrotizing dermatitis and septicemia after application of a d-limonene-based insecticidal shampoo in a cat. *Journal of the American Veterinary Medical Association* 221(2):258–62, 239–40.

49 Rosenbaum MR, Kerlin KL (1995). Erythema multiforme major and disseminated intravascular coagulation in a dog following application of a d-limonene-based insecticidal dip. *Journal of the American Veterinary Medical Association* 207(10):1315–19.

50 Elmore SA, Basseches J, Anhalt GJ, Cullen JM, Olivry T (2005). Paraneoplastic pemphigus in a dog with splenic sarcoma. *Veterinary Pathology* 42(1):88–91.

51 de Bruin A, Muller E, Wyder M, *et al.* (1999). Periplakin and envoplakin are target antigens in canine and human paraneoplastic pemphigus. *Journal of the American Academy of Dermatology* 40(5 Pt 1):682–5.

52 Neville BW, Damm DD, Allen CM, Bouquot JE (2002). In: *Oral and Maxillofacial Pathology*, 2nd edn. WB Saunders, Philadelphia.

53 McVey DS, Shuman W (1991). Use of multiple antigen substrates to detect antinuclear antibody in canine sera. *Veterinary Immunology and Immunopathology* 28(1):37–43.

54 Scott DW (1987). Pemphigoid in domestic animals. *Clinical Dermatology* 5:155–8.

55 Mueller RS, Krebs I, Power HT, Fieseler KV (2006). Pemphigus foliaceus in 91 dogs. *Journal of the American Animal Hospital Association* 42(3):189–96.

56 Olivry T, Rivierre C, Murphy KM (2003). Efficacy of cyclosporine for treatment induction of canine pemphigus foliaceus. *Veterinary Record* 152(2):53–4.

57 Khachemoune A, Guldbakke KK, Ehrsam E (2006). Pemphigus foliaceus: a case report and short review. *Cutis* 78(2):105–10.

58 Ahmed AR (2006). Use of intravenous immunoglobulin therapy in autoimmune blistering diseases *International Immunopharmacology* 6(4):557–78.

59 Daoud YJ, Kamin KG (2006). Comparison of cost of immune globulin intravenous therapy to conventional immunosuppressive therapy in treating patients with autoimmune mucocutaneous blistering diseases. *International Immunopharmacology* 6(4):600–6.

60 Rosencrantz WS (2004). Pemphigus: current therapy. *Veterinary Dermatology* 15(2):90–8.

61 Yeung AK, Goldman RD (2005). Use of steroids for erythema multiforme in children. *Canadian Family Physician* 51:1481–3.

62 Laguna C, Martin B, Torrijos A, Garcia-Melgares ML, Ferber I (2006). Stevens–Johnson syndrome and toxic epidermal necrolysis. *Actas Dermo-Sifiliográficas* 97(3):177–85.

63 Trotman TK, Phillips H, Fordyce H, King LG, Morris DO, Giger U (2006). Treatment of severe adverse cutaneous drug reactions with human intravenous immunoglobulin in two dogs. *Journal of the American Animal Hospital Association* 42(4):312–20.

64 French LE (2006). Toxic epidermal necrolysis and Stevens–Johnson syndrome: our current understanding. *Allergology International* 55(1):9–16.

65 Khalili B, Bahna SI (2006). Pathogenesis and recent therapeutic trends in Stevens–Johnson syndrome and toxic epidermal necrolysis. *Annals of Allergy, Asthma & Immunology* 97(3):272–80.

66 DiBartola SP (2000). Clinical approach and laboratory evaluation of renal disease. In: Ettinger SJ, Feldman EC (eds). *Textbook of Veterinary Internal Medicine*, 4th edn. WB Saunders, Philadelphia, pp. 1706–7.

67 Leão JC, Gueiros LA, Leite Av Jr., *et al.* (2005). Uremic stomatitis in chronic renal failure. *Clinics* 60(3):259–62.

68 Beaney GP (1964). Otolaryngeal problems arising during the management of severe renal failure. *Journal of Laryngology and Otology* 78:507–15.

69 Fischer J (2007). UCDVMC-SD Renal Dialysis Unit, San Diego, *personal communication*.

70 Jaspers MT (1975). Unusual oral lesions in a uremic patient. Review of the literature and report of a case. *Oral Surgery, Oral Medicine, Oral Pathology* 39:934–44.

71 Antoniades DZ, Markopoulos AK, Andreadis D, Balaskas I, Patrikalou E, Grekas D (2006). Ulcerative uremic stomatitis associated with untreated chronic renal failure: report of a case and review of the literature. *Oral Surgery, Oral Medicine, Oral Pathology, Oral Radiology, Endodontics* **101**(5):608–13.

72 Greene CE, Chandler FW (1998). Candidiasis, torulopsosis, and rhodotorulosis. In: Greene CE (ed). *Infections Diseases of the Dog and Cat.* WB Saunders, Philadelphia, pp. 414–17.

73 Taboada J (2000). Systemic mycoses. In: Ettinger SJ, Feldman EC (eds). *Textbook of Veterinary Internal Medicine*, 5th edn. WB Saunders, Philadelphia, p. 475.

74 Kumar BV, Padshetty MS, Bai KY, Rao MS (2005). Prevalence of *Candida* in the oral cavity of diabetic subjects. *Journal of the Association of Physicians of India* **53**:599–602.

75 Belazi M, Velegraki A, Fleva A, *et al.* (2005). Candidal overgrowth in diabetic patients: potential predisposing factors. *Mycoses* **48**(3):192–6.

76 Tapper-Jones LM, Aldred MJ, Walker DM, Hayes TM (1981). *Candidal* infections and populations of *Candida albicans* in mouths of diabetics. *Journal of Clinical Pathology* **34**(7):706–11.

77 Patton LL, Phelan JA, Ramos-Gomez FJ, Nittayananta W, Shiboski CH, Mbuguye TL (2002). Prevalence and classification of HIV-associated oral lesions. *Oral Disease* **8**:98–109.

78 Worthington HV, Eden OB, Clarkson JE (2004). Interventions for preventing oral candidiasis for patients with cancer receiving treatment. *Cochrane Database of Systematic Reviews* (Online) **18**(4):CD003807.

79 De la Rosa GR, Champlin RE, Kontoyiannis DP (2002). Risk factors for the development of invasive fungal infections in allogenic blood and bone marrow transplant recipients. *Transplant Infectious Disease* **4**(1):3–9.

80 MacDonald JM (2000). Glucocorticoid therapy. In: Ettinger SJ, Feldman EC (eds). *Textbook of Veterinary Internal Medicine*, 5th edn. WB Saunders, Philadelphia, pp. 307–17.

81 Noro R, Saito T, Suzuki J, *et al.* (2002). A case of secondary pulmonary *Cryptococcus* showing various radiographic changes during its natural course without antifungal treatment. *Nihon Kokyúki Gakkai Zasshi* **40**(6):489–93.

82 Dickerman RD, Stevens QE, Schneider SJ (2004). Sudden death secondary to fulminate intracranial aspergillosis in a healthy teenager after posterior fossa surgery: the role of corticosteroids and prophylactic recommendations. *Journal of Neurosurgical Sciences* **48**(2):87–9.

83 Fukushima C, Matsuse H, Tomari S, *et al.* (2003). Oral candidiasis associated with inhaled corticosteroid use: a comparison of fluticasone and beclomethasone. *Annals of Allergy, Asthma & Immunology* **90**(6):646–51.

84 Fukushima C, Matsuse H, Saeki S, *et al.* (2003). Salivary IgA and oral candidiasis in asthmatic patients treated with inhaled corticosteroid. *Asthma* **42**(7):601–4.

85 Lador N, Polacheck I, Gural A, Sanatski E, Garfunkel A (2006). A trifungal infection of the mandible: case report and literature review. *Oral Surgery, Oral Medicine, Oral Pathology, Oral Radiology, Endodontics* **101**(4):451–6.

86 Lai WH, Lu SY, Eng HL (2002). Levamisole aids in treatment of refractory oral candidiasis in two patients with thymoma associated with myasthenia gravis: report of two cases. *Chang Gung Medical Journal* **25**(9):606–11.

87 Hayshi M, Abe C, Nozawa RT, Yokota T, Iso T, Shiokawa Y (1986). Effects of immunomodulators on candidacidal activity of normal peritoneal cells in BALB/c mice. *International Journal of Immunopharmacology* **8**(3):299–304.

88 Barasch A, Safford MM, Dapkute-Marcus I, Fine DH (2004). Efficacy of chlorhexidine gluconate rinse for treatment and prevention of oral candidiasis in HIV-infected children: a pilot study. *Oral Surgery, Oral Medicine, Oral Pathology, Oral Radiology, Endodontics* **97**(2):204–7.

89 Elad S, Wexler A, Garfunkel AA, Shapira MY, Bitan M, Or R (2006). Oral candidiasis prevention in transplantation patients: a comparative study. *Clinical Transplantation* **20**(3):318–24.

90 Donnelly RF, McCarron PA, Tunney MM, David Woolfson A (2006). Potential of photodynamic therapy in treatment of fungal infections of the mouth. Design and characterization of a mucoadhesive patch containing toluidine blue O. *Journal of Photochemistry and Photobiology.* B, Biology: **8**.

91 Kuipers ME, Heegsma J, Bakker HI, *et al.* (2002). Design and fungicidal activity of mucoadhesive lactoferrin tablets for the treatment of oropharyngeal candidosis. *Drug Delivery* **9**(1):31–8.

92 Samaranyayke YH, Samaranyayke LP, Pow EH, Beena VT, Yeung KW (2001). Antifungal effects of lysozyme and lactoferrin against genetically similar, sequential *Candida albicans* isolates from a human immunodeficiency virus-infected southern Chinese

cohort. *Journal of Clinical Microbiology*
39(9):3296–302.

93 Plunkett SJ (1993). Toxicologic emergencies. In:
*Emergency Procedures for the Small Animal
Veterinarian*. WB Saunders, Philadelphia,
pp. 142–3.

94 Gieger TL, Correa SS, Taboada J, Grooters AM,
Johnson AJ (2000). Phenol poisoning in three
dogs. *Journal of the American Animal Hospital
Association* 36(4):317–21.

95 Martins WD, Westphalen FH, Westphalen VP
(2003). Microstomia caused by swallowing of
caustic soda: a report of a case. *Journal of
Contemporary Dental Practice* 4(4):91–9.

96 Hashem FK, Al Khayal Z (2003). Oral burn
contractures in children. *Annals of Plastic Surgery*
51(5):468–71.

97 Kruger FC (2004). Caustic injury to the upper GI
tract. *Journal of the South African Dental
Association* 59(8):335.

98 Wingfield WE (1997). *Veterinary Emergency
Medicine Secrets*. Hanley and Belfus, Philadelphia,
p. 307.

99 Howell JM (1986). Alkaline injections. *Annals of
Emergency Medicine* 15(7):820–5.

100 Friedman EM, Lovejoy FH Jr. (1984). The
emergency management of caustic ingestions.
Emergency Medicine Clinics North America
2(1):77–86.

101 Boukthir S, Fetni I, Mrad SM, Mongalgi MA,
Debbabi A, Barsaoui S (2004). High doses of
steroids in the management of caustic esophageal
burns in children. *Archives de Pédiatrie*
11(1):13–7.

Chapter 8

1 Melmed C, Shelton GD, Bergman R, *et al.*
(2004). Masticatory muscle myositis:
pathogenesis, diagnosis, and treatment.
Compendium on Continuing Education August:
590–604.

2 Harvey CE, Emily PP (1993). In: *Small Animal
Dentistry*. Mosby Year book, St. Louis.

3 Blot S (2005). Inflammatory myopathies. In:
Ettinger SJ, Feldman EC (eds). *Textbook of
Veterinary Internal Medicine*, 6th edn. Elsevier, St.
Louis, pp. 903–4.

4 Orvis JS, Cardinet GH III (1981). Canine muscle
fiber types and susceptibility of masticatory
muscles to myositis. *Muscle Nerve* 4:354–9.

5 Shelton GD, Bandman E, Cardinet GH III
(1985). Electrophoretic comparison of myosins
from masticatory muscles and selected limb
muscles in the dog. *American Journal of
Veterinary Research* 46:493–8.

6 Shelton GD, Cardinet GH III, Bandman E
(1988). Expression of fiber specific proteins during
ontogeny of canine temporalis muscle. *Muscle
Nerve* 11:124–32.

7 Shelton GD (1987). Pathophysiologic basis of
canine muscle disorders. *Journal of Veterinary
Internal Medicine* 1:36–44.

8 Evans J, Levesque D, Shelton GD (2004). Canine
inflammatory myopathies: a clinicopathologic
review of 200 cases. *Journal of Veterinary Internal
Medicine* 18:679–91.

9 Gilmour M, Morgan R, Moore F (1992).
Masticatory myopathy in the dog: a retrospective
study in 18 cases. *Journal of the American Animal
Hospital Association* 28:300–6.

10 Shelton GD, Cardinet GH III, Bandman E
(1987). Canine masticatory muscle disorders: a
study of 29 cases. *Muscle Nerve* 8:783–90.

11 Riser WH (1993). Canine craniomandibular
osteopathy. In: Bojrab MJ (ed). *Disease
Mechanisms in Small Animal Surgery*. Lippincott
Williams & Wilkins, Philadelphia, pp. 892–9.

12 Johnson KA, Watson ADJ (2005). Skeletal
diseases. In: Ettinger SJ, Feldman EC (eds).
Textbook of Veterinary Internal Medicine, 6th edn.
Elsevier, St. Louis, pp. 1976–8.

13 Montgomery R (2003). Miscellaneous
orthopaedic diseases. In: Slatter D (ed). *Textbook
of Small Animal Surgery*. WB Saunders,
Philadelphia, p. 2255.

14 Padget GA, Mostosky UV (1986). Animal
model: the mode of inheritance of
craniomandibular osteopathy in West Highland
White terrier dogs. *American Journal of Medical
Genetics* 25:9.

15 Halliwell, WH (1993). Tumor-like lesions of
bone. In: Bojrab MJ (ed). *Disease Mechanisms in
Small Animal Surgery*. Lippincott Williams &
Wilkins, Philadelphia, pp. 934–5.

16 Delahunta A (1983). Cranial nerve – lower motor
neuron: general somatic efferent system, special
visceral efferent system. In: *Veterinary
Neuroanatomy and Clinical Neurology*. WB
Saunders, Philadelphia, pp. 110.

17 Inzana KD (2005). Peripheral nerve disorders. In:
Ettinger SJ, Feldman EC (eds). *Textbook of
Veterinary Internal Medicine*, 6th edn. Elsevier, St.
Louis, p. 900.

18 Shell LG (1997). Diseases of cranial nerves. In:
Leib MS, Monroe WE (eds). *Practical Small
Animal Internal Medicine*. WB Saunders,
Philadelphia, p. 551.

19 Fossum TW (1997). Management of joint
diseases. In: *Small Animal Surgery*. Mosby Year
book, St. Louis, pp. 898–902.

20 Verstraete FM (2003). In: Slatter D (ed). *Textbook of Small Animal Surgery*. WB Saunders, Philadelphia.

21 Piermattei DL, Flo GL (1997). Fractures and luxations of the maxilla and mandible. In: *Handbook of Small Animal Orthopedics and Fracture Repair*, 3rd edn. WB Saunders, Philadelphia, pp. 669–72.

22 Wiggs RB, Lobprise HB (1997). In: *Veterinary Dentistry: Principles and Practice*. Lippincott–Raven, Philadelphia.

23 Umphlet RC, Johnson AL (1988). Mandibular fractures in the cat: a retrospective study. *Veterinary Surgery* 17:333–7.

24 Umphlet RC, Johnson AL (1990). Mandibular fractures in the dog: a retrospective study of 157 cases. *Veterinary Surgery* 19:272–5.

25 Evans HE (1993). The skull. In: *Miller's Anatomy of the Dog*, 3rd edn. WB Saunders, Philadelphia, p. 128.

26 Gracis, M, Orsini P (1998). Treatment of traumatic dental displacement in dogs: six cases of lateral luxation. *Journal of Veterinary Dentistry* 15:65–72.

27 Spodkick GJ (1992). Replantation of a maxillary canine after traumatic avulsion in a dog. *Journal of Veterinary Dentistry* 9:4–7.

28 Ulbricht, RD, Marretta SM, Klippert LS (2004). Mandibular canine tooth luxation injury in a dog. *Journal of Veterinary Dentistry* 21:77–83.

29 Sommer RF, Ostrander FD, Crowly MC (1961). *Clinical Endodontics*. WB Saunders, Philadelphia, p. 70.

30 Grossman LI (1958). Endodontics. In: *Handbook of Dental Practice*, 3rd edn. Lippincott–Raven, Philadelphia, p. 150.

31 Johnson KA (1994). Osteomyelitis in dogs and cats. *Journal of the American Veterinary Medical Association* 12:1882–7.

32 Theon AP, Rodriguez C, Madewell BR (1997). Analysis of prognostic factors and patterns of failure in dogs with malignant oral tumors treated with megavoltage irradiation. *Journal of the American Veterinary Medical Association* 15:778–84.

33 Withrow SJ (2001). Cancer of the oral cavity. In: Withrow SJ, MacEwen EG (eds). *Small Animal Clinical Oncology*, 3rd edn. WB Saunders, Philadelphia, pp. 305–18.

34 Verstraete FM (2005). Mandibulectomy and maxillectomy. *Veterinary Clinics of North America, Small Animal Practice* 35:1009–39.

35 Straw RC, Powers, BE, Klausner J, *et al.* (1996). Canine mandibular osteosarcoma: 51 cases (1980–1992). *Journal of the American Animal Hospital Association* 27:601–10.

36 Smith MM (2002). Surgical approach for lymph node staging of oral and maxillofacial neoplasms in dogs. *Journal of Veterinary Dentistry* 19:170–4.

37 Herring ES, Smith MM, Robertson JL (2002). Lymph node staging of oral and maxillofacial neoplasms in 31 dogs and cats. *Journal of Veterinary Dentistry* 19:122–6.

38 Monroe WE (1997). Diseases of the parathyroid glands. In: Leib MS, Monroe WE (eds). *Practical Small Animal Internal Medicine*. WB Saunders, Philadelphia, pp. 1078–80.

39 Bagley RS, Dougherty SA, Randolph JF (1994). Tetanus subsequent to ovariohysterectomy in a dog. *Progress in Veterinary Neurology* 5:63–5.

40 Lee EA, Jones BR (1996). Localised tetanus in two cats after ovariohysterectomy. *New Zealand Veterinary Journal* 44:105–8.

41 Greene CE (2006). Tetanus. In: Greene CE (ed). *Infectious Diseases of the Dog and Cat*, 3rd edn. WB Saunders, Philadelphia, pp. 267–73.

42 Hartman K, Greene CE (2005). Diseases caused by systemic bacterial infections. In: Ettinger SJ, Feldman EC (eds). *Textbook of Veterinary Internal Medicine*, 6th edn. Elsevier, St. Louis, pp. 628–9.

43 Barsanti JA (2006). Botulism. In: Greene CE (ed). *Infectious Diseases of the Dog and Cat*, 3rd edn. WB Saunders, Philadelphia, pp. 263–7.

Chapter 9

1 Williams LE, Rassnick KM, Power HT, Lana SE, Morrison-Collister KE, Hansen K, Johnson JL (2006). CCNU in the treatment of canine epitheliotropic lymphoma. *Journal of Veterinary Internal Medicine* 20:136–43.

2 Boy SC, Van Heerden WF, Steenkamp G (2005). Diagnosis and treatment of primary intraoral leiomyosarcomas in four dogs. *Veterinary Record* 156:510–13.

3 Brockus CW, Myers RK (2004). Multifocal rhabdomyosarcomas within the tongue and oral cavity of a dog. *Veterinary Pathology* 41:273–4.

4 Nakamura K, Ochiai K, Kadosawa T, Kimura T, Umemura T (2004). Canine ganglioneuroblastoma in the oral mucosa. *Journal of Comparative Pathology* 130:205–8.

5 Boy SC, Steenkamp G (2006). Odontoma-like tumours of squirrel elodont incisors: elodontomas. *Journal of Comparative Pathology* 135:56–61.

6 Papadimitriou S, Papazoglou LG, Tontis D, Tziafas D, Papaionnnou N, Patsikas MN (2005). Compound maxillary odontoma in a young German Shepherd dog. *Journal of Small Animal Practice* 46:146–50.

7 Boyd RC (2002). Ameloblastic fibro-odontoma in a German Shepherd dog. *Journal of Veterinary Dentistry* **19**:148–50.

8 Eickhoff M, Seeliger F, Simon D, Fehr M (2002). Erupted bilateral compound odontomas in a dog. *Journal of Veterinary Dentistry* **19**:137–43.

9 Snyder LA, Bertone ER, Jakowski RM, Dooner MS, Jennings-Ritchie J, Moore AS (2004). p53 expression and environmental tobacco smoke exposure in feline oral squamous cell carcinoma. *Veterinary Pathology* **41**:209–14.

10 Bertone ER, Snyder LA, Moore AS (2003). Environmental and lifestyle risk factors for oral squamous cell carcinoma in domestic cats. *Journal of Veterinary Internal Medicine* **17**:557–62.

11 Zaugg N, Nespeca G, Hauser B, Ackermann M, Favrot C (2005). Detection of novel papillomaviruses in canine mucosal, cutaneous and *in situ* squamous cell carcinomas. *Veterinary Dermatology* **16**:290–8.

12 Johnston KB, Monteiro JM, Schultz LD, *et al.* (2005). Protection of Beagle dogs from mucosal challenge with canine oral papillomavirus by immunization with recombinant adenoviruses expressing codon-optimized early genes. *Virology* **336**:208–18.

13 Herring ES, Smith MM, Robertson JL (2002). Lymph node staging of oral and maxillofacial neoplasms in 31 dogs and cats. *Journal of Veterinary Dentistry* **19**:122–6. Comment in: *Journal of Veterinary Dentistry* 2002;**19**:120.

14 Kafka UC, Carstens A, Steenkamp G, Symington H (2004). Diagnostic value of magnetic resonance imaging and computed tomography for oral masses in dogs. *Journal of the South Africa Veterinary Association* **75**:163–8.

15 White RAS, Jefferies AR, Freedman LS (1985). Clinical staging for oropharyngeal malignancies in the dog. *Journal of Small Animal Practice* **26**:581–94.

16 Lascelles BD, Thomson MJ, Dernell WS, Straw RC, Lafferty M, Withrow SJ (2003). Combined dorsolateral and intraoral approach for the resection of tumors of the maxilla in the dog. *Journal of the American Animal Hospital Association* **39**:294–305.

17 Felizzola CR, Stopiglia AJ, de Araujo VC, de Araujo NS (2002). Evaluation of a modified hemimandibulectomy for treatment of oral neoplasms in dogs. *Journal of Veterinary Dentistry* **19**:127–35. Comment in: *Journal of Veterinary Dentistry* 2002;**19**:120.

18 McEntee MC, Page RL, Theon A, Erb HN, Thrall DE (2004). Malignant tumor formation in dogs previously irradiated for acanthomatous epulis. *Veterinary Radiology & Ultrasound* **45**:357–61.

19 Boria PA, Murry DJ, Bennett PF, *et al.* (2004). Evaluation of cisplatin combined with piroxicam for the treatment of oral malignant melanoma and oral squamous cell carcinoma in dogs. *Journal of the American Veterinary Medicine Association* **224**:388–94.

20 Hoyt RF, Withrow SJ (1982). Oral malignancy in the dog. *Journal of the American Animal Hospital Association* **20**(1):83–92.

21 Dhaliwal RS, Kitchell BE, Marretta SM (1998). Oral tumors in dogs and cats. Part I. Prognosis and treatment. *Compendium of Continuing Education* **20**:1011–21.

22 Dhaliwal RS, Kitchell BE, Marretta SM (1998). Oral tumors in dogs and cats. Part II. Prognosis and treatment. *Compendium of Continuing Education* **20**:1109–19.

23 Ramos-Vara JA, Beissenherz ME, Miller MA, *et al.* (2000). Retrospective study of 338 canine oral melanomas with clinical, histologic, and immunohistochemical review of 129 cases. *Veterinary Pathology* **37**:597–608.

24 Shelly S, Chien MB, Yip B, *et al.* (2005). Exon 15 BRAF mutations are uncommon in canine oral malignant melanomas. *Mammalian Genome* **16**:211–17.

25 Spangler WL, Kass PH (2006). The histologic and epidemiologic bases for prognostic considerations in canine melanocytic neoplasia. *Veterinary Pathology* **43**:136–49.

26 Proulx DR, Ruslander DM, Dodge RK, *et al.* (2003). A retrospective analysis of 140 dogs with oral melanoma treated with external beam radiation. *Veterinary Radiology & Ultrasound* **44**:352–359.

27 Sulaimon S, Kitchell B, Ehrhart E (2002). Immunohistochemical detection of melanoma-specific antigens in spontaneous canine melanoma. *Journal of Comparative Pathology* **127**:162–8.

28 Spugnini EP, Dragonetti E, Vincenzi B, Onori N, Citro G, Baldi A (2006). Pulse-mediated chemotherapy enhances local control and survival in a spontaneous canine model of primary mucosal melanoma. *Melanoma Research* **16**:23–7.

29 Kinzel S, Hein S, Stopinski T, *et al.* (2003). Hypofractionated radiation therapy for the treatment of malignant melanoma and squamous cell carcinoma in dogs and cats. *Berliner und Münchener Tierärztliche Wochenschrift* **116**:134–8.

30 Freeman KP, Hahn KA, Harris FD, King GK (2003). Treatment of dogs with oral melanoma by hypofractionated radiation therapy and platinum-based chemotherapy (1987–1997). *Journal of Veterinary Internal Medicine* **17**:96–101.

31 Bergman PJ (2007). Anticancer vaccines. *Veterinary Clinics of North America Small Animal Practice* **37**:1111–19.

32 Bergman PJ, McKnight J, Novosad A, *et al.* (2003). Long-term survival of dogs with advanced malignant melanoma after DNA vaccination with xenogenic human tyrosinase: a phase I trial. *Clinical Cancer Research* **9**:1284–90.

33 Pressler BM, Rotstein DS, Law JM, *et al.* (2002). Hypercalcemia and high parathyroid hormone-related protein concentration associated with malignant melanoma in a dog. *Journal of the American Veterinary Medicine Association* **221**:263–5.

34 Poirier VJ, Bley CR, Roos M, Kaser-Hotz B (2006). Efficacy of radiation therapy for the treatment of macroscopic canine oral soft tissue sarcoma. *In Vivo* **20**:415–19.

35 Postorino Reeves NC, Turrel JM, Withrow SJ (1993). Oral squamous cell carcinoma in the cat. *Journal of the American Animal Hospital Association* **29**:438–41.

36 Carpenter LG, Withrow SJ, Powers BE, *et al.* (1993) Squamous cell carcinoma of the tongue in 10 dogs. *Journal of the American Animal Hospital Association* **29**:17–24.

37 Théon AP, Rodriguez C, Madewell BR (1997). Analysis of prognostic factors and patterns of failure in dogs with malignant oral tumors treated with megavoltage radiation. *Journal of the American Veterinary Medicine Association* **210**:778–84.

38 McCaw DL, Pope ER, Payne JT, West MK, Tompson RV, Tate D (2000). Treatment of canine oral squamous cell carcinomas with photodynamic therapy. *British Journal of Cancer* **82**:1297–9.

39 Schmidt BR, Glickman NW, DeNicola DB, de Gortari AE, Knapp DW (2001). Evaluation of piroxicam for the treatment of oral squamous cell carcinoma in dogs. *Journal of the American Veterinary Medicine Association* **218**:1783–6.

40 Ciekot PA, Powers BE, Withrow SJ, Straw RC, Ogilvie GK, LaRue SM (1994). Histologically low-grade, yet biologically high-grade, fibrosarcomas of the mandible and maxilla in dogs: 25 cases (1982–1991). *Journal of the American Veterinary Medicine Association* **204**:610–15.

41 Heyman SJ, Diefenderfer DL, Goldschmidt MH, *et al.* (1992). Canine axial skeletal osteosarcoma. A retrospective study of 116 cases (1986 to 1989). *Veterinary Surgery* **21**:304–10.

42 Stebbins KE, Morse CC, Goldschmidt MH (1989). Feline oral neoplasia: a ten-year survey. *Veterinary Pathology* **26**:121–8.

43 Salisbury SK, Lantz GC (1988). Long-term results of partial mandibulectomy for treatment of oral tumors in 30 dogs. *Journal of the American Animal Hospital Association* **24**:285.

44 Schwarz PD, Withrow SJ, Curtis CR, *et al.* (1991). Mandibular resection as a treatment for oral cancer in 81 dogs. *Journal of the American Animal Hospital Association* **27**:601–10.

45 Straw RC, Powers BE, Klausner JS, *et al.* (1996). Canine mandibular osteosarcoma: 51 cases (1980–1992). *Journal of the American Animal Hospital Association* **32**:257–62.

Chapter 10

1 Neville BW, Damm DD, Allen CM (2002). Salivary gland pathology. In: Bouquot JE (ed). *Oral and Maxillofacial Pathology*, 2nd edn. WB Saunders, Philadelphia, pp. 389–436.

2 Bellenger CR, Simpson DJ (1992). Canine sialoceles: 60 cases. *Journal of Small Animal Practice* **33**:376–80.

3 Wiggs RB, Lobprise HB (1995). Clinical Oral Pathology. In: *Veterinary Dentistry, Principles and Practice*. Lippincott–Raven, Philadelphia, pp. 104–39.

4 Waldron DR, Smith MM (1991). Salivary mucoceles. *Problems in Veterinary Medicine* **3**(2):270–6.

5 Peeters MF (1991). The treatment of salivary cysts in dogs and cats. *Tijdschrift Voor Diergeneeskunde* **166**(4):169–72.

6 Dunning D (2003). Oral cavity. In: Slatter D (ed). *Textbook of Small Animal Surgery*, 3rd edn. Elsevier Science, Philadelphia, pp. 553–61.

7 Loney WW Jr, Termini S, Sisto J (2006). Plunging ranula formation as a complication of dental implant surgery: a case report. *Journal of Oral & Maxillofacial Surgery* **64**(8):1204–8.

8 Henry CJ (1992). Salivary mucocele associated with dirofiliariasis in a dog. *Journal of the American Veterinary Medical Association* **200**:1965–6.

9 Popescu E, GogalniceanuD, Danilla V, *et al.* (2004). Plunging ranula. *Revista medico-chirurgicală a Societăii de Medici, Naturali Iasi* **8**(4):903–8.

10 Kalinowski M, Heverhagen JT, Rehberg E, Klose KJ, Wagner HJ (2002). Comparison study: MR sialography and digital subtraction sialography for benign salivary gland disorders. *American Journal of Neuroradiology* 23(9):1485–92.

11 Jager L, Manauer F, Holzknecht N, *et al.* (2000). Sialolithiasis: MR sialography of the submandibular duct: an alternative to conventional sialography and US? *Radiology* 216(3):665–71.

12 Lewis G, Knottenbelt JD (1991). Parotid duct injury, is immediate surgery necessary? *Injury* 22(5):407–9.

13 Zhao YF, Jia J, Jia Y (2005). Complications associated with surgical management of ranulas. *Journal of Oral & Maxillofacial Surgery* 63(1):51–4.

14 De Visscher JG, van der Wal KG, de Vogel PL (1989). The plunging ranula. Pathogenesis, diagnosis, and management. *Journal of Craniomaxillofacial Surgery* 17(4):182–5.

15 Yoshimura Y, Obara S, Kondoh T, Naitoh S (1995). A comparison of three methods used for the treatment of ranula. *Journal of Oral & Maxillofacial Surgery* 53(3):280–3.

16 Morita Y, Sato K, Kawana M, Takahasi S, Ikarashi F (2003). Treatment of ranula: excision of the sublingual gland versus marsupialization. *Auris, Nasus, Larynx* 30(3):311–14.

17 Baurmash HD (2002). Treating oral ranula: another case against blanket removal of the sublingual gland. *British Journal of Oral & Maxillofacial Surgery* 39(3):217–20.

18 Salvatore G, Briganti V, Cavallaro S, *et al.* (2006). Nickel gluconate-mercurius heel-potentized swine organ preparations: a new therapeutical approach for the treatment of pediatric ranula and intraoral mucocele. *International Journal of Pediatric Otorhinolaryngology* 71(2):247–55.

19 Roh JL (2006). Primary treatment of ranula with intracystic injection of OK-432. *Laryngoscope* 116(2):169–72.

20 Fukase S, Ohta N, Inamura K, Aoyagi M (2003). Treatment of ranula with intracystic injection of the streptococcal preparation OK-432. *Annals of Otology, Rhinology, & Laryngology* 112(3):214–20.

21 Kostner A, Buerger L (1965). Primary neoplasms of the salivary glands in animals compared to similar tumors in man. *Pathological Veterinaria* 2:201–26.

22 Spangler WL, Culbertson MR (1991). Salivary gland disease in dogs and cats. *Journal of the American Veterinary Medical Association* 198:465–9.

23 Hammer A, Getzy D, Ogilvie G, *et al.* (1997). Salivary gland neoplasia in the dog and cat: survival times and prognostic factors. *Proceedings Annual Conference of the American College of Veterinary Radiology and Veterinary Cancer Society* p. 87.

24 Carberry CA, Glanders CA, Harvey HJ, Ryan AM (1988). Salivary gland tumors in dogs and cats: a literature and case review. *Journal of the American Animal Hospital Association* 24:561–7.

25 Withrow SJ (2001). Cancer of the gastrointestinal tract. In: Withrow SJ, MacEwen EG (eds). *Small Animal Clinical Oncology*, 3rd edn. WB Saunders, Philadelphia, pp. 318–19.

26 Buyukmihci N, Rubin LF, Harvey CE (1975). Exopthalmus secondary to zygomatic adenocarcinoma in a dog. *Journal of the American Veterinary Medical Association* 167(2):162–5.

27 Habin DJ, Else RW (2005). Parotid salivary gland adenocarcinoma with bilateral ocular and osseous metastases in a dog. *Journal of Small Animal Practice* 36(10):445–9.

28 Evans SM, Thrall DE (1983). Postoperative orthovoltage radiation therapy of parotid salivary gland adenocarcinoma in three dogs. *Journal of the American Veterinary Medical Association* 182:993–4.

29 Chen AM, Garcia J, Bucci MK, *et al.* (2007). The role of postoperative radiation therapy in carcinoma ex pleomorphic adenoma of the parotid gland. *International Journal of Radiation Oncology, Biology, Physics* 67(1):138–43.

30 Harrison LB, Armstrong JC, Spiro RH, Fass DE, Strong EW (1990). Postoperative radiation therapy for major salivary gland malignancies. *Journal of Surgical Oncology* 45(1):52–5.

31 Parsons JT, Mendenhall WM, Stringer SP, Cassisi MJ, Million RR (1996). Management of minor salivary gland carcinomas. *International Journal of Radiation Oncology, Biology, Physics* 35(3):443–54.

32 Le QT, Birdwell S, Terris DJ, *et al.* (1999). Postoperative irradiation of minor salivary gland malignancies of the head and neck. *Radiotherapy & Oncology* 52(2):165–71.

33 Airoldi M, Pedani F, Succo G, *et al.* (2001). Phase II randomized trial comparing vinorelbine versus vinorelbine plus cisplatin in patients with recurrent salivary gland malignancies. *Cancer* 1(3):541–7.

34 Tsukuda M, Kokatsu Y, Ito K, *et al.* (1993). Chemotherapy for recurrent adeno- and adenoidcystic carcinomas in the head and neck. *Journal of Cancer Research & Clinical Oncology* 119(12):756–8.

35 Dreyfuss AI, Clark JR, Fallon BG, *et al.* (1987). Cyclophosphamide, doxorubicin, and cisplatin combination chemotherapy for advanced carcinomas of salivary gland origin. *Cancer* **60**(12):2869–72.

36 Belani CP, Eisenberger MA, Gray WC (1988). Preliminary experience with chemotherapy in advanced salivary gland neoplasms. *Medical and Pediatric Oncology* **16**(3):197–202.

37 Laurie SA, Licitra L (2006). Systemic therapy in the palliative management of advanced salivary gland cancers. *Journal of Clinical Oncology* **24**(17):2673–8.

38 Mimura M, Tanaka N, Ichinose S, Kimijima Y, Amagasa T (2005). Possible etiology of calculi formation in salivary glands: biophysical analysis of calculus. *Medical Molecular Morphology* **38**(3):189–95.

39 Grases F, Santiago C, Simonet BM, Costa-Bauza A (2003). Sialolithiasis: mechanism of calculi formation and etiologic factors. *Clinica Chimica Acta* **334**(1–2):131–6.

40 Kasaboglu O, Er N, Tumer C, Akkocaoglu M (2004). Micromorphology of sialoliths in submandibular salivary gland: a scanning electron microscope and X-ray diffraction analysis. *Journal of Oral & Maxillofacial Surgery* **62**(10):1253–8.

41 Roccia P, Di Liberto C, Speciale R, La Torretta G, Lo Muzio L, Campisi G (2006). Obstructive sialoaenitis: update of diagnosis and therapy issues. *Recenti Progressi in Medicina* **97**(5):272–9.

42 Iro H, Waitz G, Nitsche N, Benninger J, Schneider T, Ell C (1992). Extracorporeal piezoelectric shock-wave lihotripsy of salivary gland stones. *Laryngoscope* **102**(5):492–4.

43 Fokas K, Putzer P, Dempf R, Eckardt A (2002). Extracorporeal shockwave lithotripsy for treatment of sialolithiasis of salivary glands. *Laryngorhinootologie* **81**(10):706–11.

44 Zenk J, Bozzato A, Winter M, Gottwald F, Iro H (2004). Extracorporeal shock wave lithotripsy of submandibular stones: evaluation after 10 years. *Annals of Otology, Rhinology, & Laryngology* **113**(5):378–83.

45 Escudier MP, Brown Je, Drage NA, McGurk M (2003). Extracorporeal shockwave lithotripsy in the management of salivary calculi. *British Journal of Surgery* **90**(4):482–5.

46 Reimers M, Vavrina J, Schlegel C (2000). Results after shock wave lithotripsy for salivary gland stones. *Schweizerische Medizinische Wochenschrift* (Suppl) **125**:122S–6S.

9781840761726